Developmental Coordination Disorder

DEDICATION

To all who have shared this journey

*In loving memory of those
who started
but did not complete
this journey
with us.*

*Laird S. Cermak
Bob MacDonald
Gai Clarke*

Developmental Coordination Disorder

Sharon A. Cermak, Ed.D., O.T.R./L., FAOTA
Professor of Occupational Therapy
Department of Occupational Therapy
Sargent College of Health and Rehabilitation Sciences
Boston University
Boston, Massachusetts

Dawne Larkin, Ed.D.
Senior Lecturer and Director of Motor Learning Programs
Centre for Lifespan Development
Department of Human Movement and Exercise Science
University of Western Australia
Nedlands, Western Australia

DELMAR
THOMSON LEARNING ™

Australia Canada Mexico Singapore Spain United Kingdom United States

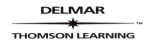

Developmental Coordination Disorder

Edited by Sharon A. Cermak and Dawne Larkin

Health Care Publishing Director:
William Brottmiller

Executive Editor:
Cathy L. Esperti

Acquisitions Editor:
Candice Janco

Project Editor:
David R. Buddle

Editorial Assistant:
Maria D'Angelico

Production Editor:
James Zayicek

Executive Marketing Manager:
Dawn F. Gerrain

Art/Design Coordinator:
Jay Purcell

Printed in Canada
1 2 3 4 5 6 XXX 06 05 04 03 02 01

For more information contact Delmar,
3 Columbia Circle, PO Box 15015,
Albany, NY 12212-5015.

Or find us on the World Wide Web at
http://www.delmar.com

For permission to use material from this text or product, contact us by
Tel   (800) 730-2214
Fax   (800) 730-2215
www.thomsonrights.com

Library of Congress Cataloging-in-Publication Data

Cermak, Sharon.
  Developmental coordination disorder / by Sharon Cermak, Dawne Larkin.
    p. cm.
  Includes bibliographical references and index.
  ISBN 0-7668-0092-8
  1. Clumsiness in children. 2. Motor abilities in children. 3. Child development. 4. Occupational therapy for children. I. Larkin, Dawne. II. Title.
  RJ496.M68 C46 2001
  618.92--dc21

                                                    2001032537

NOTICE TO THE READER

Contents

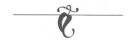

Preface

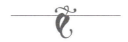

Developmental coordination disorder (DCD), commonly recognized in children because of their difficulty performing and learning motor activities, has a long history. It has been described using various terms by researchers and clinicians from different disciplines under different theoretical frameworks. In this book, we have drawn together authors from different backgrounds to enrich our understanding of DCD. These multiple frameworks are not mutually exclusive; however, they influence the language we use to define and describe the child with DCD. The chapters in this book provide different viewpoints that can enhance our understanding, influence our assessment and intervention, and contribute to increased awareness about DCD. We hope that by bringing these ideas together, we can facilitate better understanding among professionals and researchers who are committed to refining theory and practice to help children with DCD and their families.

Part I provides an introduction to DCD. In the first chapter, we provide an overview of developmental coordination disorder drawing on literature from a range of areas, disciplines, and across time. Cantell and Kooistra, in Chapter 2, emphasize the long-term effects of DCD, bringing together research that has convinced professionals that DCD may have influences into adulthood and can negatively affect a child's future. It is clear that we can no longer stand back and ignore DCD based on the unfounded presumption that the child will grow out of it. Part II deals with subtypes of DCD. Dewey addresses the complexity of DCD in Chapter 3 through the exploration of the issue of subtypes of DCD. This issue is extended in Chapters 4 and 5 where the authors use a neuropsychological framework to examine subtypes of DCD. In Chapter 4, Estil and Whiting deal with the interplay between language and motor difficulties. In Chapter 5, Sigmundsson and Whiting look at another type of mild motor difficulty, hand-eye coordination problems, and examine possible neuropsychological underpinnings.

Part III deals with assessment of DCD. In Chapter 6, we provide an overview of some of the issues that we face in the identification and assessment of DCD. One of the major considerations for our field is how we deal with the multiple frameworks that confuse and confound our assessment. How do we pull them together?

In Part IV of the book, the authors address sensory and motor mechanisms hypothesized to contribute to DCD. In Chapter 7, Rösblad employs the comprehensive perception-action framework to examine the issue of visual perception and motor control in children with DCD. Williams brings her long history of research and practice with children with motor impairment to Chapter 8, where she reviews the research on motor control and DCD. This research has drawn on different theoretical frameworks, ranging from information processing to dynamic systems, as a basis for the driving hypotheses about constructs such as timing and force control.

Part V moves to functional issues addressing personal, physical, and psychosocial implications of having DCD. In Chapter 9, May-Benson, Ingolia, and Koomar bring together a wealth of information and experience about the difficulties of dealing with activities of daily living in children and adults with DCD. Case-Smith and Weintraub focus on the development of hand function and the problems posed by DCD in Chapter 10. Hands and Larkin, in Chapter 11, describe the interplay between physical fitness and DCD, emphasizing the importance of fitness to the lifestyle and motor learning of the child with DCD.

Psychosocial issues are addressed in Chapters 12 and 13. Causgrove Dunn and Watkinson focus on psychosocial factors, especially motivation, and how these factors impact on the physical activity of children with DCD. In Chapter 13, we focus on the family and the influences of DCD on family dynamics. We also deal with the contribution of the family to the identification and the lifestyle of the child with DCD. It is clear that this is a complex area where different family dynamics dictate the interplay between the family, the child, and the professionals.

The final part of the book focuses on interventions for DCD. Practice and theory are intermingled, juxtaposing intervention approaches that emerge from different theoretical frameworks. These are working interventions that practitioners currently use to help children with mild motor difficulties interact more effectively with their environment. In Chapter 14, Kimball views intervention from a sensory integrative perspective and addresses some of the challenges still faced by this approach. In Chapter 15 Missiuna and Mandich look broadly at the influence of motor learning on praxis. In Chapter 16, Larkin and Parker look at task specific intervention for DCD. The theoretical model that drives this intervention is consistent with a broad systems framework. Finally, in Chapter 17, Benbow draws on her extensive experience to provide a very practical view of intervention for hand skills and handwriting. These interventions differ in a number of ways but generally they include one common feature, social support from a concerned and knowledgeable professional. The varied approaches raise many questions. Why is it that there is still controversy surrounding our interventions? Why is it that some children respond to one intervention better than another intervention? Is this an issue of subtypes, specific resources that the child brings, learning styles, or personal interactions and motivations?

We thank the authors for the wonderful insights and the wealth of practical and theoretical understandings that they have brought to us through their chapters. We hope that the diversity of ideas presented here will enrich your understanding of these mild motor difficulties that we call DCD. In turn, we hope that it will promote further interaction among theory, research, and practice, and contribute to future positive developments for all the children and adults with DCD who have contributed so much to our current knowledge.

Contributors

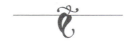

Mary Benbow, M.S., O.T.R.
Private Consultant and International Lecturer
La Jolla, California

Marja Cantell, Ph.D.
Department of Physical Education
University of Jyvaskyla
Jyvaskyla, Finland

Jane Case-Smith, Ph.D.
Division of Occupational Therapy
School of Allied Medical Professions
The Ohio State University
Columbus, Ohio

Janice Causgrove Dunn, Ph.D.
Faculty of Physical Education & Recreation
University of Alberta
Edmonton, Canada

Sharon A. Cermak, Ed.D., O.T.R./L., FAOTA
Department of Occupational Therapy
Sargent College of Health and Rehabilitation
    Sciences
Boston University
Boston, Massachusetts

Deborah Dewey, Ph.D.
Department of Pediatrics, University of Calgary
    and Behavioural Research Unit, Alberta
    Children's Hospital Research Centre
Calgary, Canada

Lise-Beate Estil, M.S.c.
Department of Sport Sciences
Norwegian University of Science and
    Technology
Trondheim, Norway

Sasson S. Gubbay, M.D., F.R.A.C.P.
Clinical Professor of Neurology
University of Western Australia
Perth, Australia

Beth Hands, Ph.D.
Department of Human Movement and Exercise
    Science
The University of Western Australia
Perth, Australia

Peg Ingolia, M.S., O.T.R./L.
Occupational Therapy Associates–Watertown,
    P. C.
Watertown, Massachusetts

Judith Giencke Kimball, Ph.D., O.T.R./L.,
** F.A.O.T.A.**
Department of Occupational Therapy
University of New England
Biddeford, Maine

Libbe Kooistra, Ph.D.
KIHU Research Centre for Olympic Sports
Jyvaskyla, Finland

Jane Koomar, Ph.D., O.T.R./L., F.A.O.T.A.
Occupational Therapy Associates–Watertown,
  P. C.
Watertown, Massachusetts

Dawne Larkin, Ed.D.
Department of Human Movement and Exercise
  Science
University of Western Australia
Perth, Australia

Angela Mandich, M.S.c., O.T.(C.)
School of Occupational Therapy
University of Western Ontario
London, Canada

Teresa May-Benson, M.S., O.T.R./L.
Occupational Therapy Associates–Watertown,
  P. C.
Watertown, Massachusetts

Cheryl Missiuna, Ph.D., O.T.(C.)
School of Rehabilitation Science
McMaster University
Hamilton, Canada

Helen E. Parker, Ph.D.
Department of Human Movement and Exercise
  Science
University of Western Australia
Perth, Australia

Birgit Rösblad, P.T., Ph.D.
Kolbacken's Child Rehabilitation Centre
and Department of Psychology
University of Umea
Umea, Sweden

Hermundur Sigmundsson, Ph.D.
Faculty of Social Sciences and Technology
  Management
Norwegian University of Science and
  Technology
Trondheim, Norway

E. Jane Watkinson, Ph.D.
Faculty of Physical Education and Recreation
University of Alberta
Edmonton, Canada

Naomi Weintraub, Ph.D.
School of Occupational Therapy
Hebrew University of Jerusalem
Jerusalem, Israel

H. T. A. Whiting, Ph.D.
Department of Psychology
University of York
Heslington, United Kingdom

Harriet Williams, Ph.D.
Department of Exercise Science
University of South Carolina
Columbia, South Carolina

Contributors' Addresses for Contact

(* indicates first author)

Mary Benbow: Chapter 17*
1440 Torrey Pines Road
La Jolla, CA 92037
Phone: 858-459-2152
Fax: 858-459-0487
E-mail: benbow@pacbell.net

Dr. Marja Cantell: Chapter 2*
Department of Physical Education
University of Jyvaskyla
P.O. Box 35 (L), 40351 Jyvaskyla
Finland
Phone: 358-14-602132
Fax: 358-14-602101
E-mail: mcantell@pallo.jyu.fi

Dr. Jane Case-Smith: Chapter 10*
Ohio State University
Division of Occupational Therapy
Ohio State University
406 School of Allied Medical Professions
1585 Perry Street
Columbus, OH 43210
Phone: 614-292-0357
Fax: 614-292-0210
E-mail: case-smith.1@osu.edu

Dr. Janice Causgrove Dunn: Chapter 12*
Faculty of Physical Education and Recreation
University of Alberta
Edmonton, Alberta T6G 2H9
Canada
Phone: 780-492-0580
Fax: 780-492-2364
E-mail: janice.causgrove-dunn@ualberta.ca

Dr. Sharon A. Cermak: Chapters 1*, 6, and 13*
Professor of Occupational Therapy
Boston University
Sargent College of Health and Rehabilitation
    Sciences
635 Commonwealth Avenue
Boston, MA 02215
Phone: 617-353-7520
Fax: 617-353-7500
E-mail: cermak@bu.edu

Dr. Deborah Dewey: Chapter 3*
Behavioural Research Unit
Alberta Children's Hospital Research Centre
1820 Richmond Road S.W.
Calgary, Alberta T2T 5C7
Canada
Phone: 403-229-7365
Fax: 403-543-9100
E-mail: deb@ach.ucalgary.ca

Lise-Beate Estil: Chapter 4*
Department of Sport Sciences
Faculty of Social Sciences and Technology
　Management
Norwegian University of Science and
　Technology
Dragvoll
N-7491 Trondheim
Norway
Phone: 47-7359-1769
Fax: 47-7359-1770
E-mail: Lise.Estil@sut.ntnu.no

Dr. Sasson S. Gubbay: Chapter 1
Clinical Professor of Neurology
Department of Medicine
University of Western Australia
Crawley, Western Australia 6009
Australia
Phone: 618-9381-7555
Fax: 618-9381-7848
E-mail: ssgubbay@cyllene.uwa.edu.au

Dr. Beth Hands: Chapter 11*
Department of Human Movement and Exercise
　Science
University of Western Australia
Crawley, WA 6009
Australia
Phone: 618-9380-2361
Fax: 618-9380-1039
E-mail: bhands@cygnus.uwa.edu.au

Peg Ingolia: Chapter 9
Senior Therapist in school and private practice-
　based intervention
OTA–Watertown
124 Watertown St.,
Watertown, MA 02472
Phone: 617-923-4410
E-mail: pegingolia@earthlink.net

Dr. Judith Giencke Kimball: Chapter 14*
Chairperson, Department of Occupational
　Therapy
Decary Hall #301
University of New England
11 Hills Beach Road
Biddeford, ME 04005
Phone: 207-283-0170 ext. 2234
Fax: 207-283-6379
E-mail: jkimball@mailbox.une.edu

Dr. Libbe Kooistra: Chapter 2
Senior Researcher
KIHU Research Centre for Olympic Sports
Rautpohjankatu 6
University Campus
Fin-40700 Jyvaskyla
Finland
Phone: 358-14-213352
Fax: 358-14-2603171
E-mail: kooistra@kihu.jyu.fi

Dr. Jane Koomar: Chapter 9
Director
OTA–Watertown
124 Watertown St.,
Watertown, MA 02472
Phone: 617-923-4410
Fax: 617-923-0468
E-mail: koomar@msn.com

**Dr. Dawne Larkin: Chapters 1, 6*, 11, 13, and
　16***
Department of Human Movement and Exercise
　Science
University of Western Australia
35 Stirling Hwy.
Crawley, WA 6009
Australia
Phone: 618-9380-2361 or 618-9335-9474
Fax: 618-9380-1039
E-mail: dlarkin@cyllene.uwa.edu.au

Angela Mandich: Chapter 15
School of Occupational Therapy
University of Western Ontario
Elborn College
London, Ontario N6G 1H1
Canada
Phone: 519-661-2111, ext. 88993
Fax: 519-661-3894
E-mail: amandich@julian.uwo.ca

Teresa May-Benson: Chapter 9*
Research Director
Occupational Therapy Associates–Watertown,
    P. C.
124 Watertown St.
Watertown, MA 02472
Phone: 617-923-4410
Fax: 617-923-0468
E-mail: tmay-ben@bu.edu

Dr. Cheryl Missiuna: Chapter 15*
School of Rehabilitation Science
McMaster University
1400 Main Street West IAHS 414
Hamilton, Ontario
Canada L8S 4K1
Phone: 905-525-9140, ext. 27842
Fax: 905-524-0069
E-mail: missiuna@mcmaster.ca

Dr. Helen E. Parker: Chapter 16
Department of Human Movement and Exercise
    Science
University of Western Australia
35 Stirling Hwy.
Crawley, WA 6009
Australia
Phone: +618-9380-2361
Fax: +618-9380-1039
E-mail: hparker@cyllene.uwa.edu.au

Dr. Birgit Rösblad: Chapter 7*
Kolbacken's Child Rehabilitation Centre and
    Department of Psychology
University of Umea
S-90187 Umea
Sweden
Phone: +46-90-786-64-22
Fax: +46-90-786-66-95
E-mail: birgit.rosblad@psy.umu.se

Dr. Hermundur Sigmundsson: Chapter 5*
Faculty of Social Sciences and Technology
    Management
Norwegian University of Science and
    Technology
NTNU, Trondheim
Norway
Phone: +47-7359-0617
Fax: +47-7359-1770
E-mail: hermundurs@sv.unit.no

Dr. E. Jane Watkinson: Chapter 12
Associate Dean, Research and Graduate Studies
Faculty of Physical Education and Recreation
University of Alberta
Edmonton, Alberta T6G 2H9
Canada
Phone: 403-492-5910
Fax: 403-492-2364
E-mail: jane.watkinson@ualberta.ca

Dr. Naomi Weintraub: Chapter 10
Associate Professor
School of Occupational Therapy
Faculty of Medicine
Hebrew University
P.O. Box 24026
Mt. Scopus
Jerusalem 91240
Israel
Fax: 972-2532-4985
E-mail: msnwei@mscc.huji.ac.il

Professor H. T. A. Whiting: Chapters 4 and 5
Department of Psychology
University of York
Heslington, York Y01 5DD, U.K.
TeleFax: 01904-433433
E-mail: htawl@york.ac.uk

Professor Harriet Williams: Chapter 8*
Department of Exercise Science
University of South Carolina
Columbia, SC 29208
Phone: 803-777-5267
Fax: 803-777-8422
E-mail: HWILLIAMS@sophe.sph.sc.edu

PART
I

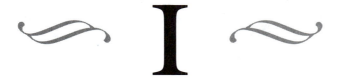

Introduction to Developmental
Coordination Disorder

CHAPTER

1

What Is Developmental Coordination Disorder?

Sharon A. Cermak, Sasson S. Gubbay, and Dawne Larkin

Developmental coordination disorder (DCD) is used to refer to the difficulty in movement skills that children have that is not primarily due to general intellectual, primary sensory, or motor neurological impairment (Gubbay, 1985; Hall, 1988). A key feature of this condition, which has been called by many different names, is difficulty in learning and performing everyday tasks in home, school, and play environments. Although there is broad agreement that the motor behavior of children with DCD is qualitatively inferior, a deeper understanding of the difficulties with motor behavior is still lacking. In this chapter, we will explore DCD through its historical antecedents, the terms and definitions used to describe the condition, and its clinical description, prevalence, recognition, etiology, and comorbid conditions.

HISTORICAL PERSPECTIVES

The concept of developmental motor problems has been discussed for over 100 years. Various groups of professionals have contributed to our current understandings in the area of DCD, including pediatric neurologists, pediatricians, physical educators, movement scientists, occupational and physical therapists, psychologists, and neuropsychologists. While each of these groups has contributed to our knowledge base, each has also approached it from its own perspective, contributing to a richness of information, unfortunately obscured by differences in terminology and a lack of communication.

At the beginning of the 20th century, an awareness of different levels of motor performance was clearly described in studies that identified the motor ability of children as "very clever, clever, medium, awkward and very awkward" (Bagley, 1900/01, p. 194). These studies often focused on the link between intellectual and motor ability rather than the effects of motor disability. Nevertheless, interest in identification and intervention for children and young adults with mild motor problems has received attention throughout the 20th century. As early as 1926, Lippitt was concerned specifically with "Poor muscular coordination in children" (p. 186) and suggested that "the root of the difficulty often lies in a condition of the nervous system which can only be corrected by patient training and care" (p. 186). Orton's (1937) discussion of "developmental apraxia" or "abnormal clumsiness" was strongly influenced by ideas about adult apraxia and damage to the "dominant" hemisphere. However, he used the term "developmental" to emphasize the interaction between hereditary and environmental factors and described the condition as "a failure in development of normal skills" (p. 204). Orton emphasized that unusual difficulties in learning complex movements could involve speech and writing as well as body movements. The relationship between language and motor impairment continues to challenge us today (see Chapter 4).

Neurology's influence continued in the use of terms inferring that minor brain damage was the etiology for the motor coordination or motor planning difficulties. The terms included "developmental apraxia and agnosia" (Walton, Ellis, & Court, 1962), "developmental apraxic and agnosic ataxia" (Gubbay, 1975), "minimal cerebral dysfunction" (Wigglesworth, 1963), "minimal brain dysfunction" (Clements, 1966), and "minimal cerebral palsy" (Kong, 1963). Pediatricians, pediatric neurologists, therapists, and neuropsychologists continue to use these terms, particularly "developmental dyspraxia" (Cermak, 1985, in press; De Ajuriaguerra & Stambak, 1969; Denckla, 1984; Denckla & Roeltgen, 1992; Dewey, 1995; Miyahara & Mobs, 1995).

In parallel with the developments in neurology and psychology, physical education has a long and varied history with children, adolescents, and college students who have coordination difficulties. Attempts were made to divide groups into homogeneous cohorts to facilitate better teaching and learning (Johnson, 1932). Programs were devised to improve performance in individuals with motor difficulties, including children (Arnheim & Sinclair, 1975; Cratty, 1975; Morris & Whiting, 1971; Oliver & Keogh, 1967) and college women (Broer, 1955; Lafuze, 1951). A variety of studies were conducted to better understand difficulties, including psychosocial concerns, experienced by children with coordination problems (Cratty, Ikeda, Martin, Jennett, & Morris, 1970; Keogh, 1968; Rarick & McKee, 1949; Symes, 1972).

Interest in perceptual deficits and perceptual-motor dysfunction was particularly prevalent during the 1960s (Ayres, 1960, 1965; Brenner, Gillman, Zangwill, & Farrell, 1967). Again, the emphasis often fell on the relationship between movement and cognitive development. There was a strong focus on remedial education, and perceptual-motor programs became popular at this time (Frostig, 1968; Kephart, 1960). The development of the sensory integration approach to the assessment and remediation of developmental dyspraxia was based on a neurobehavioral framework and emerged from Ayres' (1965) earlier work on perceptual motor dysfunction. This theory was elaborated in a series of factor analysis and cluster analysis studies that revealed a close and repeated relationship between somatosensory processing and motor planning (Ayres, 1965, 1972b, 1977, 1989; Ayres, Mailloux, & Wendler, 1987).

More recent influences from the field of motor control and learning, including information processing, dynamical systems, and ecological perspectives, are now used to address issues dealt with throughout this book (see Chapters 7 and 8). Likewise, neurobehavioral approaches continue to be applied to answer questions about DCD and highlight the issue of subtypes of DCD (see Chapters 4, 5, and 14).

The issue of subtypes of motor impairment as well as comorbid conditions has emerged over the years. Orton (1937) described damage to the dominant hemisphere as the linking agent between language and developmental dyspraxia. Annell (1949) discussed seven subtypes of motor dysfunction. Wigglesworth (1963) extended his concept of minimal cerebral palsy by breaking it into subtypes of motor disturbance, along with subtypes of sensory and perceptual dysfunctions. Gubbay, Ellis, Walton, and Court (1965) implicitly acknowledged subtypes when they noted that these children "exhibited varying degrees and types of apraxia and agnosia" (p. 296), while the description by Prechtl and Stemmer (1962) of a "choreiform syndrome" extended the pool of possible subtypes. Ayres (1965, 1972a, 1972b, 1977, 1989) addressed subtypes of sensory integration in children with learning disabilities. Developmental dyspraxia consistently emerged as a subtype. In more recent work by Ayres and her colleagues, the issue of subtypes of dyspraxia was examined (Ayres, 1985, 1989; Ayres et al., 1987; Conrad, Cermak, & Drake, 1983). Cratty (1994) summarized a lifetime of research and practice in the area of motor dysfunction and described subsyndromes within the "clumsy child syndromes," that included "ataxic syndrome," "hypotonic syndrome," "tension syndrome," "dyspraxic syndrome," "manual-graphic syndromes," and "visual-perceptual clumsiness." Like Annell (1949), Cratty also found a group of children who were too difficult to classify. More recent views of subtyping reveal that the issue is still contentious and far from resolution (see Chapters 3 and 4).

TERMS AND DEFINITIONS

"Developmental dyspraxia" is a term frequently used to describe the clumsy syndrome and is widely used by various disciplines in the United Kingdom and the United States. This term, derived from adult neurology, is more specifically used by neurologists (Denckla, 1984; Denckla & Roeltgen, 1992), occupational therapists (Cermak, 1985; Missiuna & Polatajko, 1995; Szklut, Cermak, & Henderson, 1995), and neuropsychologists (Dewey, 1995) to describe the motor learning/planning problems experienced by children with DCD. These motor planning problems are sometimes considered to be due to difficulty integrating information from the bodily senses (Ayres, 1980; Cermak, 1991) or to problems with motor sequencing and selection (Ayres, 1989; Miyahara & Mobs, 1995). Denckla and Roeltgen (1992, p. 466) define developmental dyspraxia as "a disorder of gesture" that includes meaningful or nonmeaningful acts. Although this term has often been used interchangeably with DCD, some feel that "dyspraxia" is a more specific term related in particular to the organization of movement and/or motor planning (Cermak, in press; Denckla & Roeltgen, 1992; Dewey, 1995; Dyspraxia Foundation, 1998; Miyahara & Mobs, 1995). Clarification of the definition of and consensus about the diagnostic criteria for developmental dyspraxia is difficult given the varied usage by a diverse group of professionals and parents.

Terms such as "congenital maladroitness" (Ford, 1960, p. 197), "physical awkwardness" (Keogh, 1968; Wall, 1982), and "clumsiness" are roughly descriptive of the behavior but provide no clear understanding of the condition. The terms "clumsy" and the "clumsy child syndrome" have been used frequently over a long period by many different professionals (Abbie, Douglas, & Ross, 1978; Arnheim & Sinclair, 1975; Cratty, 1994; Geuze & Kalverboer, 1990; Gubbay, 1975; Hall, 1988; Illingworth, 1963; Larkin & Hoare, 1992; Orton, 1937; Polatajko, 1999). Such descriptors are now considered unacceptable (Polatajko, Fox, & Missiuna, 1995), particularly if they are linked to the child rather than the movement. This is in keeping with current concerns about the psychological effect of terminology on children with disability (Hart, 1999).

Movement dysfunction has been described and defined in different ways. In 1962, Walton and colleagues described this dysfunction, stating that "[M]ovements are performed with an excessive expenditure of energy and with inaccurate judgement of the required force, tempo, and amplitude." Hall (1988) referred to "a deficit in the acquisition of skills requiring fluid coordinated movement" (p. 375). Although there is neither a universally agreed upon definition nor a set of characteristics, there is general agreement that the movement is dysfluent and that the child has motor learning difficulties (Lafuze, 1951; Larkin & Hoare, 1992; McKinlay, 1988; Missiuna, 1994; Wall, Reid, & Paton, 1990).

At a 1994 consensus meeting in London, Ontario (Polatajko et al., 1995), a multidisciplinary group of internationally recognized researchers who work with children with motor clumsiness agreed to use the term "developmental coordination disorder" as described by the American Psychiatric Association (APA) in DSM-III-R (APA, 1987) and revised in DSM-IV (APA, 1994). According to DSM-IV, the essential feature of a DCD is "a marked impairment in the development of motor coordination" (p. 53). Several additional criteria must be met for the diagnosis to be made.

1. This impairment must significantly interfere with "academic achievement or activities of daily living."
2. The coordination difficulty is "not due to a general medical condition (e.g., cerebral palsy, hemiplegia, or muscular dystrophy)" and the criteria are not met for a pervasive developmental disorder.
3. "If mental retardation is present, the motor difficulties must be in excess of those usually associated with it" (APA, 1994, p. 53).

The DSM-IV allows for the concomitant presence of attention deficit hyperactivity disorder and indicates that, if the criteria for both disorders are met, both diagnoses may be given (APA, 1994).

Another diagnostic system, the ICD-10 Classification of Mental and Behavioural Disorders in Children and Adolescents (World Health Organisation, 1996), uses the term "specific developmental disorder of motor function" (SDDMF; p. 193) to refer to children with DCD, developmental dyspraxia, or the clumsy child syndrome. The ICD-10 definition is very similar to the DSM-IV criteria for DCD. However, the criteria specified in ICD-10 do not require academic and/or daily living impairments for the diagnosis, although the characteristics described include impairments in activities of daily living. A unique feature of ICD-10 is that the motor dysfunction is usually "associated with some degree of impaired performance on visuo-spatial cognitive tasks" (p. 193). Similar to that found in the DSM-IV (APA, 1994), this description refers to the presence of associated speech problems in some of the children with SDDMF. Another feature of ICD-10 is that the diagnosis of SDDMF is made after an individually administered standardized test of gross and fine motor coordination. ICD-10 thus recommends a norm-referenced approach to the diagnosis of SDDMF, whereas DSM-IV uses a criterion-referenced approach.

Jongmans, Mercuri, Dubowitz, and Henderson (1998) point out some of the difficulty in definitional criteria. Both DSM-IV and ICD-10 include the qualification that the problem in motor coordination not be "due to a medical condition." We know that a high incidence of premature children show motor clumsiness, and some manifest neurological damage (Jongmans et al., 1998). When Gubbay (1975) proposed the definition for the clumsy syndrome, it included absence of known neurological damage. However, subsequent technology has enabled us to detect lesions in the brains of many of these children (Knuckey, Apsimon, & Gubbay, 1983). Henderson and Barnett (1998) asked, "Does the presence of a brain lesion, however small or transitory, constitute a medical condition?" (p. 463). With more sophisticated methods of assessment of structure and function, such as functional magnetic resonance imaging (MRI) and positron emission tomography (PET), heterogeneous neuropathological and pathophysiological lesions have been demonstrated but are not necessarily associated with motor clumsiness or intelligence (Cooke & Abernethy, 1999). Traditionally, such lesions were regarded as the basis of "medical conditions." Today, however, a number of neurologists and medical practitioners define a medical condition or disease as a state that is managed primarily by a physician; though this definition is somewhat controversial, it suggests how DCD might be seen as other than a medical condition even while it may involve neurological damage.

Another factor regarding the definition of DCD relates to the tool used to assess children. In the ICD-10, although a standardized test of fine and gross motor coordination is advocated, no specific tests are recommended (WHO, 1996). The use of different tests to identify children with DCD has resulted in different subject selection in research studies (Mæland, 1992; Tan, Parker, & Larkin, in press) and has likely contributed to the discrepant research findings. Smyth (1992) points out that, since motor ability can be expected to be normally distributed and children vary widely in their ability to perform motor skills, there is no generally accepted level of performance that distinguishes motor impairment, thus there can be no absolute definition.

Further difficulties arise from the interpretation of criteria set out in the DSM-IV (APA, 1994). For example, the criterion suggesting difficulties with "activities of daily living" needs clarification, as it has different meanings for different professionals. For some professionals, this terminology refers to a group of self-care tasks; for others, it refers to daily interactions with the environment. A narrow interpretation of this criterion might exclude children who would benefit from intervention.

As discussed in 1994 at the consensus meeting in London, Ontario, "DCD" might best be thought of as a temporary term that practitioners and researchers will use until we have a more thorough understanding of this complicated condition. The advantages of using this term are practical rather than theoretical. It does not carry a history of theoretical controversy like "dyspraxia," and it does not implicitly infer an etiology such as "minimal brain dysfunction." There is a very practical by-product of the recognition and diagnostic criteria provided by the APA (1987, 1994). In countries where there is publicly funded health care, children diagnosed with DCD might be eligible for government-funded assistance for therapy. Regardless of the term used to describe the clinical condition, most clinicians and researchers agree that difficulty with motor learning is a key feature. Even though children with DCD can learn motor skills, they usually require more practice than average, and the quality of movement may be compromised.

CLINICAL DESCRIPTION AND FUNCTIONAL IMPLICATIONS

It is important to recognize that DCD covers a heterogeneous group of children (Hoare, 1994; Sugden & Keogh, 1990), and not all children show the same clinical picture. This is due, in part, to the fact that there are different subtypes of DCD manifesting different profiles (see Chapter 3) and different children have different comorbidities. However, since one criteria for a diagnosis of DCD is that it "significantly interferes with the child's academic achievement or daily living skills" (APA, 1994), it is important to assess the impact of DCD on daily living skills and academic achievement.

Daily living skills that can be affected include dressing, feeding, self-care, and play skills, including fine and gross motor skills. Dressing includes tasks such as buttoning one's coat, shirt, or dress, zipping a jacket or pants, and tying one's shoes (Figure 1.1). As the child gets older, it includes learning how to cut one's fingernails, put on a tie, use a hair dryer, and put on make-up (Figure 1.2). Activities related to feeding may include using a spoon, fork, and knife, pouring from a container, or, in school, opening a lunch box, unwrapping one's sandwich, opening a bag of chips or a milk carton, or peeling an orange (Figure 1.3a, b, c, and Figure 1.4). Self-care activities such as blowing one's nose with a tissue, putting toothpaste on a toothbrush, and brushing one's teeth also demand motor planning and skill, as does opening the lock to one's school locker or house. Many leisure activities such as sewing, art projects, construction, and manipulative activities may also be difficult for the child.

Academic and pre-academic achievements also require motor skills. For the preschool child, fine motor skills are needed for constructive manipulatory play,

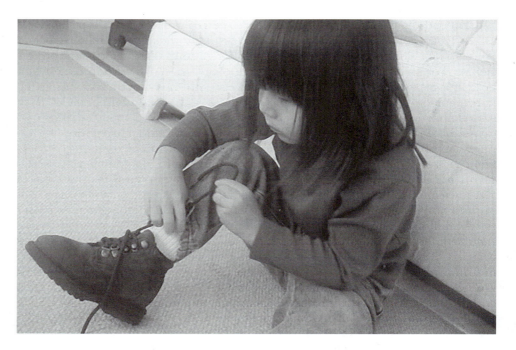

Figure 1.1   Jessa, age 4½, trying to tie her shoelaces. (Photograph taken by Bethany Cermak.)

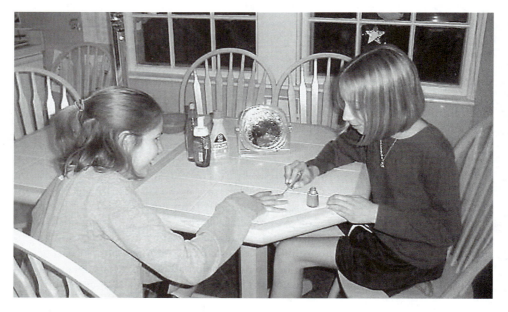

Figure 1.2   ADL activities change with age, but continue to be important through adulthood. (Photograph taken by Bethany Cermak.)

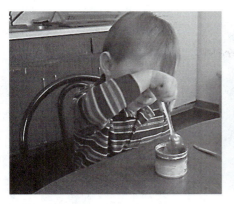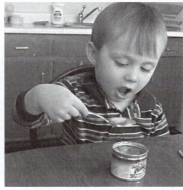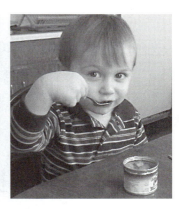

Figure 1.3   Cal, age 2½, feeds himself with a spoon. (Photograph taken by Bethany Cermak.)

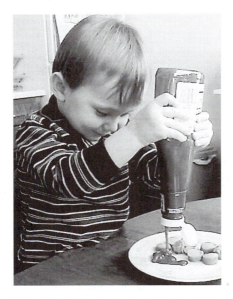

Figure 1.4   Cal is motivated to do things himself and takes pleasure in his accomplishments. (Photograph taken by Bethany Cermak.)

including building with blocks, using tinker toys, coloring, pasting, and using scissors for cutting. These activities are critical aspects of the school day and form the basis for the child's learning. As the child reaches school age, handwriting is often problematic for a child with DCD (Benbow, 1995) (Figure 1.5). Initially, learning proper letter formation and legibility may present major challenges. As the child progresses in school, he or she may have difficulty writing quickly enough to take notes in class or to complete an essay in the allotted time (Levine, Oberklaid, & Meltzer, 1981). Word processing, which is often suggested for the child with hand-

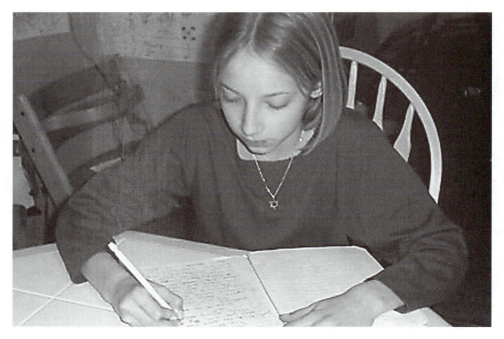

Figure 1.5   Handwriting presents a challenge for many children. (Photograph taken by Bethany Cermak.)

writing problems, may be difficult to master since problems in fine motor skills may interfere with learning keyboarding (Cermak, 1991). Difficulty in fine motor skills can also interfere with the child's participation in art, music, home economics, shop, and other classes requiring hand skills (Figure 1.6). Based on classroom observations in grades 2, 4, and 6, McHale and Cermak (1992) reported that 30–60% of a child's school day was spent in fine motor activities, with the majority of this time spent in writing. Thus, problems in fine motor skills may have a significant negative impact on school performance.

In order to participate fully in school, a child needs both fine motor and gross motor skills. Ball skills, locomotor skills, pumping a swing, and climbing are all important playground activities for the preschool child and early school aged child (Figure 1.7). For the older school aged child, gym class and playground sports are required. Primeau (1992) observed children with and without dyspraxia in a school playground. She found that children with dyspraxia participated 27% of the time, compared to 84% for control children. Bouffard, Watkinson, Thompson, Causgrove Dunn, and Romanow (1996) observed children during school recess and found that children with movement difficulties were vigorously active less often, played less often with large playground equipment, and spent less time in positive social interaction with others of their own gender. Competence in activities outside school such as riding a bicycle, rollerblading, swimming, and other sports activities is particularly important in the social arena (Figure 1.8).

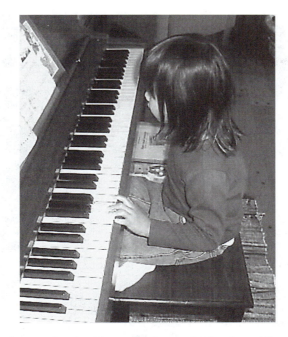

Figure 1.6   Learning to play the piano requires individuation of finger movements, bilateral integration, sequencing, and motor planning. (Photograph taken by Bethany Cermak.)

In discussing the performance of the child with DCD, it is important to consider not just whether the child is "able to perform a task," but the amount of effort and time it takes to do the task. Speed is a critical feature for school success, since limited time is allotted for each activity and transitions occur rapidly. The experiences of several children illustrate the importance of this. John, age 7, often came home with half his lunch uneaten, and complained about being "starved" all afternoon. Observation indicated that it took John 10 minutes to unwrap his lunch and get help opening his milk carton. Since the lunch period was only 20 minutes long, in effect, John had only had 5 minutes to eat his lunch before the teacher was asking the children to clean up. Mary, age 10, often did poorly on spelling tests because she did not have time to write the word before the teacher said the next word. John, age 13, was spending so much effort trying to write legibly that he couldn't understand what was being said while he was taking notes. Matthew, age 14, was highly gifted, yet his written essays in class were always short. When asked, Matthew said he intentionally wrote short essays because handwriting was so difficult. In all cases, children were frustrated by their inability to master skills. This leads to patterns of task avoidance. Based on interviews with parents of motor impaired children, Ahern (1995) reported that parents said their children often reacted to failure by giving up easily in specific areas. Some parents reported that their child was reluctant to try new things and that children avoided doing things that they felt would be difficult for them. Many parents reported that they gave

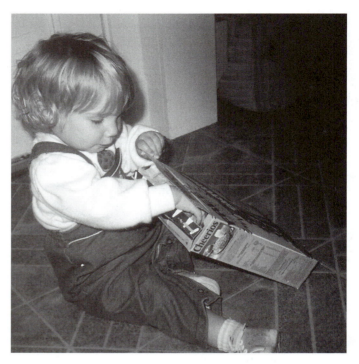

Figure 1.7   Bethany, age 14 months, uses motor planning skills to figure out how to get Cheerios™ from the box. (Photograph taken by Laird S. Cermak.)

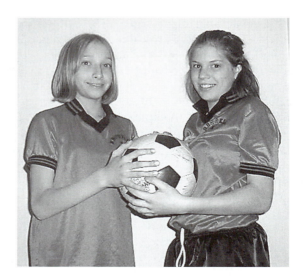

Figure 1.8   Friendships are often formed through participation in team sports. Best friends Amanda and Leah met each other playing soccer. (Photograph taken by Bethany Cermak.)

their child more time and direction to carry out activities of daily living. Some parents reported providing modifications (Ahern, 1995). One mother cut up her daughter's food, while another let her daughter eat with her fingers. Other adaptations included the use of Velcro™ fastenings rather than buttons and laces. Parents indicated that they regularly put more time and effort into teaching their child with motor impairment than they did for other siblings.

In addition to academic and daily life consequences of DCD, there are tremendous social implications. In the early years, play is largely motoric and is essential to the psychosocial aspects of development (Bundy, 1991). Play and motor skills enhance a child's feelings of self-esteem and competence (Rarick & McKee, 1949). Skill in sports and games is considered one of the best predictors of social status in childhood. Children with movement dysfunction exhibit low self-esteem, particularly in cultures that place a high value on physical ability and skill (Rose, Larkin, & Berger, 1997; Schoemaker & Kalverboer, 1994; Weingarten, 1980). In a comparison of children with learning disabilities, with and without problems in motor coordination, Shaw, Levine, and Belfer (1982) found that children with "developmental double jeopardy," that is, concomitant learning and motor problems, were at a significantly greater risk for problems in self-esteem. They also reported that children with movement difficulty were less happy than other children.

Children with poor coordination report low levels of support from classmates and best friends (Rose, Larkin, & Berger, 1994). A probable contributing factor is consistent rejection by classmates (Symes, 1972). In other research, teachers rated 41% of children with coordination problems as less popular with peers, in contrast to 13% in a control sample (Hoare, 1991). Schoemaker and Kalverboer (1994) examined the social and affective concomitants of clumsiness in children. Children with motor problems were more introverted than children without, judged themselves to be less competent both physically and socially, and were significantly more anxious. The children reported having fewer playmates and also rated themselves as less accepted by their peers. According to Schoemaker and Kalverboer (1994), 50% of the parents of a group of children with motor problems reported that their child had difficulties in making contact with other children, whereas none of the parents of controls indicated such problems. The children with motor difficulties also showed significantly more signs of anxiety. The difficulty in social skills may be both a primary and a secondary problem. Ozols and Rourke (1985) suggested that children with perceptual motor impairment might be at great risk for the development of social problems because they lack many of the perceptual and cognitive skills that are crucial in social functioning.

Longitudinal studies indicate that the presence of motor problems in middle childhood is associated with academic, cognitive, and behavioral problems at later ages (I. C. Gillberg & Gillberg, 1989). According to Fox and Lent (1996), "when children are diagnosed with DCD, physicians must have a very high index of suspicion for future psychiatric or learning disorders" (p. 1968). The social and emotional implications of DCD and the long-term consequences are reviewed in Chapter 2.

PREVALENCE

According to DSM-IV, the prevalence of DCD has been estimated to be 6% in the age range of 5–11 years. However, other estimates have varied, ranging up to 22% (Kadesjo & Gillberg, 1999; Keogh, 1968; Wright & Sugden, 1996). Population estimates for adolescents and adults also need to be established. Estimating the prevalence of DCD is difficult because there are no clear definitions and diagnostic criteria for DCD. Often, percentile cut-offs are set arbitrarily, below which a child is identified with DCD (Sugden & Keogh, 1990). In this case, each cut-off point necessarily determines the percentage of children identified with DCD. For example, Henderson and Sugden (1992) used the 15th percentile. Gubbay (1975) selected 6% of his sample of school children as clumsy after a pilot survey had suggested that this proportion of children was considered to have significant motor problems by either themselves, their parents, or their schoolteachers. Other factors influencing prevalence rates include the differences in types and methods of assessment, and cultural differences. This issue is discussed more fully in Chapter 6.

As with many other types of developmental disabilities, a higher prevalence of DCD may be found in boys than in girls (Gubbay, 1978; Henderson & Hall, 1982; Kadesjo & Gillberg, 1999; Keogh, Sugden, Reynard, & Calkins, 1979; Sovik & Mæland, 1986; Taylor, 1990), but the prevalence of movement difficulties in girls and boys has been the subject of conflicting data. Many of the samples from referred clinical populations have a higher incidence of boys with DCD; for example, Taylor (1990) reported a 3:1 ratio of males to females referred for remediation, while Missiuna (1994) found a ratio of 5:1 male/female in teacher-referred children with movement difficulties. However, some population studies report a more equal distribution (Gubbay, 1975; Mæland, 1992). Cultural influences may play a part (Stephenson, McKay, & Chesson, 1990). For example, Revie and Larkin (1993) compared rates of identification by teachers of boys and girls with poor coordination. The girls whom the teachers identified as clumsy had significantly poorer motor coordination than the boys did. The implication is that girls have to have more severe movement difficulties than boys in order to be diagnosed. Gubbay (1975) attributes the greater diagnoses of male children to possibly greater parental concerns over sons' than daughters' motor skills.

Gender differences may also be influenced by the characteristics of the tasks used to assess coordination. As early as 1933, Yarmolenko reported that children between the ages of 8 and 15 years showed gender differences in many activities. In general, girls excelled in activities that require the use of finer coordination, while boys excelled in those that require grosser movements or strength. Thus, tests that emphasize fine motor skills, where females are typically more proficient, are more likely to identify males, whereas tests that emphasize strength or gross motor skills, where males are generally more proficient, are more likely to identify females (Jongmans et al., 1998). In fact, Rarick, Dobbins, and Broadhead (1976) identified two profiles of coordination difficulty: fine motor problems and gross motor problems. The profile characterized by poor fine motor coordination consisted of mostly boys, whereas the profile characterized by gross motor difficulty consisted of mostly girls. Having separate gender norms on tests would attenuate this difference; however, most screening tools do not have separate gender norms.

RECOGNITION

Early recognition of DCD is particularly difficult, so DCD is often not identified until the child reaches school age. This may be because a particular child's lack of coordination only becomes a problem when it results in failure to satisfy his or her particular environmental demands, and it is in school where the child's inability to meet the requirements becomes problematic. Morris and Whiting (1971) point out that the problem of motor impairment relates in part to the value placed on motor skills by a child's culture. The demands for motor proficiency are a function of age, gender, environment, and culture.

Delayed motor milestones may be one of the early indicators of DCD. It has been reported that many children reach motor milestones at a later than average age. Johnston, Short, and Crawford (1987) found that 13% were delayed. Gubbay (1978) reported delays in motor milestones in 18% of his sample. Of the group of 51 children with motor problems, Knuckey et al. (1983) reported that 42 (83%) showed delayed motor milestones. Hoare (1991) looked at motor milestones in a group of 80 children with poor coordination compared to a control sample. She found that the average age of crawling was similar between two groups, although the children with poor coordination walked later (14.5 months ± 4.2 compared to 12.4 ± 2.2 months). In a study of 114 children who had attended a movement intervention program, the percentage of parents reporting delay in reaching motor milestones was as follows: riding a tricycle or bicycle, 65%; crawling, 40%; walking, 39%; and speaking, 28% (Ahern, 1995). Over half of the parents reported that they had sought help in the first place because their child's milestones were delayed. However, tricycle riding was included, and this is often not considered a motor milestone, but a more complex skill. The majority of children with DCD have difficulty learning complex motor skills, even when their motor milestones are within the average range.

There are several reasons why early recognition/diagnosis of DCD is important. The sooner movement difficulties are diagnosed, the less likely it is that associated social, emotional, and behavioral problems will develop because early identification and treatment can provide physical and emotional gains (Abbie et al., 1978; Schoemaker, Hijlkema, & Kalverboer, 1994). Short and Crawford (1984) found that self-esteem problems increase at between 5 and 7 years of age. These authors reported that poor self-concept was almost twice as prevalent in 7-year-old motor-impaired children as in unimpaired children. In contrast, the self-concept of 5-year-olds was the same for both groups.

Students with DCD often are considered lazy, overprotected, or immature. In the study by the Dyspraxia Foundation, when parents were asked about the school's attitude toward their child prior to diagnosis, 80% of parents said school staff believed that the child would grow out of the movement problem. Seventy-five percent of teachers believed the child could do better if he or she tried harder. Results from over half the schools indicated the children were "naughty," and over a third of the schools felt poor parenting contributed to the problem. In addition, 45% of parents reported that when the diagnosis of dyspraxia was made, the school reported they had never heard of it (Dyspraxia Parent Website). Nevertheless, identification can contribute to a more positive and supportive environment for the child with DCD.

ETIOLOGY

There is no single factor that causes DCD, and the etiology is unclear (Wall et al., 1990) and probably heterogeneous (Gubbay, 1975). Advances in structural and functional imaging of the brain have indicated that wide areas of the brain are involved in the planning and performance of motor actions (Rizzolatti, Luppino, & Matelli, 1998; Rowe & Frackowiak, 1999; Willingham, 1998). Additionally, research into the effect of motor skill learning on the development of the brain (Anderson, Alcantara, & Greenough, 1996; Kleim et al., 1998) and the clearly documented responsiveness of the damaged neuromuscular system to training (Liepert et al., 1998) attests to the interplay between experience and structure. Clearly, we have to explore multicausative models.

Various causes of DCD have been investigated at different levels of analysis, and a wide range of approaches has been taken to identify the source of the difficulties experienced by children with DCD (Barnett, Kooistra, & Henderson, 1998). Factors considered center around brain damage or dysfunction, genetic predisposition, impairment in information processing, or an impoverished environment (or reduced opportunities). Each of these views will be discussed individually, although it is emphasized that they are not mutually exclusive.

Brain Damage or Dysfunction

Early researchers suggested that children with motor dysfunction may be experiencing "minimal brain damage" (Gubbay et al., 1965; Walton et al., 1962). Researchers have examined neurological soft signs, and, although they found more soft signs in children with DCD than in controls (Henderson & Hall, 1982; Lundy-Ekman, Ivry, Keele, & Woollacott, 1991), the etiological significance for DCD is not clear (Touwen, 1990).

Prenatal, perinatal, or postnatal incidents affecting early brain development are thought to play an important role in developmental coordination disorders. The effects of these factors have been studied in two ways. First, birth histories and brain scans of children later identified as clumsy have been examined retrospectively. Second, children born at risk (e.g., premature, low birth weight) have been followed longitudinally. Both approaches have yielded converging evidence.

Birth Histories and DCD

Gubbay (1975, 1985) stated that a history of perinatal abnormalities is often found in children with DCD, particularly those with more severe movement problems. Similarly, Johnston, Short, and Crawford (1987) described a greater incidence of perinatal complications (especially jaundice), lower birth weights, and a higher incidence of children being premature or overdue in a sample of children with poor coordination.

Hoare (1991) studied 160 children aged 6–9 years. Eighty children were classified as poorly coordinated, and 80 had normal coordination. In the sample of children with coordination problems, 31% were born more than 2 weeks premature, compared to 13% in the normal control sample. Thirty-three percent of mothers of these children had pregnancy complications, compared to 17% in the control sample. Furthermore, 50% of parents of the sample with poor coordination reported that the birth of their child was accompanied by complications, including a greater incidence of breech birth, use of forceps, cesarean section, and vacuum extraction. This figure was lower (37%) in the control sample. Hoare also reported the birth weight of the two groups. The sample of children with coordination problems had a mean weight of 3,182 ± 739 grams at birth compared to 3,434 ± 586 grams for the control group. In addition, neonatal problems were more prevalent in the group with coordination problems (42%) than in the control group (20%), mainly due to a greater incidence of jaundice, ventilation, and other risk factors.

Few studies have examined brain images in children with DCD. In one that did, Knuckey et al. (1983) examined commuted tomography (CT) scans of 51 children with developmental clumsiness, aged 8 to 12. Overall, 39% of these children (compared to 9% of the control group) showed abnormal CT scans. When the children with movement problems were subdivided into mild and severe subgroups, approximately 50% of the children who were rated as having severe motor problems showed abnormal CT scans. These abnormalities included ventricular dilatation, peripheral atrophy, and parenchymal disruption. However, there was not a particular pattern of abnormality.

Children Born at Risk

DCD is frequently found among preterm or low birth weight children (Fox & Lent, 1996; Marlow, Roberts, & Cooke, 1993). Conditions related to prematurity are considered major predisposing factors, if not a direct cause of brain injury (Jongmans et al., 1998; Levene et al., 1992). An increasing number of studies are focusing on the relationship between brain lesions identified in prematurely born children and later outcomes.

Levene et al. (1992) examined 152 children at age 5 years, from a cohort of very low birth weight infants who had sequential ultrasound examinations in the neonatal period. As a group, the low birth weight children studied at 5 years scored significantly higher (more motor problems) on the Test of Motor Impairment (TOMI) than their matched controls. When the low birth weight children were divided into four groups on the basis of their neonatal ultrasound scans, the group with the more abnormal scans (germinal matrix haemorrhage to intraventricular hemorrhage)—that is, without parenchymal involvement and with prolonged flares—had significantly more problems with manual dexterity than the group with consistently normal CT scans.

Jongmans and colleagues (Jongmans, Henderson, de Vries, & Dubowitz, 1993; Jongmans et al., 1998) followed children born prematurely in a longitudinal study and found that some children had perceptual-motor problems at school age, while others did not. MRI scans indicated that some of these children had small lesions at birth that persisted with age, some had small lesions that resolved with age, while others had apparently normal brain scans. These authors found that, at age 6 years, the premature group scored significantly more poorly than the matched control children on all perceptual motor measures, including the Movement ABC. Half the sample of children with prematurity had perceptual-motor problems. Moreover, the children with multiple perceptual-motor problems, failing both the Movement ABC and the VMI test, had been born significantly earlier, and a greater proportion had shown brain lesions than premature children with no perceptual-motor problems. The children with perceptual-motor problems were also more likely to show co-occurring minor neurological signs and problems of cognition, reading, and/or behavior.

In a longitudinal study in Finland, more than 1,000 children with various risk factors since birth, including low birth weight, respiratory problems, Apgar score of 6 or less at 5 minutes, and hyperbilirubinemia, were followed. When children were tested at ages 5 and 9 years, the investigators found that children with motor problems were seen significantly more often in the risk group than in the control group (Michelsson & Lindahl, 1993). In a recent study, neonatal ischemic white-matter injury, identified by cranial ultrasound, was associated with poor motor performance in children with low birthweight assessed at ages 2, 6, and 9 years (Pinto-Martin, Whitaker, Feldman, Van Rossem, & Paneth, 1999). However, a study of 15–17-year-old adolescents (from a cohort of very low birthweight infants) failed to find a relationship between lesions identified with cranial MRI and problems with motor performance on the Movement ABC (Cooke & Abernethy, 1999). What now appears as an inconsistent relationship between motor dysfunction and underlying brain damage might become clearer with increased understanding of the interplay between neural plasticity and environmental stimulation (Kolb, 1999).

Family Factors

Illingworth (1968) indicated that clumsiness is often a familial feature. More often than by chance, there may be a family history of motor or related neurodevelopmental dysfunction (Gubbay, 1975). Evidence of a familial relationship comes from different sources, and the incidence varies. Gubbay (1978) reported a family history in 21% of a group with developmental apraxia. Johnston et al. (1987) reported a history of clumsiness in close relatives ranging from 20% in their 5-year-olds to 13% in their 7-year-olds. In a study of 80 children with coordination difficulties and 80 controls, 30% of children with poor coordination had another member of their family considered to be poorly coordinated, in contrast to 4% in the control group (Hoare, 1991).

Other indicators of familial contributions to coordination difficulties, particularly in conjunction with problems with speech and language, have focused on genetic links. From their study of dyslexics, Wolff, Melngailis, Obregon, and Bedrosian (1995) concluded that there was a behavioral phenotype with impaired motor timing. Kaplan, Wilson, Dewey, and Crawford (1994) reported on a subtype of reading disability, accompanied by deficits in motor coordination and balance, and suggested that this subtype was inherited. Stordy (2000) suggests a genetic predisposition as the common basis for comorbid dyslexia and DCD. Her preliminary data suggests that a problem with fatty acid conversion is linked to both disorders. Further support for heritability of motor- and language-related problems comes from a study of an English family, the K.E. family (Watkins, Gadian, & Vargha-Khadem, 1999), where the authors suggest that the disorder may be a motor learning dysfunction particularly related to articulation. Current research is also focusing on genetic links to visuospatial construction (for review, see Mervis, Robinson, & Pani, 1999), which might have implications for DCD. Knowing more about the genetic links to coordination problems should improve our understanding of subtypes of DCD and lead to earlier and better-targeted interventions for some children.

INFORMATION PROCESSING APPROACHES

Walton and colleagues (1962) pointed out that cerebral disorganization in a neuro-physiological sense rather than an anatomical sense might be a more accurate interpretation of clumsiness. They considered that it was "the pathways concerned with the organization of skilled movement, or recognition of tactile and other sensory stimuli which are poorly organized" (p. 610). Impaired perceptual-motor performance, which was often linked to known causes of brain damage, led researchers to examine the relationship between perceptual motor factors and motor impairment using information processing approaches (Morris & Whiting, 1971). Movement dysfunction has been linked to different perceptual processing (Hoare, 1994; Laszlo & Bairstow, 1983; Lord & Hulme, 1988; Mon-Williams, Wann, & Pascal, 1999; Wilson & McKenzie, 1998), defects in motor organization (Geuze & Kalverboer, 1990; Henderson, Rose, & Henderson, 1992; Lundy-Ekman et al., 1991; Williams, Woollacott, & Ivry, 1992), or both (Hoare, 1994; Smyth & Glencross, 1986; Smyth & Mason, 1997). In trying to understand the nature of DCD, many investigators have examined the mechanisms and processes that are linked to movement skill problems. Children with DCD generally perform more poorly than control children on a variety of measures reflective of motor control and motor learning (for reviews see Chapter 8), and sensory/perceptual processing (see Chapters 5 and 7). There are clear indications of heterogeneity (Hoare, 1994; Mon-Williams et al., 1999), and there is debate as to whether these information processing problems are underlying causes or emergent manifestations of DCD.

THE EFFECTS OF EXPERIENCE

Studies that have looked at experience and the effects of movement experience on the development of motor skills in children with DCD are remarkably few. An early study by Rarick and McKee (1949) did pioneering work in this area. They found that children with extremely low levels of motor competence had inferior experiences in the movement domain. As a consequence, children with movement difficulties may refrain from participation in physical activity due to a cycle of demonstrated incompetence, lack of confidence, exclusion, and withdrawal, which is based on a history of failure in the motor skill domain (Bouffard et al., 1996; Cermak, 1985). Withdrawal from movement, in turn, leads to limited interaction with the environment, which we propose could have multiple impacts on a child's optimal development in multiple domains. Specifically, a reduction in levels of participation in physical activity has an additional and negative effect on physical fitness and motor skills (Bouffard et al., 1996; see Chapter 11).

Harvey and Reid (1997) examined gross motor performance and fitness in a group of children with attention deficit hyperactivity disorder (ADHD), a group that also has been identified as poorly coordinated (Beyer, 1993). As a group, the performance of children with ADHD in fitness and fundamental gross motor skills was below average when compared to the norms of children of similar age and gender. Poor motor performance and poor physical fitness lead to a lack of sustained effort and practice, low levels of self-esteem, and, consequently, to a lack of participation, which further reduces opportunities for skill and fitness development.

It is clear from the longitudinal studies (Cantell, Smyth, & Ahonen, 1994; Gubbay, 1978; Visser, Geuze, & Kalverboer, 1998) that a proportion of children diagnosed with DCD in early years no longer manifest DCD in adolescence. The effect of their experiences with movement has received little documentation. Clearly, there is a need for further longitudinal research into the effects of movement experiences on the manifestation of DCD.

COMORBID CONDITIONS

Many medical or neurological conditions, including visual impairment, thyroid malfunction, congenital hypothyroidism, mild cerebral palsy, and early stage muscular dystrophy, can contribute to impaired motor performance (Barnett et al., 1998; Denckla & Roeltgen, 1992; Fox & Lent, 1996; Gubbay, 1975). The reader is referred to Denckla and Roeltgen (1992) for a discussion of differential diagnosis. For a diagnosis of DCD, it is important that these conditions be ruled out. For example, nonspecific abnormalities have been shown to occur in the electroencephalogram (EEG) of children with developmental dyspraxia (Gubbay, 1975). Despite its limitations, EEG may be useful in DCD for excluding an underlying or associated epileptic disorder, or where there is a suspicion of a progressive neurological condition, and sometimes when reassurance is required. DCD may occur in isolation, although it frequently coexists with a variety of other learning problems, including attention deficits, learning disability, and speech/language deficits (Gubbay, 1975; Henderson & Hall, 1982; Kadesjo & Gillberg, 1999; Polatajko, 1999; Shaw et al., 1982).

Learning Disabilities and DCD

Learning difficulties in children with motor impairments have been studied by a number of investigators, and it is possible that they can be causally linked. For example, Strang and Rourke (1985) identified a subtype of learning disability that they called "nonverbal perceptual-organizational-output disability (NPOOD). Children with NPOOD exhibit bilateral psychomotor impairment, difficulty with complex movement skills, and disability in the perception, analysis, organization, and synthesis of nonverbal information. Rourke (1989) later referred to this as "nonverbal learning disability." In other instances, the motor and academic learning difficulties may be comorbid. Certainly, the prevalence of academically based learning difficulties is high among children with DCD. Gubbay (1975) reported that 50% of children with problems in motor coordination had difficulty with schoolwork, a slightly higher prevalence than the 41% reported by Sprinkle and Hammond. Drillien and Drummond (1983) reported that 32% of children with motor impairments had moderate problems in school and 32% had severe problems. Dellen, van, Vaessen, and Schoemaker (1990) reported that one third of their sample of 31 children identified as clumsy repeated a grade, compared to one child in the control group. Although somewhat variable, all these studies indicate that many children with problems in motor coordination also show school-related problems.

A high incidence of children with learning disabilities has also been identified as having poor motor coordination and visual-motor skills. However, it is recognized that problems in motor coordination are not predictive of a learning disability and that not all children with learning disabilities have problems in motor coordination (Miyahara, 1994). A number of factors influence prevalence rates. These include differences in types and methods of testing, reliability of the instruments used, and heterogeneity of the test sample (Henderson, 1994; Johnston et al., 1987). It is difficult to determine the prevalence of motor deficits within the learning disability population and the prevalence of a learning disability within the DCD population. Measurement is confounded by inconsistencies of definition of learning disability, and the differing criteria and tests used to identify children with problems in motor coordination (Mæland, 1992; Tan et al., 2001). To date, there is no consistent correlation between motor dysfunction and learning disabilities. Moreover, the motor deficits of children with learning disabilities are quite variable, and there is not a characteristic pattern (Cermak, 1985, 1991; Miyahara, 1994).

Attention Deficit Disorder and DCD

According to Fox and Lent (1996), about half of all children with DCD also have attention deficit disorder, with or without hyperactivity. The recent study from Sweden provides support for this estimate (Kadesjo & Gillberg, 1999). Although problems in attention or hyperactivity also can contribute to poor motor performance, many children with ADHD have problems in motor coordination and fitness in addition to their hyperactivity and attentional problems (Beyer, 1993; Harvey & Reid, 1997). Gillberg and colleagues (Gillberg, I. C., Gillberg, & Groth, 1989; Rasmussen, Gillberg, Waldenstrom, & Svenson, 1983) recognized comorbidity of attentional, motor, and perceptual problems found in children and coined the acronym "DAMP" for deficits in attention, motor control, and perception. Denckla, Rudel, Chapman, and Krieger (1985) reported that children with dyslexia and attentional disorders had a significantly poorer motor proficiency than did children with dyslexia without attentional problems. More recently, Norrelgen, Lacerda, and Forssberg (1999) reported that children with combined ADHD and DCD also had a problem with phonological working memory.

Because of the frequent comorbidity between DCD and other developmental disorders, Kaplan, Wilson, Dewey, and Crawford (1998) suggest that DCD may not be a discrete disorder. They suggest that the term "atypical brain development" may be more appropriate (see Chapter 3). This suggestion is controversial, and many believe it is like going back to the "minimal brain dysfunction" concept (Clements, 1966) of the 1960s. Rispens and van Yperen (1997) point out that, in the 10th edition of the International Classification of Diseases (ICD), specific developmental disorder (SDD) serves as a conceptual umbrella, suggesting that the subsumed disorders are of the same type. However, they propose that it is premature to use the term SDD as a unifying concept in classification.

SUMMARY AND CONCLUSIONS

So what is DCD? In 1985, the Committee on Children with Disabilities stated that children "grow out of" clumsiness. This view is no longer considered accurate. Strong evidence exists that many children's motor problems persist well into adolescence and adulthood (see Chapter 2). Certain lifestyles and events can increase difficulties with motor performance. The negative impact of movement withdrawal or low levels of physical activity on the developing motor system, the musculoskeletal system, and the cardiorespiratory system can increase movement problems. Psychosocial stresses can further exacerbate the condition.

In 1971, Morris and Whiting stated that it is difficult to attribute the deficit to particular causal factors. This is still true today. The influence of ecological and dynamic systems frameworks on the field of motor control and learning is now affecting how we view DCD and might resolve some of the current puzzles. A dysfunction in any of the multiple subsystems involved in the organization of motor tasks could contribute to multiple developmental pathways and the heterogeneous profiles of children with DCD. Initial perturbations occurring at one level of a child's system might have repercussions throughout the system if other conditions are not optimal. As Gottlieb (1998) suggests, "An understanding of developmental phenomena demands a relational or coactive concept of causality as opposed to singular causes acting in supposed isolation" (p. 799).

"Developmental coordination disorder" is a fuzzy term without a precise definition. It serves to define a broad band of mild motor problems that researchers and practitioners are still struggling to refine. It is important that descriptions of DCD remain flexible until we have a better understanding of the motor learning and performance limitations of children and adolescents with movement dysfunctions and how different manifestations of DCD might interfere with optimal development.

CHAPTER

2

Long-Term Outcomes of Developmental Coordination Disorder

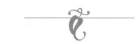

Marja Cantell and Libbe Kooistra

Motor development does not occur in isolation, but is set in a context of interrelated factors (Connolly & Forssberg, 1997) that change over time. Many so-called risk factors have no implications in isolation but become important in interaction with other factors (Kalverboer, 1988). Therefore, in the event of motor dysfunction, considering only the perceptual and physical systems does not take into account the dynamics of motor development or its interactive context (Dent-Read & Zukow-Goldring, 1997). Consequently, the purpose of this chapter is to review longitudinal studies on children with DCD, not only from the perceptual motor perspective, but also from the cognitive and social perspectives. Our goal is to give a multidimensional review on the issue of persistency of DCD by looking at the various assessments and sampling methods used in different studies, summarizing the main results, and discussing the limitations embedded in developmental studies in general. In the end, we suggest some recommendations based on our review for future follow-up and intervention studies on DCD.

FOLLOW-UP STUDIES WITH DCD POPULATIONS

Perceptual Motor Outcome

The studies chosen for this review are presented in Table 2.1. Information is included regarding the definitions, screening, follow-up procedures, and outcome measures. These studies represent different theoretical bases and were carried out by professionals from different backgrounds (physical educators, physiotherapists, occupational therapists, psychologists, neurologists, and pediatricians). Some of the included studies are based on neurodevelopmental theory (Hadders-Algra, Huisjes, & Touwen, 1988; Lunsing, Hadders-Algra, Huisjes, & Touwen, 1992; Soorani-Lunsing, Hadders-Algra, Huisjes, & Touwen, 1994; Soorani-Lunsing, Hadders-Algra, Olinga, & Huisjes, 1993); others use a neuropsychological approach (Ahonen, 1990; Cantell, Smyth, & Ahonen, 1994, 1999; Lyytinen & Ahonen, 1989), a neurological or psychiatric approach (Hellgren, Gillberg, Gillberg, & Enerskog, 1993; Hellgren, Gillberg, Bagenholm, & Gillberg, 1994; Shafer, Shaffer, O'Connor, & Stokman, 1986), or a descriptive approach (Geuze & Borger, 1993; Knuckey & Gubbay, 1983; Losse et al., 1991; van Dellen, Vaessen, & Schoemaker, 1990).

Two Views on the Developmental Course of DCD

The literature on DCD in later childhood and adolescence offers two different and sometimes contradictory views on how persistent the problems are. There is an optimistic view of DCD, which states that DCD is largely confined to childhood

Table 2.1A Longitudinal Studies on Perceptual Motor Development

Authors Country Type	Screening Sample	Definition (Examiner)	Follow-up Sample	Outcome
Henderson & Hall, 1982; Losse et al., 1991/UK/ descriptive	5–6 years 16 screened 16 control	Clumsiness (teacher)	15–17 years 17 clumsy 17 control	87% persistent DCD 8 of 14 items discriminated groups
Knuckey & Gubba, 1983/Australia/ descriptive	8–12 years 52 screened 51 control	Clumsiness (neurologist)	16–20 years 24 clumsy 31 control	35% persistent DCD 2 of 5 items discriminated groups
Van Dellen et al., 1990; Geuze & Börger, 1993/ Netherlands/ descriptive	6–12 years 31 clumsy 30 control	Clumsiness (teacher)	11–17 years 19 clumsy 24 control	50–75% persistent clumsy 3–6 tasks discriminated groups

Table 2.1B   Longitudinal Studies on Perceptual Motor Development

Authors Country Type	Screening Sample	Definition (Examiner)	Follow-up Sample	Outcome
Hadders-Algra et al., 1988; Soorani-Lunsing et al., 1992, 1993, 1994/ Netherlands/ neurodevelopmental	6 years 482 screened 322 control	MND (neurologist)	12–14 years 167 MND 169 control	**At age 12:** 78% persistent MND 24% Hypotonia 21% Choreiform dyskinesia 17% Coordination problems 48% Fine manipulative disability **At age 14:** 40% persistent MND 8% Hypotonia 8% Choreiform dyskinesia 5% Coordination problems 17% Fine manipulative disability
Lyytinen & Ahonen, 1989; Ahonen, 1990; Cantell et al., 1994; Cantell, 1998/Finland/ neuropsychological	5 years 146 screened 40 control	Motor delay (nurse)	7–17 years **At age 11:** 74 delay 40 control **At age 15:** 81 delay 34 control **At age 17:** 45 delay 20 control	**At age 11:** 62% persistent motor delay Visuo-motor and hopping problems the strongest predictors of motor delay **At age 15:** 46% persistent motor delay **At age 17:** 46% persistent motor delay
Rasmussen et al., 1983; Gillberg & Gillberg, 1989; Hellgren et al., 1993/ Sweden/neurological and psychiatric	7 years 82 screened 59 control	DAMP: 42 MPD/ADD 7 MPD (pre-school teachers)	**At age 13:** 37 MPD/ADD 5 MPD 44 control **At age 16:** 39 MPD/ADD 6 MPD 45 control	**At age 13:** 30% persistent MPD or MPD/ADD 29% overall clumsiness 6 of 13 items discriminated groups **At age 16:** 33% severe MPD/ADD 36% overall clumsiness
Shaffer et al., 1985; Shafer et al., 1986/US/ neurological	7 years 86 screened 86 control	Soft signs (neurologist)	17–18 years 82 soft signs 81 control	61% of the boys had at least one soft sign 32% of the girls had at least one soft sign 4/5 tasks discriminated groups

and that it decreases with age. Erhardt, McKinlay, and Bradley (1987), who suggested that it takes adolescents with poor coordination longer to reach a ceiling in their performance, support this. Hall (1988) proposed that motor problems disappear by adolescence and that they therefore cannot be called "long-term disabilities." Also, the results by Knuckey and Gubbay (1983) might be interpreted as falling into this optimistic category. They found that mild to moderate degrees of clumsiness improved to normality by age 16–20 years and concluded that DCD as a problem is largely confined to childhood, rather than being a long-term disability. However, they also reported a particular category of children with severe degrees of clumsiness that had a less favorable outcome. Knuckey and Gubbay (1983) suggested that maturational lag might be the etiology in mild developmental clumsiness, whereas structural lesions involving the cerebral cortex might be present in the more severely afflicted children.

The more pessimistic view of the long-term prognosis is that DCD does not disappear as a function of age. Several follow-up studies have shown that about half of the children who were motor impaired remain poorer in their motor performance than their controls until adolescence (Ahonen, 1990; Geuze & Börger, 1993; Hellgren et al., 1993; Losse et al., 1991). Cantell (1998) and Cantell et al. (1994) suggested that persistency of DCD is related to the severity of the problem; 47% of their original sample had persistent and severe DCD, and 53% had changed and become quite similar to their controls. Some researchers have considered that movement difficulties reflect performance at the lower end of the normal distribution (Hall, 1988; Latash & Anson, 1996). A viewpoint like this allows a child's movement problems to be placed on a continuum of severity, rather than categorizing children as "having" DCD or not having it.

A comparison can be made between three sets of longitudinal studies using slightly different approaches. The longitudinal studies by Hadders-Algra et al. (1988) and Soorani-Lunsing et al. (1994) focused on minor neurological dysfunction (MND), or "soft" signs, and related them to motor dysfunction. It was hypothesized that the soft signs might indicate a nervous system that is wired differently from normal, which results in increased vulnerability of the brain to exogenous influences. Soorani-Lunsing et al. (1994) divided the sample into two groups according to their follow-ups at 9 and 13 years of age: persistent MND and transient MND. The persistent type was suggested to reflect a MND that, in contrast to its transient type, cannot be moderated by the onset of puberty. Persistent MND was related not only to motor, but also to behavioral and cognitive problems. The adolescents in the transient MND group had a good outcome resembling their normative peers.

The second comparison is a longitudinal study of 11- to 16-year-old boys with and without DCD by Visser, Geuze, and Kalverboer (1998). The approach was explorative, examining the relationships among physical growth, level of physical activity, and DCD. A multilevel regression modeling produced a surprising outcome: adolescents with DCD were not as affected by the growth spurt as the adolescents in the control group. Improvement in motor competence was to some extent affected by the type and amount of physical activity undertaken during the follow-up. It seemed that the majority of children with DCD caught up with controls. Visser et al. (1998) suggested that children with DCD seem to profit from the growth spurt possibly because of enhanced maturation of some parts of the central nervous system. This suggestion agrees with Soorani-Lunsing et al. (1994), who argued that motor problems could be a sign of a differently maturing CNS.

The third group of studies used the term DAMP for describing the subgroups with deficits in attention, motor control, and perception, or both attention and motor problems (Gillberg & Gillberg, 1989). At age 13, motor perceptual problems remained in 30% of the children originally identified at 7 years of age (called "severe" in Gillberg, Gillberg, & Groth, 1989). This result was interpreted to indicate a fair prognosis. However, children with mild or moderate DAMP were also likely to suffer from academic and behavioral problems. At 16 years of age, a comparison of the pooled DAMP group ($n = 56$) had significantly more problems with balance than the control group ($n = 45$; Hellgren et al., 1993). The subgroups originally diagnosed with MPDADD (motor and attention problems) and the MPD (motor problems) had significantly longer complex reaction times than the control group. The subgroup with more severe MPDADD demonstrated a higher incidence of left-handedness, more fine motor problems, and overall clumsiness (Hellgren et al., 1993). In a later review, Gillberg (1998) concluded that DAMP is a neurodevelopmental disorder with changing clinical landmarks and that it can continue to cause difficulties throughout childhood and adolescence. Sugden and Wright (1998) have pointed out, in reference to Gillberg's studies, that the overlap between motor problems and other related ones, such as attention and hyperactivity problems, makes it difficult to disentangle a clear motor outcome.

In sum, the studies reviewed here report different amounts of persistent perceptual motor problems in adolescence. Although some children seem to have a long-term DCD, others have an improving trajectory, and a uniform pattern of problems is difficult to establish. We suggest that, by making the distinction in the degree of severity of DCD, as well as controlling the effects of growth and physical activity levels, it is possible to reveal qualitative differences in individuals with perceptual motor problems. These qualitative differences might be crucial in determining not only the long-term outcome in the perceptual motor domain, but also in the cognitive and social domains. The next sections will deal with associated problems and address whether catching up with motor development also results in disappearance of academic and social problems.

Academic and Educational Outcome

Studies on children with DCD in which the development of academic competence has been examined are relatively rare. Two follow-up studies have continued until the age of 16 (Hellgren et al., 1994; Losse et al., 1991), and four of these studies continued until 17 years of age (Cantell, Smyth, & Ahonen, 2000; Geuze & Börger, 1993; Knuckey & Gubbay, 1983; Shafer et al., 1986). The main focus of these studies has been on estimating average levels of cognitive competence without paying much attention to the severity of the underlying perceptual motor difficulties. However, the additional problems experienced by adolescents with less severe DCD are likely to be less than those experienced by adolescents diagnosed with severe DCD. Although, in both cases, academic progress might be at risk, it seems that combined perceptual motor problems, especially when associated with decreased IQ levels, may affect a whole spectrum of educational, social, and behavioral areas.

Of the studies carried out, Knuckey and Gubbay (1983) reported a favorable motor outcome in their 17-year-olds, but levels of academic achievement were lower than expected. Although, on group level, this finding was unrelated to severity of motor problems, those individual adolescents with extreme motor problems had the least skilled jobs. Further, the DCD group was found to be engaged in sports as much as the control group. Knuckey and Gubbay concluded that only a small proportion of the individuals with DCD is likely to be affected by their disability after leaving school. However, they suggested the possibility of secondary emotional disturbances occurring together with DCD.

The longitudinal study of Shafer et al. (1986) included a population of children with motor soft signs and focused primarily on the relationship between the neurological and emotional status. They also studied IQ at the ages of 7 and 17. Although IQ at age 7 was related to IQ at 17, it had almost no relationship to neurological status at age 17. When the relationship between IQ at 7 and persistency of soft signs between 7 and 17 was studied, persistent soft signs were confined to the subgroup of individuals with the lowest IQs. In further analyses, they confirmed that the relationship of persistent soft signs and low IQ did not explain the whole picture: both the lowest and the highest IQ scores were particularly related to more soft signs. Shafer et al. did not study the educational status of adolescents with DCD, but they suggested that the suboptimal neurological performance, particularly of boys, could not be explained solely in terms of a maturational lag.

Children with DCD showed problems in learning and concentration in several other follow-up studies (Ahonen, 1990; Geuze & Börger, 1993; Gillberg & Gillberg, 1989). When Gillberg and Gillberg restudied their original 7-year-old sample at age 13, school achievement problems were still common in the DAMP group. Moreover, when, at age 7, the motor problem was the only diagnosis of a child, 40% had poor school achievement at age 13; when severe combined motor and attention problems were diagnosed at age 7, 85% had poor school achievement at age 13 (compared with 30% of the comparison group). This was supported by Ahonen's follow-up (1990), in which 75% of children with stable DCD had learning difficulties at age 11, in comparison to 25% of their peers.

Losse et al. (1991) reported that by age 16 the adolescents diagnosed with DCD at age 6 had lower school achievement and IQ, although their effort ratings were similar to others. In relation to this, Cantell et al. (1994) found that at age 15 there was a relationship between IQ scores, school records, and educational plans in adolescents with DCD. The group with persistent DCD had lower IQ and school records and preferred less challenging educational choices. As a consequence, some of them were already unemployed at the age of 17 (Cantell, 1998). The group, who caught up in their motor competence, also had lower IQ, but their school records and future plans were similar to the control group. It seems that a combination of personal and environmental factors plays an aggravating role in the adolescent educational/academic outcome of DCD.

In sum, the majority of longitudinal studies on DCD report some degree of cognitive and academic underachievement in adolescents with early-diagnosed DCD. It may be suggested that IQ has prognostic value for those children with DCD with borderline intellectual functioning. However, in those studies in which the effects of IQ were controlled, the perceptual deficits in DCD persisted (Ahonen, 1990; Cantell, 1998). Further research is needed to understand the role of catching up, the possible adaptability of the CNS in some individuals, and the lack of it in others.

Social and Emotional Outcomes

A few studies on DCD have investigated the issue of associated social and emotional problems related to atypical motor development. The majority of the studies used questionnaires, either with children or adolescents with DCD, or with their parents and teachers. Three studies also conducted interviews.

Self-Perceptions

Recent studies on self-perception in children with DCD have applied the multifaceted approach and, thus, have provided a profile for various dimensions of self-perceptions. Although most of these studies are not longitudinal, their results can contribute to the understanding of the development and the long-term outcome of self-perception. For example, Maeland (1992) studied Harter's (1982) cognitive, social, and physical dimensions of self-perception in 10-year-old children with and without DCD. In addition, she compared them on Harter's Global Self-Worth component. Only differences in the physical domain were found. Children with DCD perceived themselves as being poorer in sport and outdoor games. However, results also revealed that the difference was no larger than could be explained by differences in actual performance. It was concluded that children were realistic about their physical skills and that their motor problems did not affect their self-esteem. Willoughby and Polatajko (1995), in a comparable study, reported slightly more negative findings. Six-year-old children with DCD and learning difficulties had lower scores in both the perceived physical and perceived cognitive competence domains as compared with controls, but did not differ on the perceived social acceptance scale. Piek, Dworcan, and Coleman (in press) compared 9- to 11-year-old children with and without DCD on the same self-perception dimensions. They found differences on all the three dimensions—cognitive, social, and physical—but, again, no differences on the Global Self-Worth scale.

It seems, thus, clear that children with DCD do have lower perceptions of physical competence. They do not feel as competent in games and sports as their age peers do. With respect to academic and social competence, however, results are more equivocal. No agreement exists on whether perceived competence in the non-motor domains of self-concept is affected. Since no differences were found on global self-worth measures, it might be argued that poor perceived physical competence does not generalize to self-esteem.

Only two studies used the Harter model to study self-perception in adolescence. Losse et al. (1991) found that 16-year-old adolescents with DCD not only suffer from poor perceived physical competence, but also from low perceived social and academic competence. However, no differences were found on General Self-Worth. Cantell and colleagues (Cantell et al., 1994; Cantell, 1998) provided some confirmation of these findings. They compared the self-perceptions of DCD and control groups at the ages of 15 and 17, and found in both assessments that perceptions of athletic and scholastic competence were lower in the DCD group. In addition, an Intermediate group, which had caught up in their perceptual motor competence, did not differ from the controls. All the groups involved, that is the control, the persistent DCD, and the Intermediate group, had similar self-esteem.

Another study, with an adolescent population and a multidimensional perspective (Larkin & Parker, 1997), explored differences in global self-worth and physical competence using Marsh's Physical Self-Description Questionnaire (Marsh, Richards, Johnson, Roche, & Tremayne, 1994). Adolescents with DCD had higher self-perceptions in the passive domains of physical self (e.g., physical appearance) and lower self-perceptions in the active aspects of the physical self (e.g., sports competence). Moreover, their global self-worth was lower when compared to controls.

Although the studies on self-perception of adolescents with DCD used different instruments, they all found that the adolescents with DCD had lower perceptions of physical competence than the controls. This similarity was not reflected unitarily in the perception of global self-worth, since only Larkin and Parker (1997) found differences between the DCD group and the controls. Fitting in with the findings by Larkin and Parker, lack of competence in one area of self-perception can generalize to other domains, and finally results in low perceptions of global self-worth (Harter, 1987). According to this view, various cognitive, behavioral, and social problems co-occur with the "main" problem, lacking motor skills (Gillberg, 1998). Further, Henderson, May, and Umney (1989), discussing the secondary consequences of lower global self-worth in children with DCD, found them to be helpless and unrealistic in the way they set goals for themselves.

Parents' and Teachers' Reports

Similar trends have been found in parents' and teachers' reports. Children with DCD were rated as being less confident (Schoemaker & Kalverboer, 1994) and being more embarrassed or anxious while being observed (Smyth & Anderson, 1999). Parents and teachers in Cantell's study (1998) reported that the 15-year-old adolescents with DCD were less sociable and more passive, and their behavior could be described as "socially negative." This supports Geuze and Börger's study (1993) in which the adolescents with DCD were also found to have less developed social contacts and friendships. In contrast to these findings, which seem to show a passive (internalizing) behavioral pattern for the adolescents with DCD, Losse et al. (1991) found behavioral problems that varied from bullying to police offences.

Psychiatric Assessments

Psychiatric or clinical assessments of children and adolescents with DCD are scarce. To our knowledge, there are three longitudinal studies, each of which uses a different instrument. They all seem to report some symptoms of psychiatric problems in the adolescent DCD population. Shafer et al. (1986) reported a strong association between the existence of neurological soft signs at age 7 and measures of affective or anxiety disorder at age 17. This finding is consistent with the longitudinal study by Gillberg and Gillberg (1989), which showed that by age behavioral problems became more complex, ranging from antisocial behavior to depression. Gillberg and Gillberg concluded that there was still a considerable overlap between problems of behavior and school achievement. In a further follow-up at 16 years of age, Hellgren et al. (1994) found that more than half of the adolescents with DAMP had a psychiatric or personality disorder, while the same was true only for one-tenth of the control group. Many psychiatric symptoms were found, ranging from affective and anxiety disorders to personality disorders, including social negativism or withdrawal.

In the follow-up study by Ahonen (1990), the DCD group at age 11 was described as more immature, socially isolated, and passive than the control group. As mentioned above, when the same sample was 15 years old, parents and teachers reported a similar pattern. In addition, measured with a psychiatric symptoms questionnaire (Goldberg, 1981), somatic symptoms were more common in the DCD group than in the control group (Cantell, 1998).

Another way to look at behavioral and emotional outcome is to measure personal feeling of control, that is "locus of control" (Nowicki & Strickland, 1973). In Cantell's study (1998) with the 15-year-olds, the DCD group experienced more external than internal control in their life. However, by the age of 17, this difference had disappeared. The reason for perceptions of external control might be related to cumulative experiences of lacking personal control in the perceptual motor domain—which might explain findings on passivity and social withdrawal or less challenging educational routes in the DCD group. As a function of age, when the educational and vocational choices are made, adolescents might feel more in control of their life. It should be noted, however, that this kind of an experiential sequence is only hypothetical and hard to show, since there are so many interrelated factors acting simultaneously on development.

Engagement in Activities

The issue of engagement in spare time and social activities has been addressed in some DCD studies. The results suggest that children and adolescents with coordination disorders engage in fewer hobbies (Cantell et al., 1994), be it physically active or social hobbies. To some degree, individuals seem to be able to adjust their interests according to their abilities. For example, playing computer games seems to be more common in the DCD group (Larkin & Parker, 1999). Other studies do not necessarily link DCD to a nonactive life style, and similar engagement in various interests is found, but suggest that less enjoyment might be involved (Losse et al., 1991).

In sum, studies on emotional and social outcomes of DCD suggest that the long-term prognosis includes some notable differences in comparison to age-normative comparison groups. Independent of the instrument used, adolescents with DCD themselves report lower physical competence than do their peers. Some studies have also found that cognitive and social domains, as well as the overall self-esteem, are affected by the DCD. Perceptions of others, that is, of parents and teachers, seem to confirm that children and adolescents with DCD have some problems in the development of sociability that might reflect maturational differences between the DCD and their peers. Also, psychiatric assessments show more behavioral and social problems in the adolescent population with DCD than in the comparison group. The behavioral tendency most likely to be related to DCD is withdrawal, passivity, and isolation, rather than conduct disorder or acting out. However, the interpretation of all these assessments has to be done with caution since only a few of these studies are longitudinal, and, the instruments used in studies are different, thus making it difficult to compare them.

ASSESSMENTS AND LIMITATIONS OF LONGITUDINAL STUDIES ON DCD

Contradictory findings in longitudinal studies on DCD might be due to methodological and procedural inconsistencies. In this section, several critical issues will be discussed: sampling, assessment, and analysis of change.

Sampling and Assessment

Proper identification of children with DCD for longitudinal studies is hampered by several factors, including poor screening criteria and diagnostical definitions. The literature shows several labels on the basis of which children are selected: minimal brain dysfunction (MBD), deficit in attention, motor control, and perception (DAMP), minor neurological dysfunction (MND), and dyspraxia, to name a few (see Chapters 1 and 6). Although labels initially do not seem to have much in common, closer examination reveals overlap. Their shared variance consists of mild motor impairment (Henderson, 1993).

Identification of children with DCD is further impeded by the heterogeneous nature of movement difficulties. Instruments covering the entire range of motor competence do not exist. The agreement between different identification instruments is reported to be low. Assessments seem to identify about the same number of children with motor coordination problems, about 5–6%, but each measure can screen a somewhat different set of children (Sövik & Maeland, 1986). Therefore, Sugden and Wright (1998) proposed a two-step procedure to identify children with DCD. A two-step procedure would also comply with the definitions and identification given by DSM-IV (APA, 1994) and ICD-10 (WHO, 1996). In this kind of procedure, the teachers would do the first stage of assessment by filling out a questionnaire related to any feature that "significantly interferes with academic achievement or activities of daily living"—criteria included in the DSM-IV. The second stage would include the motor testing of those children who showed problems in the first stage. This is best assessed on the basis of individually administered standardized tests of fine and gross-motor coordination. It is notable, however, that this procedure is based on vague guidelines and on a complex questionnaire, requiring classroom teachers to observe gross-motor behavior. Therefore, it is likely that the children screened vary as a function of the teacher's ability to make motor observations.

Although such a multiple measurement design may be ideal to identify children with DCD before the onset of puberty, it is not clear whether the same design can be applied to identify children with DCD during adolescence. The current diagnostic criteria for developmental disorders in the DSM-IV do not take into account the possible change in the manifestation of a disorder with age. Longitudinal data on several developmental disorders have shown that symptom patterns often change during development (Spreen, 1989). Primary manifestations of the disorder abide, and more subtle problems appear. In addition, secondary manifestations of the disorder, such as social or emotional problems may become more manifest. Consequently, criteria to diagnose the disorder during primary school age may not be valid anymore. What is needed are proper diagnostic criteria for the identification of children during adolescence that will take the changes in the manifestations of the disorder into account (Rutter, 1998).

Measuring Change

Studies on long-term outcome in DCD differ in the way they report failure and change. Descriptive studies often use standardized motor tests or neuropsychological test batteries to report change in motor skills as a function of age (Cantell et al., 1994; Geuze & Börger, 1993; Knuckey & Gubbay, 1983). Neurodevelopmental studies concentrate on changes in the occurrence of soft signs, measured during neurodevelopmental examination (Shafer et al., 1986; Soorani-Lunsing et al., 1993). In some studies, both descriptive motor tests as well as neurodevelopmental measures are combined (Gillberg & Gillberg, 1989; Losse et al., 1991). The usefulness of both types of measures to study long-term outcomes of DCD will be discussed.

A neurodevelopmental examination is designed to supplement the classical neurological examination in order to reveal subtle deficiencies in neurological functioning. Examples are Touwen's examination (1979), which was used in the studies by Soorani-Lunsing et al. (1994) and Gillberg and Gillberg (1989). These examinations are used primarily to evaluate the developmental trajectory and predictive power of so-called "soft signs" (Shafer et al., 1986). The presence of soft signs indicates that the nervous system of a child may be wired differently from that of normal children. It does not mean that a child has a developmental delay or a handicap. However, children with soft neurological signs may be at risk for behavioral and cognitive problems. Although some children with soft signs may be diagnosed to have DCD, others have been found to move competently. In general, puberty is related to a decrease in soft neurological signs (Soorani-Lunsing et al., 1994; Gillberg et al., 1989).

Descriptive motor tests, such as the Movement ABC (Henderson & Sugden, 1992) and the Bruininks-Oseretsky Test (Bruininks, 1978), are aimed at assessing functional performance in everyday actions, using chronological age as the criterion against which performance is judged. The tests often lack a sound theoretical base. Test items are chosen because they might be revealing of relevant problems in a particular age range. Although several descriptive motor tests have been developed to assess motor performance during primary school age, so far well-standardized motor tests for older populations are limited (Losse et al., 1991). As a consequence, in studies on long-term outcome, such as that by Knuckey and Gubbay (1983), tests have been used that were primarily designed to measure motor functioning during primary school age. One might question whether those tests are valid and sensitive to measure deviations in motor performance in adolescence. When the same motor tests are used across different age ranges, one assumes that development is merely characterized by quantitative changes in motor skill performance. Although quantitative changes are seen across ages, qualitative changes occur as well. During primary school age, children first attempt to master fundamental movement skills such as stabilizing, locomotor, and manipulative movements (Gallahue & Ozmun, 1995). From 7 years onward, the fundamental skills are progressively refined, combined, and applied in increasingly demanding task situations. The items of descriptive motor tests are usually examples of closed skills, such as ball throwing, which are skills performed in a stable environment. In contrast, during adolescence, individuals have to participate in advanced games during sport and recreational activities. These activities ask for open skills, which are performed in an environment where the conditions are constantly changing, requiring the individual to adjust the movements to suit the demands of the situation. Open skill performance is rarely measured by existing motor tests used to identify DCD. As a consequence, qualitative differences that appear during development are not captured by these motor tests. Therefore, the validity of descriptive motor tests designed for primary school children for describing long-term outcome in DCD might be questioned.

Apart from the validity of the tests, the items of descriptive motor tests need to be sensitive to measure change. Although improvement in motor functioning has been reported in several studies (Cantell et al., 1994; Geuze & Börger, 1993; Gillberg & Gillberg, 1989; Knuckey & Gubbay, 1983; Losse et al., 1991), the apparent improvement may be an artifact of the tests used rather than a product of real recovery (Cantell, 1998). In contrast to measures of IQ or social functioning, there are very few tests of motor performance, which provide normative data on children in the teenage years. The items of motor tests designed for primary school children are probably too easy to reveal differences. Data from several follow-up studies confirm this expectation as the discriminative power of some of the items of the Neurodevelopmental Test Battery (Stokman et al., 1986) and the Test of Motor Impairment (Stott, Moyes, & Henderson, 1984) did decrease during adolescence. Visser et al. (1998) studied the development of motor skills in adolescent boys from 11 up to 16 years of age using the test items and norms of the Movement ABC for 11- and 12-year-old children. Significant improvements in both ball skills and balance skills were found in this age range. By the age of 16, mean performance on these skills almost reached a ceiling. The majority of children accomplish many motor skills by the age of 14 or 15. The changes that do occur during puberty are usually associated with maximum performance variables, such as size, speed, strength, and stamina (Sugden & Wright, 1998). Therefore, we may conclude that the proper assessment of children with DCD older than 12 years of age is seriously hampered. In addition, the vague definition and the lack of sensitive and valid, age-appropriate instruments hinder the generalization and comparability of findings from follow-up studies.

QUALITATIVE RESEARCH REFLECTING THE OUTCOME OF DCD

This chapter has described several longitudinal studies on DCD. The methods used so far have been quantitative and based on describing group differences. It remains a challenge for longitudinal studies on DCD to introduce more individually based studies using, for example, case studies and participatory observations. Next, we discuss some preliminary findings from studies, which used an interview and/or an observational approach.

Interviews

In addition to different kinds of questionnaires, interviews have been used in several follow-up studies on DCD. They have concentrated either on psychiatric symptoms (Hellgren et al., 1994; Shafer et al., 1986) or on personal interests (Cantell et al., 1994; Losse et al., 1991), and provide a more qualitative picture of children and adolescents with DCD. As a research tool, an interview can offer a reflection of the everyday life and the self-understanding of an individual with DCD. It can capture not only the language but also "real" examples describing the experiential world of an individual in the representative group (Mulderij, 1996). The individual stories can show something specific about the whole group and reveal important information not found through the questionnaires (van Manen, 1990).

Cantell (1998) employed a semi-structured interview developed by Damon and Hart (1988). The approach in the "Self-Understanding Interview" is social-cognitive, which means that, during development, the cognitive capacity to understand oneself helps individuals to form psychological identities and allows them to communicate these identities to others. Self-understanding is a qualitative self-description of the individual's past, present, and future. Compared with self-esteem, self-understanding is more broadly defined as the cognitive representation of the self, self-interest, and personal identity (Damon & Hart, 1988).

Table 2.2 presents the development of self-understanding that, according to Damon and Hart (1988), consists of four increasingly complex and differentiated stages from early childhood to late adolescence. The "Self-Understanding Interview" consists of seven core areas or schemas. What is measured is the capacity to think in increasingly differential levels. As a developmental model, the framework provides a way of estimating the relative maturity or immaturity of children's self-understanding. Viewed from this perspective, childhood psychopathology may include either delay in the growth of self-understanding or specific deviations from a normative pattern (Damon & Hart, 1988).

In Cantell's longitudinal study (1998), two hypotheses were made: (i) it was expected that adolescents with persistent DCD might show specific delays or deviations in self-understanding, because of their atypical perceptual motor, cognitive, and social development; and (ii) the self-understanding of the ("Intermediate")

Table 2.2   Development of Self-Understanding (Damon & Hart, 1988)

Age Group (Level of Self-Understanding)	Description
Early childhood (categorical identifications)	The individual describes his/her typical behavior, momentary moods, or material possessions. Focus is on physical qualities.
Middle and late childhood (comparative assessment)	The subject refers to capability-related physical attributes and to abilities relative to others, self, or normative standards. Focus is on active qualities.
Early adolescence (interpersonal implications)	The respondent uses active or physical attributes that influence social appeal and social interactions. Focus is on social qualities.
Late adolescence (systematic beliefs and plans)	It is common for the fourth level to use physical or active attributes that reflect volitional choices, personal, and moral standards. Focus is on psychological qualities.

adolescents who had caught up with their motor development would be more similar to their age peers in the control group than to those in the DCD group. Both hypotheses were confirmed. As expected, the DCD group seemed to function on a younger developmental level, using self-explanations from "late childhood." The adolescents in the Intermediate group were able to describe themselves quite similarly to the control group; that is, they used self-explanations associated with "early or late adolescence." Based on the social-cognitive theory of Damon and Hart (1988), the interview data indicated that the adolescents with DCD were able to make simultaneous comparisons, but that they were less competent in making interconnections than their age peers. That means for example that they were more likely to make overgeneralizations from their own evaluations. A possible limiting factor to these findings, however, concerned the measured levels of intelligence. Although in the normal range, they were significantly lower in the DCD group. Therefore, the immaturity might be partly explainable by the inability to comprehend the full meaning of the interview and its social requirements.

Kirby and Drew (1999) have also presented some preliminary qualitative data on the long-term outcome of DCD. They collected 22 case histories based on interviews and questionnaires from adolescents and adults with the diagnosis of DCD. Answers to the question "what do you see as your main problem?" showed that the key concerns were in the areas of social skills and in personal life management, rather than in the area of motor skills. In addition, the study showed lack of suitable services and intervention for adults with DCD. They concluded that the issues for children with DCD are not relevant for this population, and therefore the best diagnostic label for this adult group is unclear.

Observations

Direct observation is at the core of child behavioral assessment. It is the process by which observers, using operational definitions as their guide, record the overt motor and/or verbal behavior of others (Barton & Ascione, 1984). It is introduced here as an indication of future directions, since studies on children with DCD where systematic longitudinal observations are made have not yet been done. However, some preliminary research projects have been carried out, and one is presented here.

In the follow-up by Cantell et al. (2000), an observation sheet, the "Interview and Test Behavior Rating Scale" by Spreen (1988), was employed. The rating was carried out during an interview by a blind rater. The scale was originally developed to study constancy and change in children with learning disabilities. Cantell (1998) found that, at age 15, the adolescents in the DCD group seemed less motivated, less self-confident, and less mature in their behavior than their age peers. This finding seemed to confirm findings on the self-perception scale (Harter, 1988) and the Self-Understanding Interview (Damon & Hart, 1988). The observation of individuals with DCD as being more "immature" and insecure in their social contact are issues that are often mentioned in qualitative observations but are hard to show in research.

Although observational scales for motor testing (Henderson & Sugden, 1992; Kalverboer, De Vries, & van Dellen, 1990) and playground activities (Smyth & Anderson, 1999) do exist, there is a need for observational scales specifically designed for observing everyday activities in children, adolescents, and adults with DCD. This would allow the development of more specific guidelines for teaching and everyday support for this population at risk.

SUMMARY AND CONCLUSIONS

Longitudinal studies on the developmental outcome in DCD have tried to address whether DCD is a temporary or a persisting disorder. In this chapter, we have reviewed the perceptual-motor outcome as well as the social emotional and educational outcome in children with DCD. A picture emerged in which children, particularly those with minor motor problems, seem to grow out of their problems, while the more severely affected ones remain clumsy and at risk for developing associated problems. So far, the question why some improve and others stay behind has been a difficult one to settle. Although research to date has only begun to explore the underlying mechanisms, there is a growing consensus that the multidimensional nature of the DCD construct does not warrant explanations in terms of single unitary factors. As in many other developmental disorders, the long-term behavioral consequences of DCD are much more likely to arise from multiple interacting factors and cannot be understood in isolation from normal age-related developmental processes. Neurodevelopmental, cognitive, environmental, and experiential processes are all considered to play a role in shaping individual developmental pathways. Insight into the dynamics of these processes and knowledge about their timing and sequencing is essential to understand outcome differences in DCD, both in terms of inter-and intraindividual variability.

As we discussed, up to this point, research in DCD has emphasized the perceptual-motor and academic outcome rather than the long-term emotional and behavioral consequences. However, it is necessary to follow the emotional and behavioral consequences as, particularly in interaction with unfavorable social circumstances, they may prove to be of critical importance in maintaining the DCD status into adolescence. Concretely, this would allow dealing with important issues such as (i) how the experiential impact of DCD changes from childhood to adolescence and (ii) why some adolescents, even in the absence of overt motor symptoms, are still struggling with the experiential aftereffects of a childhood with atypical motor development.

Regarding directions for future research, it seems clear to move beyond the mere task of establishing levels of motor performance and correlated parameters. We would like to suggest a two-track approach in which a practice of more refined and reliable measurement goes hand in hand with the use of longitudinal designs in which the multiple dimensions of interest can be tested against a background of ongoing development. Recently developed statistical techniques such as latent growth curve analysis (Duncan, Duncan, Strycker, & Alpert, 1999) would thereby provide the necessary tools to model developmental pathways to outcome from a multilevel perspective.

In sum, a number of factors have been shown to be associated with outcome in DCD. In the search for outcome predictors, a developmental approach is suggested in which individual variability in outcome status is associated with differentially weighted combinations of neurodevelopmental, cognitive, and social-emotional factors.

PART
II

Subtypes and Comorbid Conditions

CHAPTER
3

Subtypes of Developmental Coordination Disorder

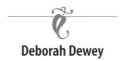

Deborah Dewey

An increasing number of children are coming to the attention of health care professionals, presenting with awkward, clumsy movement and poor coordination. Their motor problems can affect their gross motor skills, their fine motor skills, or both, as well as related functional skills. Frequently, these children also have organizational and planning difficulties that affect not only motor performance but also other areas of function. This disability has been referred to by a number of different names, including developmental coordination disorder (DCD), developmental dyspraxia, clumsy child syndrome, minimal cerebral palsy, minimal brain dysfunction, sensory integrative dysfunction, and mild motor problems (Missiuna & Polatajko, 1995).

HISTORICAL PERSPECTIVE ON DCD SUBTYPES

Although the concept of developmental motor disorder was first introduced in the early 1900s, it was not until 1937 that the idea of different *types* of motor disorders in children was first discussed. Orton (1937), in his discussion of developmental disorders of childhood, suggested that different types of

Support for the preparation of this chapter was provided by the Albert Children's Hospital Foundation and the Ruth Rannie Memorial Endowment and the David and Dorothy Lann Foundation fund.

developmental motor disorders may exist and that disorders in praxis and gnosis might result in motor skills deficits that were different from those arising from pyramidal, extrapyramidal, or cerebellar dysfunction. The results of case studies carried out by Walton, Ellis, and Court (1962) and Gubbay, Ellis, Walton, and Court (1965) suggested that children with developmental motor disorders displayed varying types of problems. Some of these children were described as evidencing an apraxic (motor planning) disorder, whereas others were described as agnosic (visuospatial recognition disorder). In addition, several other types of praxic disorders were identified in these children: constructional apraxia, dressing apraxia, and articulatory apraxia. De Ajuriaguerra and Stambak (1969), in their discussion of developmental dyspraxia, also identified several different types (i.e., apraxia involving motor performance, constructional apraxia, spatial dyskinesis, facial apraxia, ocular apraxia, postural apraxia, object apraxia, and verbal apraxia). It should be noted that these early investigations of developmental motor problems were based on models drawn from adult neurology. However, even at that time, it was acknowledged that classifying developmental disorders using the same terms as those used in adult neurology was problematic (De Ajuriaguerra & Stambak, 1969).

Early research that investigated children's visual and kinesthetic processing has also had a significant impact on subtyping research. Studies by Brenner and colleagues (Brenner & Gillman, 1966, 1968; Brenner, Gillman, & Farrell, 1968; Brenner, Gillman, Zangwill, & Farrell, 1967) reported that clumsiness was found to be present in a high proportion of children with visuomotor disability. Frostig (1963), Zangwill (1960), and more recent studies by Hulme and Lord (Hulme, Biggerstaff, Moran, & McKinlay, 1982; Hulme, Smart, & Moran, 1982; Lord & Hulme, 1987b) reported significant associations between clumsiness and disturbances in visual perception. Disturbances in kinesthetic perception were also reported in children with DCD (Bairstow & Laszlo, 1981; Hulme, Biggerstaff et al., 1982; Hulme, Smart, Moran, & McKinlay, 1984; Laszlo & Bairstow, 1983). Because of this early research, many recent investigations have focused their attention on identifying subgroups of children with DCD that display specific deficits in visual-perceptual skills and/or kinesthetic processing.

PREVALENCE AND PROGNOSIS

Initially, problems in motor coordination in childhood were thought to be of minor importance, typically outgrown in adolescence or adulthood. It is now recognized that children are not likely to outgrow their clumsiness (Geuze & Borger, 1993; Losse et al., 1991). Research suggests that the prevalence of motor disorders in children is estimated to be 5–8% of all school-aged children (American Psychiatric Association, 1994; Gubbay, 1975a; Henderson & Hall, 1982). Further, investigators have reported a higher prevalence in children with other developmental or learning problems (Fox & Lent, 1996; Kaplan, Wilson, Dewey, & Crawford, 1997). Similarly, large epidemiological studies have estimated that the prevalence of attention deficit/hyperactivity disorder ranges from 4–6% (Szatmari, 1992). Thus, relative to other developmental disorders, DCD has a similar rate of occurrence in the pediatric population.

The academic and social impact of this chronic condition can be significant (Cantell, Smyth, & Ahonen, 1994; Henderson & Hall, 1982; Henderson & Sugden, 1992; Kalverboer, de Vries, & van Dellen, 1990; Schoemaker & Kalverboer, 1994). These findings attest to the legitimacy of a separable disorder of movement skills acquisition, requiring etiological, diagnostic, and remedial attention. This stance is supported by the fact that the DSM-IV (American Psychiatric Association, 1994) has developed a relevant entry headed "developmental coordination disorder" which they define as "a marked impairment in the development of motor coordination . . . [which] significantly interferes with academic achievement or activities of daily living" (American Psychiatric Association, 1994, p. 48).

ARE THERE SUBTYPES OF DCD?

Although the condition has had many names over the years, many investigators agree that children with DCD display deficits in motor coordination that are not due to any identifiable neurological disorder (Hall, 1988). They are distinguished from their normally developing peers by a pervasive slowness in the easy acquisition of everyday motor skills, in spite of normal intelligence and freedom from diagnosed neurological disorders (Polatajko, Fox, & Missiuna, 1995). As a result, their motor performance is significantly impaired so that daily activities at school (e.g., handwriting, participation in sporting activities, social interaction) and at home (e.g., self-care activities) are adversely affected (Walton et al., 1962).

It has been noted that children with DCD form a heterogeneous group (Lord & Hulme, 1987b) and that there is no typical case (Gordon & McKinlay, 1980). This point is illustrated by the fact that recent studies that have examined the performance of children with DCD have drawn their participants from populations referred due to significant motor problems (Lord & Hulme, 1987a, 1987b, 1988a, 1988b), nominated by physical education teachers (Murphy & Gliner, 1988) or by regular classroom teachers (Dewey, 1991, 1993; Dewey & Kaplan, 1992, 1994; Henderson & Hall, 1982; Losse et al., 1991; Missiuna, 1994), screened from a population of school children on the basis of a test of motor performance (Erhardt, McKinlay, & Bradley, 1987; Gubbay, 1975b; Iloeje, 1987; Johnston, Short, & Crawford, 1987; Roussounis, Gaussen, & Stratton, 1987), or with suspected sensory integrative dysfunction (Ayres, Mailloux, & Wendler, 1987) or learning disabilities (Cermak, Coster, & Drake, 1980; Cermak, Trimble, Coryell, & Drake, 1990; Horak, Shumway-Cook, Crowe, & Black, 1988; Kaplan, Wilson, Dewey, & Crawford, 1998; Lennox, Cermak, & Koomar, 1988; O'Brien, Cermak, & Murray, 1988).

Because of the heterogeneity of children with DCD, the question that arises is whether DCD is one unitary syndrome or whether identifiable subtypes of DCD exist. Studies that are intent on finding the underlying causes of DCD have tended to proceed as if they were dealing with a single, unitary disorder (Geuze & Kalverboer, 1987; Horak et al., 1988; Murphy & Gliner, 1988; Smyth & Glencross, 1986; van Dellen & Geuze, 1988). Often these studies are based on a theory as to what underlies the motor coordination problems of children with DCD. One theory that has been suggested is that motor planning problems are due to an impairment of sensory integration (Ayres, 1972; Ayres et al., 1987). It has also been suggested that deficits in visual perception (Gubbay, 1975a; Henderson & Hall, 1982; Hulme, Biggerstaff et al., 1982a; Hulme, Smart et al., 1982; Lord & Hulme, 1987b, 1988b; O'Brien et al., 1988; Wilson & McKenzie, 1998) or deficits in kinesthetic perception (Bairstow & Laszlo, 1981; Laszlo & Bairstow, 1983; Laszlo, Bairstow, Bartrip, & Rolfe, 1988; Wilson & McKenzie, 1998) underlie poor motor coordination. Smyth and Glencross (1986) suggested that children with DCD were deficient in speed of processing kinesthetic information but not in speed of processing visual information. Other investigators have found that children with DCD are slow but not inaccurate in the process of response selection (Rosblad & von Hofsten, 1994; van Dellen & Geuze, 1988). Finally, it has been suggested that children with DCD display deficits in the timing of action (Lundy-Ekman, Ivry, Keele, & Woollacott, 1991; Piek & Skinner, 1999; Williams, Woollacott, & Ivry, 1992). Although all of the above studies have shown that children with DCD differ from non-DCD control children on a number abilities, none of these studies has provided us with any clear evidence as to whether DCD is a unitary disorder or whether identifiable subtypes of DCD exist. This can only be done by investigating the various differences exhibited within the population of children diagnosed with DCD.

Approaches to Subtype Identification

Various approaches have been used to investigate subtypes of DCD. Some studies have used a clinical/descriptive approach (Ayres et al., 1987; Dewey, Kaplan, Wilson, & Crawford, 1999; Henderson & Hall, 1982; Wann, Mon-Williams, & Rushton, 1998). Specifically, they have looked for similar patterns of behavior on a range of preselected variables. The children's performance on these variables are then investigated for similarities, and any identified subgroups are described (Hoare, 1994). Such an approach can be useful in identifying subgroups of children with DCD; however, it is difficult to use with large data sets and may be influenced by the a priori biases of the investigator (Fletcher & Satz, 1985; Hooper & Willis, 1989).

In contrast to the clinical approach, other studies have used a statistical clustering approach to identify subtypes of DCD (Ahonen, 1990; Dewey & Kaplan, 1994; Hoare, 1994; Miyahara, 1994; Taylor, 1990; Wright & Sugden, 1996). "Cluster analysis" is a generic term for a variety of procedures (e.g., Ward's, k-means iterative partitioning, average linkage) that can be used to create a classification scheme. These procedures empirically form clusters or groups of highly similar subjects. There are a number of important issues to consider when using cluster analysis. The first is the initial selection of the variables that are to be used in the cluster analysis. The variables that are chosen should be based on theoretically relevant dimensions and should maximize subtype differences. Further, repetition of information from similar variables should be avoided and all variables must be valid and reliable (Hoare, 1994; Wright & Sugden, 1996). The second issue that must be considered is that a clustering algorithm finds clusters even in random data (Milligan & Cooper, 1987). Further, different clustering algorithms (i.e., Ward's method, k-means iterative partitioning, average linkage) using the same similarity measure (i.e., Euclidean distance) can generate different groupings when applied to the same data set. Therefore, it is important to demonstrate that the clusters are stable and that they actually exist by demonstrating the reliability of the cluster solution across different clustering methods. Additional procedures that can be utilized to assess the internal validity (reliability) of the cluster solution are a split-sample design and multivariate analysis of variance on dependent measures not used to generate the cluster solution (Morris, Blashfield, & Satz, 1981).

Subtyping Studies

Initial Studies

Gubbay and colleagues (1965) proposed the idea that there were subtypes of children with developmental motor problems. He suggested that there were two subtypes of motor problems in children, one being developmental apraxia or agnosia and the other being dysfunction in pyramidal or cerebellar pathways. No empirical evidence in support of these subtypes has been published.

Henderson and Hall (1982) divided the "clumsy" children in their sample into three groups based on motor and academic abilities and behavior. Their first group included children whose motor impairment was an isolated disability. The second group consisted of children who had generally low abilities in motor and academic areas and who also displayed behavioral problems. The third group was described as an intermediate group whose performance fell between the other two groups. No further efforts were made to investigate these groups; however, as Henderson and Hall state, these findings show that these children do not form a single group but vary widely in their characteristics.

Subtypes of Children with Learning Disabilities

Ayres et al. (1987) investigated whether different types of developmental dyspraxia could be identified in children with learning problems. Correlational analyses and factor analyses indicated strong associations between praxis, tactile processing, visual perception, and repeating of sentences in these children. They concluded that these findings did not provide support for the existence of different subtypes of developmental dyspraxia. They also stated, however, that their study did not justify the existence of a unitary praxis function. However, the analyses used by these investigators are not appropriate to address the issue of whether there are different types of developmental dyspraxia.

Miyahara (1994) used a k-means iterative partitioning method to identify possible subtypes of students with learning disabilities based on the gross motor subtests of the Bruininks-Oseretsky Test of Motor Proficiency (Bruininks, 1978). The analysis identified four subtypes of children: one was free of any motor problems, a second subtype performed poorly on all of the gross motor subtests, a third displayed good balance but performed poorly on running speed, strength, and ball skills, and a fourth subtype displayed extremely poor balance, average performance on running speed and bilateral coordination, and very good performance in the areas of strength and ball skills. The external validity of these four subtypes was verified by a teacher's rating of the children's physical behaviours. However, the fact that this sample of children was selected on the basis of learning problems and not motor problems limits the generalizability of these findings to children with DCD.

Subtypes Based on Developmental History

Taylor (1990) used 21 items from the Developmental History Questionnaire to examine the heterogeneity of physical awkwardness in children ranging in age from 4 to 9 years. She administered this questionnaire to the parents of children who were referred to the Motor Development Clinic at the University of Alberta. Using a PK Means clustering technique, she identified three subtypes. The first subtype included children who displayed general delays in motor abilities such as late walking, late talking, difficulty in learning to ride a bike, marking time on stairs, avoidance of playground equipment, and a history of medical problems. The second subtype was characterized by an absence of medical problems, while the third subtype displayed a positive medical history such as neurological signs, hyperactivity, and sensory problems. All three groups were found to evidence poor motor performance, and social and behavioral problems.

Planning/Executive Subtypes

Cermak (1985) stated that sensory integration theory makes a distinction between problems in planning and problems in execution (Ayres, 1985, 1972). She also noted that therapists in clinical practice distinguished between children who show motor planning deficits and those with deficits in the execution of motor tasks (i.e., coordination). The former group has problems in organizing and planning their approach to tasks, while the latter group appears to know how to plan their approach to a motor task but are clumsy in the execution of the task. However, research studies have provided only equivocal support for these subtypes.

Conrad, Cermak, and Drake (1983) found that some children with developmental dyspraxia evidence a deficit in motor planning due to difficulties in sequencing movements, while others evidence similar deficits due to optic-spatial problems. Dewey and Kaplan (1994) investigated whether subtypes of children who demonstrated a specific deficit in motor planning or a specific deficit in the execution of motor tasks could be identified. Results of their hierarchical agglomerative and iterative partitioning cluster analyses revealed four subtypes: one with severe deficits in all motor skill areas, a second with deficits in balance, coordination, and gestural performance, a third group with deficits in motor sequencing, and a fourth group without motor deficits. Examination of performance on measures of academic, language, visual-perceptual, and visual-motor skills revealed that these four subtypes displayed different patterns of nonmotor performance.

Although Dewey and Kaplan (1994) did not find just two subtypes of DCD (i.e., execution, planning), the results of this study can be interpreted within the framework proposed by Cermak (1985, 1991). First, the results revealed that some children with DCD show a generalized impairment in all areas of motor abilities. In other words, they display motor deficits in both execution and motor planning.

Second, the findings of this study revealed a group of children who displayed deficits on tasks designed to assess motor execution (i.e., balance, coordination) but whose motor planning abilities appeared to be intact. The deficits in gestural performance displayed by this group appeared to be the result of problems in executing single gestures, instead of problems in motor planning (Cermak, 1985). Third, they revealed a group of children who displayed a specific deficit in motor planning (i.e., motor sequencing) but whose performance of single gestures was intact. Thus, the results of this study provide some support for subtypes of DCD that may be associated with a planning deficit versus an execution deficit.

Additional support for this distinction is provided by a recent study completed by Dewey et al. (1999). In this study, we investigated motor planning skills in three groups of children: DCD, suspect DCD, and non-DCD. Children were assigned to one of these three groups based on their performance on the Bruininks-Oseretsky Test of Motor Proficiency (BOTMP; Bruininks, 1978), and the Movement Assessment Battery for Children (M-ABC; Henderson & Sugden, 1992). Results indicated that children with DCD performed less well on tests of motor planning compared to children in the suspect DCD and the non-DCD groups. We then examined the proportions of children with DCD, suspect DCD, and non-DCD who displayed deficits in motor planning. Results revealed that some children in each of the three groups displayed deficits in motor planning. These findings indicate that it is possible for children to evidence disorders of coordination without also displaying deficits in motor planning. Further, children may also display deficits in motor planning but have intact motor coordination skills. On the basis of the above findings, it was concluded that DCD could be conceptualized as either a planning disorder or coordination/execution disorder. Planning disorders would be characterized by problems in knowing what to do and how to move, while coordination/execution disorders would be characterized by poorly coordinated performance in children who know what to do. More research is needed, however, to confirm these possible subtypes.

Perceptual-Motor Subtypes

Using a hierarchical agglomerative cluster analysis approach, Hoare (1994) identified five distinct subtypes of children with DCD using measures that assessed kinesthetic acuity, visual perception, visual-motor integration, manual dexterity, static balance, and running speed. The first subtype consisted of children who had below average scores on running speed and kinesthetic acuity, but above average scores on static balance and manual dexterity, suggesting that the idea of a subtype of children with an overall gross motor difficulty may be too general. Good visual perception and visual-motor skills but poor kinesthetic and balance skills characterized the second subtype. Hoare (1994) suggested that this subtype provides evidence against the notion of generalized visual dysfunction in children with DCD (Hulme, Biggerstaff et al., 1982; Hulme, Smart et al., 1982). Subtype three was below average on all the tasks, but particularly on both visual and kinesthetic tasks. Hoare (1994) concluded that this subtype supported the idea that some children with DCD display a generalized perceptual dysfunction. The fourth subtype consisted of children who displayed a significant discrepancy between their kines-thetic processing and their visual processing, suggesting that visual processing may have a significant and specific role in movement dysfunction. Subtype five was composed of children who experienced motor execution problems. Their per-formance on the motor tasks (i.e., Purdue Pegboard, static and dynamic balance) were well below average and significantly lower than their scores on any of the perceptual tasks. Thus, the results of this study provide further support for the idea that different subtypes of DCD exist.

Recently, Macnab, Miller, and Polatajko (1999) examined the five subtypes of DCD identified by Hoare (1994) using three measures that were the identical to Hoare (i.e., kinesthetic acuity, visual perception, visual motor integration) and three measures that were that were different but comparable (manual dexterity, balance, gross motor ability). Further, they used a cluster analysis approach that was identical to Hoare to obtain their subtypes of children with DCD. Although Macnab et al. (1999) did not replicate Hoare's (1994) five subtypes, there were a number of areas of agreement. In both studies, a subtype of children with DCD was found who evidenced a generalized visual dysfunction. Macnab et al. also found support for Hoare's conclusion that a subtype based on overall gross motor difficulty may be too general; she found a discrepancy in performance on static balance and a complex gross motor task. Consistent with Hoare, a subtype of chil-dren who experienced difficulties in all areas was also identified. In addition to the above three subtypes, Macnab et al. identified two additional subtypes: one with visual motor and fine motor problems, and another with poor performance on running, and good performance on kinesthetic acuity. Although both of these sub-types resembled Hoare's subgroups in terms of the pattern of deficits, they were not as impaired. Thus, the results of the Macnab et al. study provided clear sup-port for Hoare's subtypes one, two, and three. Further, some support for Hoare's subtypes four and five was found; however, the children in Hoare's subgroups displayed a greater degree of impairment than the children in Macnab's sub-groups. These differences between the two studies in terms of the subtypes of chil-dren identified could be due to differences in the two samples recruited for these studies, and differences in the measures that were used to assess manual dexterity, balance, and gross motor ability.

Motor Subtypes

Wright and Sugden (1996) investigated the nature of DCD in a select group of Sin-gaporean children aged 6–9 years using two methods: an intergroup comparison of children with DCD and matched controls, and an intragroup study that investigated whether subtypes of children with DCD could be identified. In terms of intergroup differences, results revealed that the children with DCD displayed significantly poorer motor abilities than the matched controls. Before completing a hierarchical agglomerative cluster analysis to investigate subtypes of DCD, the variables avail-able from the M-ABC Checklist and the M-ABC test (Movement ABC); (Henderson & Sugden, 1992) were subjected to a factor analysis. Five factors emerged: factor one, changing environment; factor two, fast hands; factor three, catching; factor four, dynamic balance; and factor five, control of self. The standardized scores of the five factors were then used in the cluster analysis, which revealed four clusters. Cluster one consisted of children who showed little impairment on any of the factors. Their lowest score was on the control of self factor. Cluster two consisted of children who performed very poorly when asked to adapt to external forces, particularly catching. Children in cluster three scored poorly on factor one, changing environment, and also on factors three and five, catching and control of self. Overall, they exhibited the lowest scores. Wright and Sugden concluded that this third cluster might have represented a group of children who have difficulties on all spheres of movement. Cluster four exhibited the greatest difficulty in manipulating their hands at speed and also scored poorly on dynamic balance. Wright and Sugden concluded that their results confirm the heterogeneous pattern of DCD. Further, they state that specific information about the difficulties experienced by children with DCD can only be found if one investigates subtypes of DCD. Just looking at intergroup differences (i.e., DCD versus non-DCD) does not provide enough information about the different patterns of difficulties these children experience.

A recent study by Wann et al. (1998), which investigated postural control in children aged 10–12, used the "swinging-room" paradigm (Lee & Aronson, 1974). They found that children with DCD could be separated into two groups on the basis of their postural stability. One group of children with DCD had postural control problems identified by the M-ABC and displayed a reliance on vision in the maintenance of posture in the swinging room context equivalent to that of nursery school children. The other group with DCD passed the postural control assessment (i.e., M-ABC) and did not differ from age-matched controls in the swinging room context.

Longitudinal Follow-Up Studies

Ahonen (1990) examined subtypes of DCD in a 6-year longitudinal study of 106 children who were initially seen at age 7, and reassessed at ages 9 and 11. The different motor and neuropsychological tests used could be grouped into six factors: motor control, gross motor coordination, fine motor coordination, inhibition, kinesthesia, and visual-spatiality. Using cluster analyses methods, six reliable subtypes were identified at 7 years of age: the first group displayed a general delay in motor and cognitive functions; the second was cognitively normal but had gross motor difficulties; the third group had problems in motor control; the fourth subtype had deficits in visual-spatial skills; the fifth group had similar difficulties to group four but in a milder form; the main feature of the sixth subtype was kinesthetic problems. Examination of these subtypes over the different ages indicated that, among the first subgroup, the profile of their performance on the various factors remained stable and the level of problems remained significant. The performance profiles of subgroups four and five also displayed relative stability over the different ages. In the second subgroup, however, 40% of the children displayed significant improvements in motor skills over the course of the study. Further, among the children in the third subgroup, difficulties in motor control were the central distinguishing feature at 7 years of age. By 9 years of age, problems in motor control did not consistently distinguish the third subgroup from the others. Finally, at age 11, children in the sixth subgroup no longer displayed kinesthetic difficulties, which was the main problem of this group at 7 years of age. Of note is the finding that children in third and sixth subgroups displayed visual-spatial difficulties at age 7 and that, in both of these groups, visual-spatial difficulties were still in evidence at age 11. The findings of this study suggest that, although young children with different types of motor problems can be identified, the characteristic features of these different subtypes of DCD may change and evolve over different ages. Thus, the different subtypes of DCD, which are identified, may be influenced not only by the measures that are used to assess motor problems but also by the age of the children that are being assessed.

In an extension of the previous longitudinal study, Cantell et al. (1994) found that children identified at 5 years of age as having delayed motor development fell into two groups 10 years later (see Chapter 2). One group, the stable clumsy group, continued to display motor and perceptual problems compared to the control group. The second group was made up of an intermediate group who could no longer be clearly distinguished from the control group or the stable clumsy group. At age 15, however, children in the stable clumsy group had lower academic ambitions and fewer social hobbies than children in the intermediate and control groups.

COMPARISON OF SUBTYPES

The results of the above studies do suggest that different subtypes of DCD exist; however, it is difficult to draw any specific comparisons and conclusions from these studies. As most of these studies have used different measures of motor and/or perceptual skills, the subtypes that have been identified demonstrate different patterns of skills and deficits. Careful examination of the above studies, however, does reveal some consistent patterns. Both Hoare (1994) and Macnab et al. (1999) found subtypes of children who displayed good performance on a measure of static balance. Miyahara (1994) also identified a subgroup of children with learning disabilities and motor problems who performed well on the balance subtest of the BOTMP. Further, Dewey and Kaplan (1994) identified a group of children who were characterized by good performance on the balance subtest of the BOTMP, but poor performance on a motor sequencing test. The findings of Wann et al. (1998) also provide support for a subgroup of children with DCD who display good performance on tests of balance. Most of the subtyping studies also found support for the concept of a subtype of children with DCD who display severe deficits in all areas of motor ability (Ahonen, 1990; Dewey & Kaplan, 1994; Hoare, 1994; Macnab et al., 1999; Miyahara, 1994; Taylor, 1990; Wright & Sugden, 1996). Hoare (1994) found a subtype of children with DCD who had significant difficulties with the Purdue Pegboard (a measure of manual dexterity) and with their static and dynamic balance. Similarly, Wright and Sugden (1996) also identified a subgroup of children who displayed difficulties in both manual dexterity and dynamic balance; however, this subgroup of children did not show any obvious difficulties with static balance. Subgroups of children with DCD who were characterized by general visual-perceptual difficulties have also been identified by a number of investigators (Ahonen, 1990;

Hoare, 1994; Macnab et al., 1999). Finally, both Hoare (1994) and Macnab et al. (1999) found support for the concept that a subtype based on overall gross motor difficulty may be too general. Specifically, they both found a subgroup that displayed good balance skills but poor performance on running.

SUGGESTIONS FOR FUTURE RESEARCH

Although the consistency of the findings of the above studies is interesting, more research is needed to confirm whether subtypes of DCD actually exist. It is extremely difficult to draw any clear conclusions from the empirical evidence, because the studies that have investigated subtypes of children with DCD have used various assessment instruments, some with questionable reliability, to measure motor functions. Further, before any conclusions can be made regarding the existence and validity of specific subtypes of DCD, studies will need to be done to determine whether members of identified subtypes respond differently to treatment interventions that are specific to their deficits versus a more general treatment intervention for "motor problems." For example, with a subtype of children identified as evidencing visual-perceptual deficits, one would need to examine the effects of visual-perceptual treatment versus a more general motor intervention on the specific visual-perceptual deficit, as well as the more general motor coordination problems. If these different treatment approaches resulted in different outcomes for these children, the existence of a subtype of children with DCD with visual-perceptual difficulties would be supported. No studies that have investigated subtypes of DCD have taken this approach. Thus, based on our current knowledge, we simply do not have enough evidence to draw any definite conclusions regarding the existence of subtypes of DCD.

SHOULD WE BE LOOKING FOR SUBTYPES OF DCD?

Medical classification systems such as DSM-IV (American Psychiatric Association, 1994) and ICD-10 (World Health Organization, 1992) divide specific developmental disorders into distinct categories, of which motor skills disorder (i.e., DCD) is one subtype. DCD, however, shares symptoms with a number of other conditions. Clumsiness, or poor coordination, can be indicative of DCD. These symptoms can also be indicative of neurological, intellectual, or sensory impairments (Cratty, 1994; Fox, 1995; Hall, 1988). While the descriptors are the same, the conditions are quite different (American Psychiatric Association, 1994; Cratty, 1994; Gordon & McKinlay, 1980). Children with DCD do not show any of the hard neurological signs (i.e., clear-cut evidence of neuropathology) diagnostic of a neurological condition and do not have any diagnosable sensory deficits (Hulme & Lord, 1986). Children with DCD can, however, demonstrate what has been referred to as neurological "soft signs." Neurological soft signs are thought to reflect subtle evidence of abnormality, not otherwise detectable (Cratty, 1994). Included under the designation of soft signs are such symptoms as abnormal movements, abnormal reflexes, awkwardness, associated movements, delayed motor milestones, poor coordination, and general clumsiness (Cratty, 1994; Sugden & Keogh, 1990).

Investigations of children with DCD have also noted the frequent co-occurrence of motor problems with impairments in attention, language, and reading (Cantell et al., 1994; Dewey & Wall, 1997; Gordon & McKinlay, 1980; Kadesjo & Gillberg, 1998; Kaplan et al., 1998; Losse et al., 1991; Roussounis et al., 1987; Snow, Blondis, & Brady, 1988). These studies have found that children who display DCD perform significantly poorer on tests of academic skills (i.e., reading, spelling, mathematics) and tests of writing speed, and are more likely to display problems in attention and concentration compared to normal comparison children.

The level of overlap or comorbidity among DCD, learning disabilities (LD), and attention deficit/hyperactivity disorder (ADHD) is clearly greater than could be expected by chance alone. The estimates of overlap vary greatly. For example, Kaplan et al. (1998) reported that 56% of the children with DCD also had LD and 41% had ADHD. Further, as many as 42% of children with LD also had ADHD and 63% of the children with ADHD had LD. Sugden and Wann (1987) found 29–33% of children with LD to have coordination difficulties, and Silver (1992) reported that approximately 20% of children with LD had perceptual-motor problems and almost 75% had attention deficits (Kavale & Nye, 1985–86). Kadesjo and Gillberg (1998) reported that there was a considerable overlap between DCD and ADHD, with about half of each diagnostic group also meeting the criteria for the other diagnosis. Thus, the comorbidity of LD, ADHD, and DCD is quite significant. In fact, a number of investigators have suggested that, in the case of specific developmental disorders, comorbidity is the rule rather than the exception (Gilger & Kaplan, 1999; Henderson & Barnett, 1998; Kadesjo & Gillberg, 1998; Kaplan et al., 1998; Powell & Bishop, 1992).

This has led to much debate in the literature about how developmental disorders in children should be classified (Gilger & Kaplan, 1999; Hill, Bishop, & Nimmo-Smith, 1998; Kadesjo & Gillberg, 1998; Kaplan et al., 1998; Rispens & van Yperen, 1997). Two positions have been presented. The first is that there are clear distinctions between the various developmental disorders (i.e., DCD, ADHD, LD) and that the similarities in motor, reading, and attention impairments are only superficial. According to this view, a more detailed examination of the qualitative differences in the motor, reading, and attention skills displayed by children who meet the criteria for DCD and children diagnosed with other developmental disorders would reveal differences in these abilities (Hill et al., 1998). However, recent research with children with DCD and specific language impairment (SLI) does not support this position. Hill and colleagues (1998) found that the performance of children with DCD and children with SLI on a test of gesture production was comparable. They concluded that these findings were suggestive of overlapping rather than distinct disorders.

An alternative view regarding the classification of developmental disorders is that rather than discrete groups of children, some with motor problems, some with attention problems, and some with reading problems, there is one group of children with heterogeneous, atypical brain development (ABD) (Gilger & Kaplan, 1999; Kaplan et al., 1998). This view is supported by the fact that these problems tend to co-occur in children with developmental disorders (Biederman, Faraone, Keenan, Steingard, & Tsuang, 1991; Biederman, Newcorn, & Sprich, 1991; Cantwell & Baker,

1991; Dykman & Ackerman, 1991; Kaplan et al., 1997; Shaywitz & Shaywitz, 1991). Additional support is provided by the finding that the brains of children with developmental learning disabilities, including DCD, evidence a higher incidence of abnormality compared to normally developing children, but no identifiable lesions (Bergstrom & Bille, 1978; Chase, Rosen, & Sherman, 1996; Knuckey, Apsimon, & Gubbay, 1983; Riccio & Hynd, 1996; Rourke & Tsatsanis, 1996). Thus, as Powell and Bishop (1992; p. 762) have suggested, "it seem likely that a wide range of learning disabilities can be caused when early development of the brain is disrupted, but the specific pattern of the cognitive deficits will depend on the extent and the location of the underlying neurological abnormality."

ABD differs from the concept of Minimal Brain Dysfunction (MBD) in that ABD is not a unitary syndrome, as was originally suggested for MBD, where a fairly specific collection of symptoms was required for diagnosis (Clements & Peters, 1962). Rather, ABD is meant to serve as a unifying concept regarding the etiology of the various developmental disorders (Gilger & Kaplan, 1999). It does not itself represent a specific disorder or disease, but is a concept that describes the developmental variation of the brain and subsequent brain-based skills on either side of the real or hypothetical norm. Thus, children with ABD may exhibit a variety of symptoms; however, the symptoms that they display will depend upon their specific profile of brain-based strengths and weaknesses.

IMPLICATIONS FOR SUBTYPING RESEARCH

What are the implications of a conceptual shift to thinking of DCD as an expression of ABD? While we may continue to speak of DCD, such a conceptual shift acknowledges that DCD is one of a variety of developmental learning problems (i.e., math disability, reading disability, specific language disabilities, spelling disabilities, writing disabilities, ADHD) that fall under the general classification of LD and that all of these disabilities are due to some type of neural dysfunction. This idea also acknowledges the fact that comorbidity of symptoms in developmental disorders is the rule rather than the exception and that there is a great deal of variation in the profile of strengths and weakness in children diagnosed with developmental disorders such as DCD. Thus, instead of *just* investigating subtypes of children with DCD, it may be more useful from both a research and a clinical perspective to investigate groups of children with comorbid problems, some of whom display DCD. Such investigations may result in the identification of *subtypes* of children with a developmental disorder such as DCD and other kinds of comorbid problem who are more homogeneous than the whole group of children with DCD (Kadesjo & Gillberg, 1998). On a practical level, the identification of these more homogeneous groups of children may result in the development of interventions that are more effective in improving the motor/learning skills of children with DCD.

SUMMARY AND CONCLUSIONS

Our efforts over the past decade to classify children with DCD into discrete subtypes have met with limited success. Although the subtyping literature is useful in understanding the patterns of motor functions that may be impaired in children with DCD, it does not take into account the heterogeneity of the population of children with DCD or the comorbidity of other developmental disorder. Thus, instead of focusing our efforts on trying to find subtypes of DCD based on performance on motor and/or perceptual-motor measures, it may be more useful for researchers to refocus their efforts on the investigation of combinations of problems (i.e., motor, attention, learning) displayed by children with developmental disorders. Such an approach can help us to better describe the variation in the DCD population and perhaps identify how and why this variation arises. Further, it can have important beneficial effects in terms of diagnosis and treatment.

CHAPTER

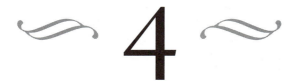

4

Motor/Language Impairment Syndromes—Direct or Indirect Foundations?

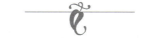

Lise-Beate Estil and H. T. A. Whiting

In most industrial countries, increasing emphasis is being placed on education, and young people are required to spend a significant part of their lives in school. The mastery of basic academic skills such as reading and writing is considered fundamental to their success. Nevertheless, much of their play and leisure time involves physical activity of one kind or another. In this context, the playground and sport field are important arenas for socialization and the development of those social skills that are needed to function in a complex society.

Children who are below the normal level of development in motor and language skills, here referred to as motor and language impaired,[1] may fail to meet the performance-related academic standards of their school environment, but may also lack the necessary physical competence to be accepted as equals in play activities demanding motor competence. This, in turn, may have detrimental effects

---

[1]Impairment is a loss or abnormality of body structure or of a physiological or psychological function (World Health Organization, 1997).

on personal development, that is, the impairments become a handicap (World Health Organization, 1980).

There are a variety of opinions about the bandwidth of normal development. This makes it difficult to identify impairments in children—particularly at an early age—and to establish meaningful identification criteria and cut-off points. This has resulted in different studies showing a range of 5–15% of school children (5–12 years) as exhibiting motor skill problems that are well below the norm (American Psychiatric Association, 1994; Brenner, Gillman, Zangwill, & Farrell 1967; Gubbay, 1975; Henderson & Hall, 1982; Mæland, 1992; Rutter, Graham, & Yule, 1970). According to most of these studies, the incidence is higher in boys than in girls (Gubbay, 1978; Henderson & Hall, 1982; Keogh, Sugden, Reynard, & Calkins, 1979; Mæland, 1992). Motor impairment in children has, over the years, been assigned a variety of labels, for example, developmental apraxia, or disturbances in motor planning (Orton, 1937); ataxia, or unsteady or uncoordinated movement (Gubbay, 1975); clumsiness (Henderson, 1977); developmental dyspraxia, or disorder of gesture (Dewey, 1995); and developmental coordination disorders (DCDs), or motor impairment in the absence of neurological signs (American Psychiatric Association, 1994). Many of these terms have also been divided into subgroups. Apraxia, for example, has been classified as ideational when defective performance of sequences of gestures is the observed deficit and as ideomotor when the disturbance is confined to isolated gestures (Dewey, 1995).

It has also been estimated that some 2–10% of similar age groups (but not necessarily the same children) exhibit different kinds of language problems, manifested in speech, reading, and writing[2] (American Psychiatric Association, 1994; Gaddes, 1985; Rutter, 1978; Stein, 1994; Stevenson, 1984). Once again, boys would seem to be more affected than girls (Bjørgen, Undheim, Nordvik, & Romslo, 1987; Edwards, Ellams, & Thompson, 1976; Gjessing, Nygaard, & Solheim, 1988; Lambe, 1999; Rutter & Yule, 1975; Silva, McGee, & Williams, 1985; Stein, 1994). Some of these children experience problems related to both motor and language skills. An overlap of 40–70% in this respect has been indicated in the literature (Nickisch, 1998; Paul, Cohen, & Caparulo, 1983; Rintala, Pienimäki, Ahonen, Cantell, & Kooistra, 1998; Wolff, Melngailis, Obregon, & Bedrosian, 1995). Given that such an overlap is unlikely to be fortuitous, it is this group of children who will be the particular focus of this chapter.

In some cases, the coexistence of motor and language problems may be related to the overall condition. For example, a general problem in the organization of movements may also manifest itself in the fine coordination required for speech, resulting in articulation problems. Yet, other language difficulties may exist that are less obviously related to the motor problems per se, for example, putting thoughts into words or finding the right words and organizing them into coherent sentences. The picture becomes even more complex when problems related to, for example, phonological dyslexia are shown to go hand-in-hand with certain kinds of motor problem, for

---

[2]The language problems referred to in the literature are fairly diffuse, encompassing problems in speech, reading, and writing as well as diverse kinds of dyslexia.

example, bimanual coordination (Moore, Brown, Markee, Theberge, & Zvi, 1996). Where such problems occur together, they may be mediated directly or indirectly.

The notion of a direct mediation implies that both problems are simply different manifestations of one underlying substrate, for example, a dysfunctional neurological system brought about by a maturational delay or damage to the central nervous system. Indirect mediation, in contrast, implies that there is one primary problem, either motor or language, and the secondary related problem, either language or motor, arises as a consequence of social constraints to which the primary problem gives rise.

INDIRECT/DIRECT MEDIATIONS

Indirect Mediations

The play arena is important for the development of both motor and language skills. Children who have poor motor skills often experience difficulty in being accepted as participants in play with other children (Schoemaker & Kalverboer, 1994). Similar problems are also reported in children who are inadequate in language skills (Brinton, Fujiki, Spencer, & Robinson, 1997). When children are excluded from interacting with other children, for either reason, this may have a negative effect on the development of both motor and language skills. In such cases, motor and language problems may be indirectly linked via social constraints. The result is a vicious circle where isolation due to motor or language incompetence leads to reduced participation and diminished opportunities for practicing both motor and language skills. This, in turn, exacerbates both the motor and language problems.

One of the mediating factors, in this respect, may be self-esteem. The negative effect of motor and/or language impairments on self-esteem has been well documented (Henderson, May, & Umney, 1989; Kalliopuska & Karila, 1987; O'Dwyer, 1987; Shaw, Levine, & Belfer, 1982; Van Rossum & Vermeer, 1990). Again, a vicious circle may be in operation. Low self-esteem stemming from problems with motor and language skills may deter such children from engaging in social situations because of fear of failure, which, in turn, leads to further delay in the development of either/or both (Harter, 1978). This chapter will not pursue the issue of indirect mediation further; at the same time, it is appreciated that it is an issue with many social consequences that are of crucial importance.

Direct Mediation

Direct mediation between motor and language skills is, perhaps, easier to document. Although, on the surface, motor and language skills would seem to fall into quite distinct categories, they share some basic characteristics that suggest that they are closely related in a number of ways. In the first place, language skills demand highly sophisticated movement skills that manifest themselves in speech, reading, and writing. For example, speech requires fine coordination of muscles in tongue, lips, jaw, larynx, and respiratory organs. The complexity of this coordination is exemplified by the fact that, for a baby to say "ba," for example, it takes the coordinated action of about 40 muscles (Kelso, 1995). Motor processes are also fundamental to reading and writing. Reading requires finely controlled movements of the eyes, while writing requires fine well-coordinated movements of both the writing hand and the eyes.

However, it has to be appreciated that the terms "motor skills" and "language skills" are very general categorizations that subsume a variety of subskills. To that extent, they are too general to be of much help in coming to an understanding of why impairments in the performance of these skills should arise in the first place and why they might occur together in some children. For this reason the subcategorizations "speech/motor impairment" and "dyslexia/motor impairment" will be two subcategories that will need to be separately invoked from time to time in what follows. In so doing, the limitations of such a division have also to be kept in mind based as it is on the traditional view that dyspraxia (speech impairment) and dyslexia (reading impairment) are distinct clinical syndromes. More recent research findings have demonstrated that the vast majority of children identified in preschool as developmentally language (speech) impaired exhibit inordinate difficulty in learning to read when they reach elementary school (Plaza, 1997; Tallal, Curtiss, & Kaplan, 1988). The speech impairment of those children who develop dyslexia is typically recognized as stemming from a phonological deficiency, which might be related to a more fundamental information processing deficit. Thus, in many cases, younger children with phonological dyslexia are likely to be members of the same subgroup, while the speech-impaired children who grow out of their problems represent yet another subgroup.

Evolutionary Perspective

From an evolutionary perspective, the development of both motor and speech skills are closely interrelated. For example, Rizzolatti and Arbib (1998), drawing on the earlier work of Kimura (for a review, see Kimura, 1993),[3] argue that speech has developed from a sequence of events that began with gestural communication. The gist of their argument is as follows. The oro-facial gestures of primates were those most likely to be used in communication between individuals.

> The open-closed alternation of the mandible that is typical of oro-facial communication in monkeys . . . appears to persist in humans where it forms the syllable "frame" in speech production . . . if manual gestures are associated with oro-facial communication, the sender's possibilities dramatically increase. . . . These considerations suggest that, at a certain stage, a brachio-manual communication system evolved complementing the oro-facial one. . . . An object or event described gesturally (such as, large object—large gesture of the arms) could now be accompanied by vocalisation. If identical sounds were constantly used to indicate

---

[3]According to Corballis (1998), this idea had already been proposed by Bonnot de Condillac during the 18th century and was simply revived by Hewes in 1973.

identical elements (such as large object, large opening of the mouth—vowel "a" and small object, tiny opening of the mouth—vowel "i"), a primitive vocabulary of meaningful sounds could start to develop. . . . The evolutionary pressure for more complex (combinatorial) sound emission, and the anatomical possibility for it, were thus the elements that moved language from its manuo-brachial origins to sound emission. Manual gestures progressively lost their importance whereas, by contrast, vocalisation acquired autonomy, until the relation between gestural and vocal communication inverted and gesture became purely an accessory factor to sound communication." (Rizzolatti & Arbib, p. 193)

Rizzolatti and Arbib (1998) invoke Liberman's (1993) motor theory of speech and positron emission tomography (PET) scan data (Schlaug, Knorr, & Seitz, 1994) in suggesting that both manual gestures and speech are related to different motor fields (hand, mouth, and larynx) represented in Broca's area of the brain. Thus, Broca's area would appear to play a mediating role in both motor and speech skills and, could, therefore, be involved in impairments in either or both of these domains.

Identifying invariances in motor and language skills (whether these involve speech or reading), as Rizzolatti and Arbib have done, is one way to explore their relation more deeply. Another way that has been well documented in the literature and that has particular relevance for the subcategory of speech/motor impairments is the putative common etiology underlying aphasia and apraxia.

Aphasia and Apraxia

The link between speech and gestural abilities is reflected in the neurological disorders aphasia and apraxia. Disruptions in speech that are experienced by individuals who have suffered damage to the central nervous system are called "aphasias" and usually result from damage to the left cerebral hemisphere (Kimura, 1993). Another symptom of left hemisphere damage is manual apraxia, commonly defined as inability to carry out specified movements, despite good strength and mobility in the muscles or limbs that are affected. It is recognized that most apraxic patients are also aphasic, and the apraxia is commonly inferred from the failure to make the required movements to a verbal command (Kimura, 1993). Liepmann (1908) has suggested that aphasia and apraxia are essentially similar and that both are manifestations of the loss of an ability to make certain kinds of movements.

The notion of a relation between gestural and language (speech) skills in children is supported by research findings of deficits of praxis in speech-impaired children (Dewey & Wall, 1997). For example, Dewey and Wall (1997) studied gestural performance in 35 children, within the age range of 6.0–10.11 years, of whom

---

[4]A child was defined as speech and language impaired if he/she demonstrated an impairment in speech articulation, voice or fluency, or deviant development of comprehension, or use of spoken, written or other symbol system that adversely affect educational performance. Children who demonstrated deficits only in articulation were not included.

15 (11 boys, 4 girls) were identified as speech and language impaired[4] and 20 children (11 boys, 9 girls) served as a control group. These groups were compared on gestural performance, such as transitive limb gestures (i.e., brush teeth with a toothbrush), intransitive gestures (e.g., wave goodbye), transitive orofacial gestures (e.g., drink from a straw), and intransitive orofacial gestures (e.g., whistle) to command. Results showed that the speech- and language-impaired group performed significantly poorer than the control group on limb intransitive and orofacial intransitive gestures. The finding that the speech- and language-impaired children were also significantly poorer than the controls on memory tests led to the proposition that children with both speech and language impairments may be deficient in their motor acts because they lack both the language and verbal memory skills needed to encode motor acts into memory.

Similar studies of gestural hand and arm movements carried out by Hill (Hill, 1998; Hill, Bishop & Nimmo-Smith, 1998) revealed a dyspraxic deficit in children (age range of 7–13 years) with specific language impairments (SLI) only, children with both SLI and motor impairments, and in children with motor impairments only (DCD). One could question whether the problems of these three subgroups of children were due to the same basic deficit related to the left hemisphere, as they all showed similar praxic problems, or whether, despite this commonality, they suffer from slightly different underlying dysfunctions.

Fine Motor Skills

Motor skills have been commonly subdivided into fine and gross. In the present context, this is a useful subdivision, as problems in the performance of fine motor skills, in particular, have more often been associated with language problems whether these be in the speech or reading domains.

With respect to SLI, for example, a number of studies have identified a diversity of fine motor skill problems in a variety of different groups of speech-impaired children involving: speed of peg-moving (Bishop & Edmundson, 1987; Owen & McKinlay, 1997; Powell & Bishop, 1992); threading beads and fastening buttons (Owen & McKinlay, 1997); posture production using hand and arm movements (Hill, 1998); and associated movements accompanying hand and finger movements, for example hand-patting, hand pronation/supination, index-thumb opposition, sequential finger-opposition, and diadokinesis (Notherdaeme, Amorosa, Ploog, & Scheimann, 1988). Although some of these studies (e.g., Powell & Bishop, 1992) provide evidence for a common etiology, what is missing are detailed discussions about which neurological abnormalities might underlie such behaviors.

Where attempts have been made to highlight a common etiology in motor and speech impairment, more consistency in the findings is apparent when the focus has been on fine motor coordination of hand and finger movements (Bradford & Dodd, 1996; Preis, Bartke, Willers, & Müller, 1995; Preis, Schittler, & Lenard, 1997). For example, Preis et al. (1995) found that even children with linguistically well-defined grammatical SLI without significant articulatory deficits (11 children: 6–11 years) were impaired in complex fine motor skills. In a pegboard moving task, eight of the SLI children needed significantly more total time with the right hand (all children were right-handed) than the control group. Motor problems in the SLI children also increased with the complexity of the motor task. What might be the neurological implications of such deficits? Preis et al. (1995) concluded that the fine-motor skill problems might signal a sequencing and temporal order deficit, as SLI children not only experience temporal and sequencing problems related to motor tasks, but also have difficulties in processing successive stimuli presented rapidly in the auditory modality. They invoke the idea that both language and motor processes might be dependent on neuronal elements, which are not specific to only one kind of process, but are responsible for modulation of specific components of different processes. They suggested further that the supplementary motor area might be involved. Functional imaging studies having shown that this area is highlighted both in complex planning of sequenced motor processes (Deiber et al., 1991; Roland, Larsen, Lassen, & Skinhoj, 1980; Seitz et al., 1996) and during speech processes (Tamas, Schibasaki, Horikoshi, & Ohye, 1993).

Attempts of this nature have also been apparent in the context of dyslexia/motor impairments exemplified, particularly, in the so-called "cerebellar hypothesis."

Cerebellar Hypothesis

Traditionally, the cerebellum has been considered to be a motor area (Eccles, Ito, & Szentagothai, 1967; Holmes, 1917, 1939; Stein & Glickstein, 1992). However, Ivry and colleagues (for a review, see Ivry, 1993) have suggested that it plays an important role, not only in motor control but also in perception of time. Cerebellar patients have been shown to be impaired in the performance of auditory time perception tasks as well as in repetitive finger tapping tasks (Ivry & Diener, 1991; Ivry & Keele, 1989; Keele, Ivry, & Pokorny, 1987; Keele, Pokorny, Corcos, & Ivry, 1985). They put forward the hypothesis that the predominant role of the cerebellum in motor control is the control of fine timing, and that the computational capabilities of this structure are not restricted to the motor domain, but are also accessible to nonmotor tasks that are dependent on precise timing. They further proposed that there is no single timing mechanism in the cerebellum, but rather that this computational ability is distributed, with different regions being involved with the particular category of temporal information utilized in different tasks.

Based on this hypothesis, Fawcett and Nicolson (1995) suggested that both the motor and language impairments observed in dyslexic subjects could be two different expressions of a single neurological deficit in the cerebellum. They found that groups of dyslexic children (N's ranging between 8 and 16 subjects and differing in age from 8 to 17 years) were significantly slower than their matched (age and IQ) controls. Instead, they were equivalent to their reading age controls in placing pegs and articulation rate, while for bead threading they were significantly slower than even their reading age controls. Referring to these findings and other studies that have shown a significant relation between balance deficits, motor skill deficits, and timing deficits in dyslexic children, they suggested that children with dyslexia might suffer from minor damage to the cerebellum. Fawcett and Nicolson's hypothesis of a cerebellar deficit was supported by a later study (Fawcett, Nicolson, & Dean, 1996) in which dyslexic children showed highly significant impairments on a battery of clinical tests designed to detect cerebellar impairment (the test battery is described in Dow & Moruzzi, 1958). The tests included maintenance of posture (balance time and postural stability), hypotonia (reduced muscle tone), and complex movements (pointing to a bull's eye with a marker pen, finger to finger pointing, adiadokinesis, toe tap speed, placing the index finger and thumb of one hand onto the index finger and thumb of the other hand). Out of 29 dyslexic children, all were impaired on arm displacement, 28 on postural stability, and 23 on finger/thumb opposition. Despite the strong suggestive evidence of cerebellar impairment, these authors were well aware of the limitations of their findings, pointing to the fact that the evidence is only indirect and nonspecific and to the possibility that research with different samples of children with dyslexia and control children might lead to lower estimates of effect size and incidence rate.

In an attempt to establish the generality of the results obtained in the 1996 study, a replication was recently carried out using larger samples of dyslexic and control children (Fawcett & Nicolson, 1999). The subjects in this study showed similar impaired performance. The cerebellar hypothesis was further supported by another recent study (Nicolson et al., 1999) in which brain activation was monitored by PET in matched groups of six dyslexic adults and six control subjects as they carried out either a prelearned sequence or learned a novel sequence of finger movements. They found that brain activation was significantly lower for the dyslexic adults than for the controls in the right cerebellar cortex and the left cingulate gyrus when executing the prelearned sequence, and in the right cerebellar cortex when learning the new sequence.

In the case of both speech/motor impairments and dyslexia/motor impairments, the hypothetical neural explanations put forward still beg the question as to whether the neurological impairments peculiar to such areas are the consequence of neural damage, abnormal neural development, or delayed maturation (a so-called "developmental lag"). The latter two kinds of explanation also give rise to questions about the relevant contributions of nature and nurture.

Developmental Lag

The notion of a developmental lag builds on the maturational perspective of a delay in the acquisition of age-related skills and implies that poor performance in language and motor skills are simply due to a genetically determined, slow maturation of the nervous system. If the language/motor impairments in children were due to a developmental lag, it would be expected that they would overcome their problems as they grow older, as has been observed in children with motor impairments (Barnett & Henderson, 1992; Losse et al., 1991). However, if the problems should persist into adulthood (as is usually the case with dyslexia), an abnormal neural development, rather than a developmental lag per se might be assumed.

Some authors (Hill, 1998; Powell & Bishop, 1992) have suggested that the coexistence of speech and movement problems may simply be the result of a developmental lag, since the motor performance (gesture production) of motor- and speech-impaired children is qualitatively similar to that of normally developing younger children. This standpoint, however, was not supported by an earlier study of Notherdaeme et al. (1988), who found, in a sample of 17 speech-impaired children[5] (16 boys and 1 girl), in the age range of 7–12 years, evidence for a deviant neural development, rather than a developmental lag per se, as associated movements in their speech-impaired children were shown to be qualitatively different from those of younger control children (10 girls and 7 boys, 4–5 years). The fact that higher rates of left-handedness and ambidexterity are reported in children with speech impairment (Bishop, 1990) also strengthens the credibility of a deviant neural development hypothesis. At the same time, it has to be recognized that there are also many studies that have shown no association between handedness and speech impairment (Bishop, 1990; Preis et al., 1997). The reasons for this incongruency are difficult to pinpoint. They could be due to different characteristics of the groups involved in the studies, differences in the methods used for measuring laterality, or different subtypes.

Denckla and Rudel (see Denckla, 1985) have suggested that a maturational lag in relation to visual and perceptual abilities may be involved in dyslexia. This proposition was based on results from studies of dyslexic, otherwise learning disabled, and normal children on the task of map-walking (Denckla, Rudel, & Broman, 1980). Dots were placed on the floor, and subjects were required to follow a path mapped out in ink on a handheld piece of cardboard, the route corresponding to that on the floor. They found that the younger dyslexic children (below the age of 10) had the worst performance of the three groups, whereas, surprisingly, the teenage dyslexic group demonstrated superiority on this test. They concluded that the most parsimonious explanation was a maturational lag in that part of the "motor analyzer" that is dependent on the left hemisphere and has been found to be important for timed, sequential, detailed movements.

Although, as might be inferred from this study, reading-disabled children may grow out of their motor problems (Denckla, 1985), there are reports of increasing differences with age between reading-impaired and control subjects on tests of language (Wolf, 1982). Denckla's (1985) explanation of this finding was that even when there is lifelong deficiency of certain left-hemisphere–subserved capabilities, "those that are part of the motor analyser system in the left hemisphere may improve sufficiently to act as means of expression for the adequate or even above average functioning of a presumably right hemisphere-subserved set of capabilities, such as athletics and perception of spatial relationships and visual design" (pp. 190–191).

An attempt to explain a retarded development of the left hemisphere, which might contribute to deviant laterality profiles, language, and other learning disorders in children, is provided by the testosterone hypothesis of Geschwind and Galaburda (1985). This hypothesis holds that high testosterone levels *in utero* may slow down the development of the left hemisphere, and may also explain why language impairments and other learning disorders are more often observed in boys than in girls.

---

[5]The children were diagnosed as developmental speech and language disordered by a team of experienced speech/language therapists. All children, 15 right-handed and 2 left-handed, attended the special school at the Max Planck Institute for Psychiatry, had IQs within normal range, and had no major neurological deficits.

With respect to motor impairment, Sigmundsson, Ingvaldsen, and Whiting (1997b) found evidence indicative of a developmental lag as the performance of 8-year-old children with hand-eye coordination problems was similar to 5-year-old controls in inter- and intrasensory modality matching. However, when scores for the preferred and nonpreferred hands were analyzed separately, only the children with hand-eye coordination problems showed significant performance differences, in favor of the preferred hand in both conditions where proprioception was involved. They suggested that the developmental lag exhibited by these children might have pathological overtones related to the development of the corpus callosum, which generally is considered to reach its final stage of maturation between 5 and 12 years of age.

Neurological Impairment

In the context of dyslexia/motor impairment, support for a common underlying neurological impairment comes from those studies that report higher rates of left-handedness and ambidexterity in children with dyslexia (Annett, Eglinton, & Smythe, 1996; Annett & Turner, 1974). Deviant laterality profiles have also been observed in children with motor impairment, manifested by a higher incidence of crossed dominance, but not a higher incidence of left-handedness (Armitage & Larkin, 1993). As deviant laterality profiles are observed in both dyslexic and motor-impaired children, this might not only be a general characteristic of the syndrome, but it might also provide a useful lead into the search for answers to the question as to why some children experience problems related to both motor and language skills.

Olson and colleagues found that phonological coding in children with reading disabilities was substantially lower than in younger nondisabled children (Olson, Wise, Conners, Rack, & Fulker, 1989). This was taken as an indication of a developmental deficit in phonological coding rather than a developmental lag per se. That this might be genetically determined was inferred from data on identical and fraternal twins that suggested that phonological coding was highly heritable.

What other evidence is available that might support the idea of neurological impairment underlying language/motor disorders whether these relate to speech or dyslexia?

Inter/Intrahemispheric Lesion/Disconnection

In a number of the studies already referred to in this chapter, it has been shown that particular samples of motor- and speech/reading-impaired children experience quite severe problems in bimanual coordination (Fawcett & Nicolson, 1995; Fawcett et al., 1996; Owen & McKinlay, 1997). Given that the distal finger movements of the right and left hand, respectively, are controlled via the contralateral hemisphere (Bogen, 1993) such coordination requires efficient transfer of information between the hemispheres via the corpus callosum (Jeeves, 1990; Preilowski, 1972, 1990; Quinn & Geffen, 1986). This has been supported in a series of studies carried out by Sigmundsson et al. (Sigmundsson, 1999; Sigmundsson, Ingvaldsen,

& Whiting, 1997a, 1997b; Sigmundsson, Whiting, & Ingvaldsen, 1999; for further details about these studies, see Chapter 5). They addressed inter and intrahemispheric problems in 7–8-year-old children with motor impairment diagnosed as having hand-eye coordination problems; speech/reading disorders were not an issue addressed at that time. They proposed that the problems exhibited by these subgroups of children with motor impairment could be behavioral manifestations of neurological impairment interpreted within a framework of an intrahemispheric lesion/disconnection affecting the transfer of information within the hemispheres or an interhemispheric disconnection.

Within the context of speech/motor impairment, Owen and McKinlay (1997) found that a group of 16 developmental speech and language disordered children[6] (age range of 4–7 years) had significantly greater problems in bimanual tasks such as threading beads and fastening buttons compared to their controls (matched on age, sex, and nonverbal intelligence). Although these researchers did not apply neurological interpretations to their data, the nature of these tasks suggests a problem in the interhemispheric transfer of information. Whether this reflects a callosal problem per se or the indirect effect of a left or right intrahemispheric lesion is open to question. As the left hemisphere, traditionally, is considered to be dominant for both motor and speech (Kimura, 1982; Kimura & Archibald, 1974), this could be a plausible interpretation. It is perhaps more surprising to the reader that a putative right hemispheric dysfunction is also being suggested as an alternative to problems in the callosum per se. Although the evidence is limited, findings by Powell and Bishop (1992) of a balancing deficit specific to the nonpreferred (left) leg in children with speech impairments could be indicative of an involvement of the right hemisphere.

That callosal dysfunction might be an underlying pathogenetic factor in children with developmental dysphasia and dyslexia is a position put forward by Njiokiktjien, Valk, and Ramaekers (1988). This proposition builds on the earlier finding of Badian and Wolff (1977) that dyslexic males (8–26 years of age) performed significantly worse with their left hand than controls in tapping to a metronome when the requirement was to alternate hands but performed equally as well when required to tap with the right and left hand separately. They argued, on the basis of evidence from patients with surgical commissurotomies, that the motor deficiency in synchronising left and right hands might be due to a disturbance in interhemispheric cooperation. More recently, Moore et al. (1996) found that dyslexia, particularly phonological dyslexia, is associated with deficits in interhemispheric interactions mediated by the corpus callosum.

The notion of an intra–left hemispheric disconnection gains support from a PET scan study of five adults with developmental dyslexia of a phonological kind and their controls (Paulesu et al., 1996). For the dyslexics, a subset of the brain regions

---

[6]They made up a complete cohort for this age group of those children considered to have the most severe "developmental speech and language disorders" in the Salford district (3,300 births per annum). The nature of their language problems was not further described.

normally involved in phonological processing was activated: Broca's area during the rhyming task and the temporo-parietal cortex during a short-term memory task. In controls, both these areas were activated simultaneously. They proposed that the defective phonological system of the dyslexic is due to weak connectivity between anterior and posterior language areas (i.e., an intrahemispheric problem).

Some support for an intra–right hemispheric disconnection is provided by Denckla (1985) who investigated performance of rapid repetitive and alternating movements in a group of 40 pure dyslexic children. She found a tendency towards large right-left differences, that is, a tendency for the left side, normally somewhat slower in a right-preferring population, to be even more so in this population. However, Denckla attributed this, and other findings of large left-right differences, to a deficiency in the "callosal system," arguing that this need not be due to a defect in the fibers of the callosum, but that callosal transmission might be impaired by lesion in the cells of origin of the callosal fibers in the cortex or in the cortical cells on which the callosal fibers synapse.

Dyslexia Timing Hypothesis

An attempt to be more specific about the nature of such putative inter/intrahemispheric problems comes from research on temporal variables in timing precision and serial ordering in bimanual coordination. Wolff and colleagues (Wolff, 1993; Wolff, Cohen, & Drake, 1984; Wolff, Michel, & Ovrut, 1990; Wolff, Michel, Ovrut, & Drake, 1990) argued that temporal problems underlie the apparent interhemispheric problems observed in many dyslexics. The gist of his argument was that it is not impaired motor coordination that causes reading retardation, but that there is probably a third factor of impaired temporal resolution that expresses itself outwardly in both the manual motor and language skill performance of dyslexic individuals.

In an extension of an earlier study, Wolff et al. (1984) turned their attention to aspects of timing control for motor speech and explored the possible links between impaired motor coordination and reading retardation. Twenty reading-retarded 12–13-year-old male volunteers of above average intelligence were compared to normal controls on synchronous finger tapping (single hand 92 bpm, alternating hand 184 bpm, alternating hand 92 bpm), asynchronous intermanual tapping, motor speech, and rapid automatized naming. They found that both groups could perform the manual and motor speech tasks adequately when movement speed was scaled to a sufficiently slow rate but that both groups showed a breakdown in coordinated movements at fast entrainment rates. While the bimanual tapping tasks were correlated with the reproduction of single syllables (both groups), reading achievement and spelling, and rapid naming (reading retarded group), unimanual tapping proficiency was not correlated with any outcome measure. They argued that the greater impairment on tasks of interlimb coordination (asynchronous tapping in particular), but not in unimanual performance, is consistent with the hypothesis that impaired motor performance and reading retardation are both related to a reduced efficiency of interhemispheric communication. Given that the retarded readers had difficulty preventing the momentarily inactive or nonleading hand from moving in unison with the active, or leading hand, Wolff et al. argued that the presumed inefficiency of interhemispheric communications may be associated with a failure to transmit motor inhibitory rather than motor excitatory impulses. Such a failure, they suggest, would have a relatively greater disruptive effect on coordinated bimanual trials than unimanual or synchronous bimanual tapping. The retarded readers also showed speech articulation difficulties on tasks requiring a rapid switching back and forth across different articulation patterns. Given that motor speech does not involve interlimb coordination and probably does not depend on efficient interhemispheric cooperation, it was argued that deficits in the temporal organization of motor inhibitory commands may account for some of the performance deficits in both domains of motor function.

Based on this and later studies (for a review, see Wolff, 1993), Wolff put forward three possible hierarchical explanatory models: (1) information processing within the left hemisphere (i.e., growing up with grossly intact but dysfunctional cerebral commissures might, for example, be associated with the adequate transmission of degraded information, as in the case of left or right hemisphere anomalies); (2) reduced efficiency of interhemispheric communication (i.e., a slow rate of information transfer for time-distributed functions that require precise temporal integration between the hemispheres); or (3) selective dysfunction of the cerebellar hemispheres (i.e., a failure to suppress redundant or conflicting information between the hemispheres). The latter model is in line with other studies that have focused particularly on cerebellar dysfunction and to which reference has been made earlier in this chapter.

However, Wolff did not regard these models as sufficient in themselves. In fact, he pointed to their limitation in the light of the plasticity of the neuromotor system, which allowed individuals with localized brain lesions or abnormal patterns of neurological development to frequently achieve the same intended goal by alternative pathways when the usual flow of information is blocked or dysfunctional. He drew attention to a different theoretical perspective for this purpose, namely dynamic systems theory (Kelso, Holt, Rubin, & Kugler, 1981), which focuses on how new patterns of behavioral coordination are formed during development from antecedent conditions that do not exhibit such novel properties. Research within this theoretical framework (Kelso & Tuller, 1981; Kelso et al., 1981) has demonstrated that the frequency at which tasks of bimanual coordination are performed is a critical variable or control parameter in spontaneous pattern formation. Given the paradigmatic changes to which this approach has given rise in the fields of motor learning and control, its extension to the kinds of problem being addressed in this chapter is awaited with much anticipation.

Magnocellular Deficit

Another interesting link to temporal insufficiency in children with dyslexia (Galaburda & Livingstone, 1993; Stein, 1993) is the proposition that a magnocellular deficit might be the neural basis of problems in processing rapidly changing signals by the central nervous system. From their studies of contrast sensitivity and visual temporal resolution of normal and dyslexic adults, Galaburda and Livingstone

(1993) have drawn the conclusion that dyslexics are less sensitive to low-contrast, fast visual stimulation and that the characteristics of the abnormalities are suggestive of a defect in the transient, or magnocellular, subdivision of the visual pathway. In postmortem studies, they also found significant anatomical differences in the lateral geniculate nuclei between dyslexic brains and controls, with the magnocellular bodies being generally smaller and more variable in size and shape, while the parvocellular layers appeared similar in the two groups. In further extrapolation of this work, they suggest that rapid information processing may not be limited to the visual modality, but may also be limited in the ability to discriminate rapid auditory transitions. This proposition was based on evidence from studies showing that language- and reading-impaired children have difficulty in distinguishing both consonant-vowel phonemes and nonlinguistic cues if they involve rapid (around 40 ms) auditory transitions (Tallal, 1980). Additionally, reading-disabled children who show defects in rapid visual information processing also do poorly on tests of phonological skills (Tallal, Stark, Kallman, & Mellits, 1981). To date, studies on magnocellular deficits have only been performed in relation to dyslexia, but, given the importance of visual perception in motor coordination, in particular hand-eye coordination tasks, this could be an interesting hypothesis also with relation to subgroups of motor and language impairments.

Vestibular Hypothesis

In the previous sections, the main focus has been on fine motor problems, in particular related to bimanual coordination and temporal sequencing. Postural problems have also figured prominently in the literature (Fawcett & Nicolson, 1992; Nicolson & Fawcett, 1990). These need also to be explained. For example, Fawcett and Nicolson (1992) showed that the balance performance of 11-year-old and 15-year-old groups of dyslexic children was significantly impaired by the introduction of a secondary task, while the balance of the control groups of children (matched for age and IQ) without language problems was unaffected, that is, the dyslexic children needed to invest more attention to maintain adequate balance. In a similar vein, Kohen-Raz (1981) has shown "trainability" of static balance to be significantly associated with level of reading ability. Given the growing body of evidence of a significant relation between poor balance and different kinds of language problems, such as SLI, reading ability, and dyslexia, it is surprising that few attempts have been made to specify the nature of this link, that is, to go from description to explanation, particularly with respect to underlying etiology.

One exception was that of Levinson (1988), who concluded that both dyslexia and other typically associated problems, such as learning disabilities, attention deficit disorders, poor balance and coordination, and speech problems, are all due to a signal-scrambling disturbance of inner-ear (cerebellar-vestibular) functioning. He claimed to have found an inner-ear dysfunction that characterized over 96% of a large dyslexic sample (Levinson, 1973). He expressed concern that the differing patterns of cerebral functioning in dyslexics versus normals observed by the use of active imaging and electrophysiological techniques should be misinterpreted as causal factors of dyslexia, rather than the result of dyslexia. He put forward the hypothesis that such observations might be due to poor input owing to a dysfunction in the vestibular system (inner ear). In support of a vestibular explanation is his own research (Levinson, 1991; based on four case studies, drawn from a sample of 100) showing that motion sickness medication may relieve many of the problems experienced by learning-disordered and dyslexic children, such as reading, drawing, handwriting, ball-catching, balance, and coordination.

Except for the studies mentioned above, there appears to have been little interest in the vestibular theory in the literature. One reason may be the rather speculative nature of the theory and the limited evidence on which it was based. Not the least of the concerns is the credibility of a single explanation for a potpourri of learning disabilities that include dyslexia, motor impairment, and attention deficit disorders. As different subgroups of children with impaired language have been shown to exhibit different patterns of performance in a range of motor tasks, it is more likely, as suggested by Bradford and Dodd (1994), that their different surface production errors reflect different underlying deficits.

SUMMARY AND CONCLUSIONS

In many instances, motor and language impairments in children may be highly correlated. Direct and indirect explanations for this overlap have been proposed. An indirect explanation would invoke social constraints associated with one of these forms of impairment adversely affecting the other, giving rise to a vicious circle of cause and effect. While this form of mediation is an interesting line to pursue, it begs the question as to what gave rise to the motor and/or language impairments in the first place.

Direct effects would attribute both forms of deficiency to a developmental lag or to abnormal neural development (which may or may not have genetic overtones). Interpretations of this kind would, however, have to be qualified when it is recognized that there is no easily definable group of language/motor-impaired children but rather a number of subgroups for which the correlations observed may require different, or at least modified, causal interpretations. Even the subcategories on which attention has been focused in this chapter, namely, speech/motor impairment and dyslexia/motor impairment are probably too coarse to provide more than suggestions as to a common etiology.

The fact that many speech-impaired children, particularly those with phonological deficits, develop dyslexia, can probably account for the findings of similar motor problems in dyslexic and speech-impaired groups of children.

Clearly, there is some way to go before the neurological implications of motor and language impairments, where they occur together, can be teased out. What is clear, however, is that there is no shortage of putative explanations for either phenomenon. It is the considered opinion of the present authors that research directed towards those groups of children who exhibit both motor and language impairments will, in the long run, lead to new methodological approaches that will clarify the nature of the etiology, particularly with respect to the question of the relative contributions of nature and nurture.

CHAPTER
5

Neural Constraints on Motor Behavior in Children with Hand-Eye Coordination Problems

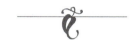

Hermundur Sigmundsson and H. T. A. Whiting

This chapter focuses on a subgroup of children whose motor impairment is expressed, primarily, in hand-eye coordination problems (HECP). In contrast to more traditional studies, which have been characterized by a focus on test outcomes (i.e., a product-based approach) that simply describe the problem but cannot explain it, an attempt is made here to explore the nature of putative neural constraints that might give rise to inefficient motor behavior. Attention is primarily directed towards the concept of sensory-motor integration, particularly with respect to vision and proprioception, an ability deemed to underlie many real-life motor skills. In this way, it has proved possible to draw parallels between behavioral manifestations of motor impairment and potential underlying neurological information-processing disorders, particularly as these relate to hemispheric competence.

DEFINITIONS AND ETIOLOGY

A variety of terms have been used to describe the movement coordination problems of children. For example, these children have been described as exhibiting evidence of clumsiness (Dare & Gordon,

1970; Orton, 1937), motor impairment (Morris & Whiting, 1971), developmental dyspraxia (Denckla, 1984), developmental apraxia and agnosia (Gubbay, 1975), and, most recently, developmental coordination disorder (American Psychiatric Association, 1987). The concept of developmental "clumsiness" has been discussed in the literature for at least 60 years (e.g., Gordon & McKinlay, 1980; Gubbay, 1975; Henderson & Hall, 1982; Morris & Whiting, 1971; Orton, 1937; Sigmundsson, Pedersen, Whiting, & Ingvaldsen, 1998; Walton, Ellis, & Court, 1962), yet it remains as unclear now as it did in the 1930s.

Clumsiness is defined by Morris and Whiting (1971) as "maladaptive motor behaviour in relation to expected or required movement performance," thus, bringing the notion of norms into the equation. Henderson and Hall (1982) had similar norms in mind when they proposed a more qualified definition: "Generally the term is used to describe children whose level of competence in motor skills is significantly below the norm, but who show no evidence of disease of the nervous system" (p. 448).

In the interim period, there has been considerable debate about the nature of the syndrome and, consequently, a definition that would adequately embrace the problems with which such children are confronted in everyday life. This has led to the adoption in some quarters of the recent American Psychiatric Association label "developmental coordination disorder" (DCD) to indicate a marked impairment in the development of motor coordination that is not explainable by mental retardation and is not due to a known physical disorder (APA, 1987). In effect, this definition differs little from many others (Gubbay, 1975; Henderson & Hall, 1982; Hulme, Biggerstaff, Moran, & McKinlay, 1982) other than, perhaps, to add the additional constraint about the absence of physical disorders. The central point in these definitions is that motor performance is impaired, but this impairment cannot be attributed to any identifiable physical or intellectual disorder. In brief, the child with motor impairment can be described as one who is clumsy in motor behavior, but otherwise normal (Smyth, 1992). In this chapter, the term "motor impairment" (clumsiness) will be adhered to.

While there is consensus about the nature of the motor impairment syndrome, there is no consensus about causation. The etiology has generally been couched in terms of nature versus nurture, with most theoretical positions assigning at least some role to both but varying in the emphasis placed on each (Berk, 1997; Haywood, 1993). Where these issues have been pursued, causation has been attributed to pre-, peri-, and postnatal factors (for a review, see Morris & Whiting, 1971). A focus on perinatal problems in the earlier medical literature led to the introduction of the terms "minimal brain damage"(MBD) and "minimal brain dysfunction." At that time, these kinds of default argument (i.e., in the absence of convincing evidence) were not considered to be very helpful and probably counterproductive with respect to tackling the problem. Nevertheless, Dare and Gordon (1970) pointed out that "there is no doubt that in many instances brain damage is present" (p. 178), and Gubbay (1975) later argued that a continuum of neurological damage underlies the motor impairment and that there is some overlap between cerebral palsy and clumsiness. These kinds of issues will be returned to from time to time in what follows.

PREVALENCE AND CHARACTERISTICS

The 6% estimate of the number of school-age children in Norway manifesting the motor impairment syndrome (Mæland, 1992; Søvik & Mæland, 1986) is very similar to the estimates made in other countries (Brenner, Gillman, Zangwill, & Farrell, 1967; Gubbay, 1975; Henderson & Hall, 1982). The importance of recognizing the syndrome and not dismissing it as within the norm is that difficulties experienced by the child can be expected to have an additive effect in a wide range of skills—motor, social, and linguistic. The focus in this chapter, however, will be on motor skills. In this respect, a lack of manual dexterity in one or more tasks such as tying shoelaces, doing up buttons, using scissors, managing a knife and fork, dressing, handwriting, and drawing are frequently noted. Problems in the performance of gross motor tasks may manifest themselves in relatively "open" skills involving, for example, the interception of moving objects such as catching a ball, as well as on relatively "closed" skills such as jumping, running, and hopping (Henderson, Rose, & Henderson, 1992; Smyth, 1992).

Given such a broad-based syndrome, there is universal agreement that motor-impaired children do not constitute a homogeneous group (Henderson & Sugden, 1992; Søvik & Mæland, 1986).

PERCEPTUAL DEFICITS IN CHILDREN WITH MOTOR IMPAIRMENTS

Over the last 30 years, some of the attempts of psychologists have been directed towards providing explanations for inadequacies in motor performance in such children by a search for deficits in the various cognitive processes involved in the planning and execution of movements (Henderson, 1992).

In the clinical literature, following Fleishman's (1966) approach, attempts have also been made to establish causal links between surface manifestations of motor impairment and underlying perceptual abilities. Two lines of enquiry have dominated this literature: visual-perceptual and/or visual-motor deficits (Dare & Gordon, 1970; Gubbay, Ellis, Walton, & Court, 1965; Henderson & Hall, 1982; Hulme, Biggerstaff et al., 1982; Hulme, Smart, & Moran, 1982; Hulme, Smart, Moran, & McKinlay, 1984; Powell & Bishop, 1992) and proprioceptive[1] deficits (Bairstow & Laszlo, 1981; Laszlo & Bairstow, 1985; Laszlo, Bairstow, Bartrip, & Rolfe, 1988; Smyth, 1991, 1994).

---

[1]Proprioception is considered those receptor mechanisms, most noticeably in the joints, muscles, and tendons, that signal information about the posture and movements of the body as a whole (Sherrington, 1906).

Theoretical Problems

Exploring the perceptual deficiencies underlying movement coordination problems has been an encouraging line of inquiry, but limitations in the theoretical frameworks in which they have been formulated have mitigated against the usefulness and applicability of the findings. Those studies, which have signalled perceptual deficiencies in samples of motor-impaired children (e.g., Hulme, Biggerstaff et al., 1982; Hulme, Smart et al., 1982; Hulme et al., 1984; Laszlo, 1990; Laszlo & Bairstow, 1985; Laszlo et al., 1988; Laszlo & Sainsbury, 1993; Smyth, 1991, 1994), have been confined to the level of description with no consensus of opinion as to the underlying causal agencies.

For example, with respect to visual-perceptual deficits, Hulme and colleagues (Hulme, Biggerstaff et al., 1982; Hulme et al., 1984) concluded that for many children their "clumsiness" stemmed from a difficulty in processing visual information (e.g., size consistency; visual discrimination; for review, see Henderson, 1993). Unfortunately, they did not explore the nature of the putative "visual deficits." Did the problem reside in the sense organs, the visual perceptual system, decision-making based on limited visual information, a deficient effector system, or combinations of all of these? Other researchers, claiming that difficulties in processing proprioceptive information are largely responsible for impaired perceptuo-motor performance (Laszlo & Bairstow, 1985; Laszlo et al., 1988), in a similar way, have been confined to the level of description. In their kinesthetic sensitivity test (KST), for example, Bairstow and Laszlo (1981) and Laszlo and Bairstow (1985) take no account of a possible lateralization effect, which may, as will be discussed later, be an important factor in relation to causality. One of the reasons might be that the "kinesthetic deficits" hypothesis they have pursued (for review, see Laszlo & Bairstow, 1985) takes no cognizance of the findings from, for example, the literature (for a review, see Heilman & Rothi, 1993) in which neurological lesion/disconnection has been linked to apraxia.

Methodological and Analytical Problems

Henderson (1993) goes so far as to argue that the visual perceptual deficits hypothesis of Hulme and his colleagues, justified only by correlational studies, is less well supported by experimental findings than the proprioceptive deficits put forward by Laszlo and her colleagues. Be that as it may, Doyle, Elliott, and Connolly (1986) have also questioned the procedures, i.e., using the method of constant stimuli as a means of measuring kinesthetic acuity (for more detailed information, see Doyle et al., 1986) used by Bairstow and Laszlo (1981) in developing their KST. Furthermore, Elliott, Connolly, and Doyle (1988) and Sugden and Wann (1988) have presented data that are inconsistent with their findings.

It is evident from this short critical overview that there are many discrepancies in the literature, some of which may be attributed to the absence of suitable theoretical frameworks into which the findings can be fitted, others to methodological problems or a failure to pursue group differences in depth. In the light of this critique, therefore, it is reasonable to explore the concept of perceptual deficit further, but in the context of "inter- and intrasensory modality matching" along the lines initiated by Hofsten and Rösblad (1988). Their argument that inter- and intramodal matching permits the study of the integration of sensory information directly related to the control of hand movements is well stated.

Inter- and Intramodal Matching

Hofsten and Rösblad (1988) pointed out that coordinative actions usually demand close inter- and intrasensory integration:

> In most cases of manual behaviour, both vision and proprioception will affect the outcomes of manual movements. In fact, if such movements are to be smooth and well co-ordinated, it is of crucial importance that visual and proprioceptive means of controlling them are in correspondence. This implies that the parameters of space defined by each of these systems are in fine agreement. If both hands are involved in an act, it is also important that the proprioceptive space defined by one limb is in correspondence with the proprioceptive space defined by the other limb. (p. 806)

Lee, Daniel, Turnbull, and Cook (1990) supported this standpoint, arguing that this linking of information (inter- and intramodal) is crucial to the development and maintenance of motor competence.

That intermodal (visual space–proprioceptive space) and intramodal (proprioceptive space–proprioceptive space) matching might provide insight into the nature of the motor impairment syndrome was proposed in an investigation (unpublished) carried out by Jongmans (1989) and cited in Henderson (1993). Using a paradigm that Hofsten and Rösblad (1988) originally used with normal children, they investigated the performance of children exhibiting clumsy behavior on a manual matching task to locate a target when the availability of vision and proprioception were systematically manipulated. Matching the located target was always carried out without vision. Given that the movements required were minimal, success on the task depended to a large extent on the ability to match visual/proprioceptive and proprioceptive information in locating targets.

The results showed that, while the target remained visible, the motor-impaired group performed as accurately as their control peers. Moreover, the addition of proprioceptive information in locating the target did not improve the performance of either group. However, when only proprioceptive information about target location was available, both groups were less accurate, but the decrease for the motor-impaired group was much more striking.

It is this kind of finding (i.e., possible underlying intramodal matching problems) that suggested the usefulness of formulating a neurobehavioral model of inter- and intramodal matching into which the available data could be fitted and which might give rise to further predictions that could be tested in the laboratory.

NEUROBEHAVIORAL MODEL OF INTER- AND INTRAMODAL MATCHING

Establishing the Context for the Model

"The great commissure forms at once a bond of union and a band of separation" (Wigan, 1844, in Bogen, 1990). Bogen (1990) points out that, while Sperry was awarded the Nobel Prize as long ago as 1981 for his work with human split-brain subjects, the implications of this work have yet to be fully appreciated: "The principle of cerebral duality, first demonstrated in cats and monkeys and then confirmed in humans has so far had insufficient recognition" (p. 215). This, by way of example, is what Sperry said about human subjects in 1974:

> Although some authorities have been reluctant to credit the disconnected minor hemisphere even with being conscious, it is our own interpretation—based on a large number and variety of nonverbal tests—that the other hemisphere is indeed a conscious system in its own right—perceiving, thinking, remembering, reasoning, willing, and emoting—all at a characteristically human level, and that both the left and right hemisphere may be conscious simultaneously in different, even mutually conflicting, mental experiences that run along in parallel. (p. 11)

With respect to somatosensory information processing in the tactile and proprioceptive modes, it soon became clear that, if a commisurotomized human was allowed to blindly feel a stimulus, then only the hemisphere contralateral to that hand was aware of the identity of the stimulus (for a review, see Bogen, 1993). This kind of exercise illustrated that the pathways for the transmission of such somatosensory information are almost completely crossed (Geffen, Nilsson, & Quinn, 1985; Kolb & Whishaw, 1996) with the corpus callosum serving a mediating role in interhemispheric transfer of information (Jeeves, 1990; Kalat, 1995; Preilowski, 1972, 1990; Quinn & Geffen, 1986).

Intermodal Matching

Sandström (1953) and Sandström and Lundberg (1956), using groups of normal adults, and later Hofsten and Rösblad (1988), using groups of normal children in their experimental work, introduced an intermodal condition (vision/proprioception), which, for success, demands congruency between the visual space and the proprioceptive space of the matching hand (for a review, see Hofsten & Rösblad, 1988). The hypothetical information-processing route when subjects are required to match information from visual space with the proprioceptive space of the left hand would, on the basis of current knowledge, appear to be as illustrated schematically in Figure 5.1. For the right hand, the projections would need to be mirror-imaged.

From the right visual field (RVF) to the visual cortical projection area V1 in the left hemisphere and the left visual field (LVF) to a similar projection area (V1) in

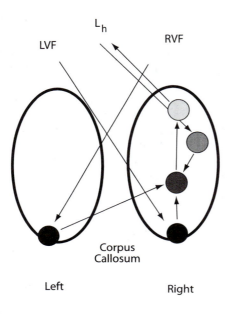

Figure 5.1   Schematic diagram of the human brain viewed from above, showing interhemispheric callosal pathway and intrahemispheric cortical connections used in carrying out movements with the left limb in response to visually defined positional information.

the right hemisphere, thereafter to area PG (Brodmann's area 7) in the posterior parietal cortex (PPC; Brodmann's area 7)—a polysensory, "intermodal mixing area" considered to have a role in controlling spatially guided behavior (Kolb & Whishaw, 1996; Mishkin, Ungerleider, & Macho, 1983; Mountcastle, Lynch, Georgopoulos, Sakata, & Acuna, 1975; Robinson, Goldberg, & Stanton, 1978). From area PG, information projects onto the precentral gyrus (primary motor cortex) in the same hemisphere as that which controls the left hand (output). Feedback from the left hand, in turn, projects to the right postcentral gyrus (primary somatosensory cortex; Brodmann's area 3-2-1), to area PG, and is important for matching that is congruency between the visual space reference (system goal) and proprioceptive space of the matching hand (system output).

Intramodal Matching

If both hands are involved in an act, it is important that the information space defined by the one limb is in correspondence with the information space defined by the other (intramodal matching). An example was provided by Laszlo and Bairstow (1980), using groups of both normal children and adults and, later, by Hofsten and Rösblad (1988) using groups of normal children in their study of proprioceptive-proprioceptive matching. The hypothetical route for such matching, based on current knowledge, is presented schematically in Figure 5.2 Information picked up via the right hand projects onto the postcentral gyrus (primary somatosensory cortex) in the left parietal lobe and is transmitted to the left PPC (Brodmann's areas 5

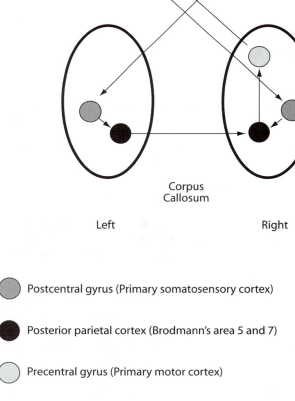

Postcentral gyrus (Primary somatosensory cortex)

Posterior parietal cortex (Brodmann's area 5 and 7)

Precentral gyrus (Primary motor cortex)

Figure 5.2 Schematic diagram of the human brain viewed from above, showing interhemispheric callosal pathway and intrahemispheric cortical connections used in carrying out movements with the left limb in response to proprioceptively defined positional information from right hand.

and 7; Kolb & Whishaw, 1996) via the corpus callosum, to the PPC of the opposite hemisphere; it traverses a pathway from there to the precentral gyrus (primary motor cortex) in the right hemisphere, which controls the left hand (Geffen et al., 1985; Quinn & Geffen, 1986). The left hand is, in this case, used as a haptic[2] perceptual system (Gibson, 1966)—feedback from the hand projecting onto area PPC via the right postcentral gyrus providing the other input necessary for determining the congruency between the proprioceptive space of the right and the left hand in this comparator area.

For the right hand matching, the projections would need to be mirror-imaged. Intramodal matching might also be mediated "intrahemispherically." This, however, would require ipsilateral matching. As this cannot be done using the two hands, one solution would be to use the foot and hand of the same side. There would, also, be the possibility to locate the target in combination, that is, felt and seen. In the case of left hand matching, for example, the model would need to be a combination of Figures 5.1 and 5.2.

Neurobehavioral models of the kind put forward lend themselves to questions about the effects that might be expected when communication between particular projection areas is impaired because of brain lesion or retardation in the establishment of the interconnections. Such impairment can be attributed to a "delay" (developmental lag) and/or "deviancy" (neurological lesion/disconnection). Perturbations and predictions in this respect have been evident in the literature for almost 100 years (for a review, see Bogen, 1993).

DEFICIT MODELS

Delay Versus Deviancy

A recurring theme within the field of motor impairment has been the notion that discrepancies between the motor behavior of motor-impaired and normal children can be seen as either manifesting delayed development or deviancy. The apparently simple phrase "motor delay" implies something quite different from the term "developmental agnosia and apraxia" (Gubbay, 1975). Whereas the first seems to imply a rather benign condition that will disappear over time the second implies a condition that mirrors one which occurs in adults with known and irreversible brain damage (Losse et al., 1991; Barnett & Henderson, 1992). The opposition of these two alternatives will be recognized here as the "delay" (developmental lag) versus "deviancy" (neurological lesion/disconnection) dichotomy.

---

[2]"This apparatus consists of a complex of subsystems. It has no 'sense organs' in the conventional meaning of the term, but the receptors in tissue are nearly everywhere and the receptors in the joints co-operate with them. Hence the hands and other body members are, in effect, active organs of perception. . . . Touch and vision in combination often yield a redundant, double guaranteed input of information" (Gibson, 1966, p. 53).

Developmental Lag (Delay)

Developmental lag theories imply that there is a maturational delay in the acquisition of age-related skills. Rutter (1984) has summarized this "maturational lag" explanation in the context of speech and language development as follows:

> It seems reasonable to regard some of the more extreme forms of developmental delay as no more than very marked exaggerations of this general trend for children to mature at different rates. . . . It is normal for different brain systems to develop at different rates, with each system "out of step" with others. (p. 584)

Further Stark, Mellits, and Tallal (1983) point out that, while the timing of "language" milestones may be delayed, the interval between one milestone and the next may be normal: such children would be aptly described as having a maturational lag. Although they were discussing other areas of development, their thinking can be applied to problems in movement skill development. Thus, the motor behavior of children with motor impairment may be similar to that of younger children, the prediction being that most of these children will outgrow their problems (Losse et al., 1991; Barnett & Henderson, 1992; Mæland, 1992). Beech and Harding (1984) also pointed to the neutrality of the term in the sense that no causal implications were being drawn in terms of either genetic or environmental factors.

Hulme et al. (1984) found in their study that 10-year-old children, diagnosed with motor impairment, showed a level of motor skill performance that was no better than that of a group of normal children some 4.5 years younger. Developmental delays of this order are rather unusual (Hulme et al., 1984). For example, in studies of children with reading retardation or dyslexia, it is common for reports to deal with groups of children whose reading lags behind that expected on the basis of their age and IQ by between two and three years (Hulme, 1981). Hulme et al. (1984) further point out that the results from the perceptual measures of visual and kinesthetic sensitivity show that children who have motor difficulties and young normal children do not differ in accuracy.

More recently, Barnett and Henderson (1992) found, in their study of the drawings of motor-impaired children, evidence for delays when comparisons were made with those of well-coordinated children of the same age and verbal ability. By following the development of some of the children over an 18-month period, they also found that there were indeed some who, over time, continued to fall further and further behind their peers; that is, they demonstrated not only an absolute lag but also a reduced rate of progress (Barnett & Henderson, 1992).

Neurological Lesion/Disconnection (Deviancy)

Many researchers have pointed out that their findings with motor-impaired children could be behavioral manifestations of putative neurological disorders. Dare and Gordon (1970) interpret clumsiness as part of the continuum of cerebral palsy.

Gubbay (1975) also pointed out that motor-impaired children often have minor or uncertain neurological abnormalities, and Dunn (1986) considered their impaired motor behavior to be an aspect of the MBD syndrome.

At the beginning of the century, Liepmann ventured an hypothesis linking neurological disconnection to apraxia, the inability to organize movements purposefully (cited in Bogen, 1993, and Heilman & Rothi, 1993). According to this concept, apraxia followed disconnection of motor areas from sensory areas. The problem with this concept is that deficits resulting from a putative disconnection of areas are difficult to distinguish from similar deficits resulting from damage within one or other of the areas involved. Kolb and Whishaw (1996) pointed out in this respect that, "As a result strict localisation of function becomes unworkable" (p. 12). It is not surprising, therefore, that Liepmann's hypothesis has more recently been related both to intrahemispheric lesion/disconnection (Faglioni & Basso, 1985; Geschwind, 1975; Heilman & Rothi, 1993) and interhemispheric disconnection (Bogen, 1993).

The idea that inter- and intramodal matching might provide insight into the nature of the motor impairment syndrome was the departure point for the series of studies to be reported utilizing the neurobehavioral models put forward in Figures 5.1 and 5.2.

PUTATIVE NEUROLOGICAL DISORDERS IN HECP CHILDREN

In the literature, there is universal agreement that children who are clumsy do not constitute a homogeneous group (Henderson & Sugden, 1992; Søvik & Mæland, 1986). It would, therefore, seem much more meaningful and productive to focus on more clearly defined subgroups of children exhibiting clumsy behavior and, at the same time, to go beyond the level of description to more explanatory frameworks.

With this in mind, Sigmundsson and his co-workers in a series of related studies turned their attention to a specific subcategory of motor-impaired children attending normal schools, namely, those exhibiting HECP. Test procedures developed in the authors' laboratory for this purpose, in contrast to those that focus only on surface behavior, have been directed towards those sensory integration abilities deemed to underlie the way in which these children carry out a range of everyday motor tasks (Hofsten & Røsblad, 1988; Laszlo & Bairstow, 1985; Lee et al., 1990; Lee, Hofsten, & Cotton, 1997; Røsblad & Hofsten, 1992). In this way, it has been possible to draw parallels between behavioral manifestations of "clumsiness" and possible underlying neurological information-processing disorders, particularly as these relate to hemispheric competence. This research was facilitated by the elaboration of an earlier developed testing instrument for sensory integration (Hofsten & Røsblad, 1988; Sandstrøm, 1953; Sandstrøm & Lundberg, 1956).

Sensory-Motor Integration Tests

Manual Matching Task: Inter- and Intramodal Matching

Basically, the testing procedures require the sensory matching of targets located visually (seen target), with the hand (felt target), or in combination (felt and seen).

Matching of the position of located targets is normally carried out without vision—an exception being the Sigmundsson (1999) study.

Studies carried out using these testing procedures (see Table 5.1; Sigmundsson, 1999; Sigmundsson, Ingvaldsen, & Whiting, 1997a, 1997b) produced evidence of significant differences in inter- and intrasensory modality matching between children with HECP and control children (age ranges of 5–8 years) when combined scores for both hands were analyzed. Analysis of the scores achieved with the right and left hand separately, however, demonstrated that the differences between the HECP and the control groups could, in the main, be attributed to lowered performances when the left hand (nonpreferred hand) was used for matching the located target position. Further, intragroup analyses produced evidence of significant asymmetrical differences in intrasensory modality matching. The condition in which they were required to locate targets with the left hand and match with the right hand was superior to the condition where they located targets with the right hand and matched the located target's position with the left hand.

When the children with HECP were required to use the left hand (right hemisphere mediation) to match the located target, their error scores under the visual, as compared to the proprioceptive condition, were 20 and 36 mm, respectively. However, when using the right hand (left hemisphere mediation) to match the located target, their error scores under the visual, as compared to the proprioceptive condition, were 22 and 25 mm, respectively. These findings strongly suggest that the HECP children have input/planning problems when they are made dependent upon proprioceptive information picked up via the right hand (Sigmundsson, Whiting, & Ingvaldsen, 1999).

One of the limitations of the "manual matching task" is that ipsilateral matching without vision is not possible making it difficult to pinpoint more precisely the nature of the problem and to be able to speculate about the cortical projection areas which may mediate in the transfer of information. Is it a left hemisphere input problem, an asymmetrical interhemispheric transfer problem, or a deficit in processing information within the right hemisphere? This question led to the development of a new version of the task using toe-hand rather than hand-hand matching.

HEMI Task: Toe-Hand Matching

This task, in principle, provides the possibility to distinguish between intra- and interhemispheric competence in "on-line" target location matching. Using the foot rather than the hand to locate targets allows the possibility of examining performance when the information processing is within a hemisphere as well as between hemispheres. This possibility is not afforded when the hand is used for location and the other hand for matching (Sigmundsson et al., 1999). Such a procedure, it was thought, might provide a window into information processing in the brain. The findings from a study (Sigmundsson et al., 1999) carried out on a different group of 7-year-old children with HECP (right hand preferent) showed that they manifest inferior performance to the control children in three of the four conditions where the right hemisphere was involved and/or information had to be transported across the corpus callosum (Table 5.1).

Table 5.1 Overview of Studies on Inter- and Intramodal Matching by 7- and 8-Year-Old Children Diagnosed As Having Hand-Eye Coordination Problems (HECP) and a Control Group of Children

Study	Input	Output	P*	Possible Explanations of Differences
Sigmundsson et al., 1997a,b	Vision Vision	Right hand Left hand	s (mean AE) s (mean AE)	Visual-perceptual and/or visual-motor deficits
Sigmundsson et al., 1997a,b	Vision/right hand	Left hand	s (mean AE)	Visual-perceptual and/or visual-motor deficits, problem which modality to rely on
Sigmundsson et al., 1997a,b	Vision/left hand	Right hand	ns	
Sigmundsson et al., 1997a,b Sigmundsson, 1999 Sigmundsson et al., 1999	Right hand Right hand Right foot	Left hand Vision/left hand Left hand	s (mean AE) s (mean AE) s (mean AE)	Right hemisphere insufficiency with or without dysfunctional corpus callosum
Sigmundsson et al., 1997a,b Sigmundsson, 1999	Left hand Left hand	Right hand Vision/right hand	ns ns	—
Sigmundsson et al., 1999	Left foot	Right hand	s (mean VE)	Right hemisphere insufficiency with or without dysfunctional corpus callosum
Sigmundsson et al., 1999	Left foot	Left hand	s (mean VE)	Right hemisphere insufficiency
Sigmundsson et al., 1999	Right foot	Right hand	ns	—

*Significant (s) differences between the HECP** and the control group of children on the mean absolute error (AE) score and mean variable error (VE) score (within subject variability).

**In order to ensure that the findings were not the consequence of a particular selection of subjects, two different samples of HECP and controls were selected.

ns, not significant.

These findings could be accounted for by right hemispheric insufficiency (lesion/disconnection; Faglioni & Basso, 1985; Geschwind, 1975; Heilman & Rothi, 1993) with or without a dysfunctional corpus callosum that, in turn, might be attributable to slow maturation (Galin, Diamond, & Herron, 1977; Kalat, 1995; O'Leary, 1980; Quinn & Geffen, 1986; Trevarthen, 1974; Yakolev & Lecours, 1967) or an interruption of transcallosal interhemispheric communication—the so-called "callosal concept" of Bogen (1993). The findings from another experiment (Sigmundsson, 1999) in which the real-life skills of "threading nuts onto a bolt" and "threading beads" were the paradigm tasks support these interpretations. These tasks form a part of the well-known Movement ABC test battery (Henderson & Sugden, 1992).

Visual-Motor Task

Threading Beads Task

Threading beads is a bimanual task (the hands coordinate in performing separate aspects of the same task) that demands interhemispheric transfer of information for its successful performance, that is, continuous use of feed-forward as well as feed-back information about component movements (Jeeves, 1990; Kalat, 1995). The results, significant differences between the HECP and control group, provide further support for a dysfunctional corpus callosum. The results obtained in this task could, however, have been influenced by right hemisphere insufficiency (for a review, see Banich, 1995).

Threading Nuts on Bolt

This task can be useful in the discussion of the concept of hemispheric competence. In the ABC test battery, children are required to hold the bolt with their non-preferred hand and provide the action with their preferred hand. Sigmundsson (1999) developed this task further, with the children being tested with both left and right hand as the active member (screwing nuts on), a procedure not previously adopted in this kind of testing. The finding of significant differences on this task between the HECP and the control groups (ages 8 years) when the left hand was used for screwing the nuts on supports the proposition that right-hand preferent children with HECP have, mainly, a left hand (right hemispheric) competence problem (Sigmundsson, 1999). It has to be remembered that the "threading nuts on bolt" task, in the manner prescribed, is a predominantly distal task and, dependent upon which hand is being used for the action, controlled by the contralateral hemisphere (Jeannerod, 1988; Shafer, 1993).

Asymmetry in performance was shown between the hands in the HECP group of children when the left hand was required to provide the action and the right hand the postural control (Sigmundsson, 1999) but not in children with no apparent hand-eye coordination problems. These findings, it might be speculated, suggest that insufficiency within the right hemisphere with or without a dysfunctional corpus callosum could be one possible factor contributing to the problems that children with motor impairment encounter in the real world—for example, when children are required to carry out tasks demanding a high level of coordination, such as needlework, dressing, and doing up buttons and shoelaces (for a review, see Smyth, 1992), and in almost every task when temporal constraints are imposed.

Analyses using lateralization-dependent variables showed there to be marked differences between the performance of the two hands in the HECP groups only, in favor of the right hand (preferred hand). This lateralization effect has only received minimal attention by research workers in this field, one of the exceptions being that of Armitage and Larkin (1993), who showed a higher prevalence of crossed dominance for children with motor impairment. Thus, the results of earlier studies in which scores derived from only the preferred hand or a combination of both hands were used (Bairstow & Laszlo, 1981; Henderson et al., 1992; Henderson, Barnett, & Henderson, 1994; Hulme, Biggerstaff et al., 1982; Hulme, Smart et al., 1982, Hulme et al., 1984; Laszlo & Bairstow, 1985; Lord & Hulme, 1987; Murphy & Gliner, 1988; Smyth, 1991, 1994; Williams, Woollacott, & Ivry, 1992) might, on the basis of the findings reported here, need to be qualified.

NATURE VERSUS NURTURE

The findings from this series of studies, it is suggested, could be behavioral manifestations of a putative neurological abnormality. The question then arises about causation. The etiology of motor impairment has, generally, been couched in terms of nature versus nurture: that is, pre- or perinatal brain damage, versus limitations in postnatal experience. Dare and Gordon (1970) pointed out that children with motor impairment are often classified as having minimal cerebral dysfunction or MBD. That view is supported by Gubbay (1975), who argued that a continuum of neurological damage underlies motor impairment and that there is some overlap between cerebral palsy and clumsiness. In the studies reported, the children with HECP have particular problems in using the left hand (nonpreferred hand) in both the sensory integration task and visual motor task (threading nuts onto a bolt), so the default argument (minimal brain damage) considered by Dare and Gordon (1970) and Gubbay (1975) may need to be taken up once again.

Lack of experience may also be a reason why the functioning of these children might be deficient (Bairstow & Laszlo, 1989; Henderson, 1992). If, for example, the children with HECP use their left hand only minimally, one of the consequences might be that the right hemisphere will not develop in the same way as the left hemisphere (for an overview, see Bogen, 1990). What is cause and effect here is difficult to determine; it is likely a vicious circle. Because of inherent processing difficulties in the hemisphere controlling the left hand, use of the hand is avoided where possible. This, in turn, may further delay or limit the development of intercallosal communication (Jeeves, 1990; Kalat, 1995; Preilowski, 1972, 1990).

SUMMARY AND CONCLUSIONS

While many questions about the motor impairment syndrome still remain to be answered, the findings from the research reported here, as well as the methodological implications discussed, have implications for the next step forward in this line of research.

The kind of behavioral studies carried out by Sigmundsson and co-workers which gave rise to the neurobehavioral models of inter- and intrasensory functioning presented here might, for example, be used to formulate hypotheses about motor-impaired children (e.g., right hemisphere insufficiency, dysfunctional corpus callosum) that can be explored further in positron emission tomography (PET) scan studies. The qualification, however, would have to be made that, even if parallelism were to be shown between behavioral and neurological events, this would only be one step towards providing the kind of evidence in which the field is ultimately interested. That a start has been made is evident from the recent studies of Njiokiktjien, de Sonneville, and Vaal (1994) in the context of learning disabilities and Paulesu et al. (1996) in the context of dyslexia. Paulesu et al. pose the question, "Is developmental dyslexia a disconnection syndrome?" PET scanning techniques were used to examine the disconnection hypothesis that they had postulated in relation to this syndrome.

In the context of motor impairment, on which this chapter has focused, an obvious next step forward will be to attempt to validate (using neuromodeling and fMRI techniques) the neurobehavioral models put forward here. There is every indication from the existing PET and fMRI literature that this support will be positive (Mima et al., 1999). Of course, even if the model should be validated in this way, it still begs the question as to why this information processing deficiency should have arisen in the first place. Questions of this nature are likely to resurrect old controversies about MBD and minimal brain dysfunction that were the cornerstone of many of the earlier medical studies in this area.

PART
III

Assessment

CHAPTER
6

Issues in Identification and Assessment of Developmental Coordination Disorder

Dawne Larkin and Sharon A. Cermak

Children with developmental coordination disorder (DCD) have difficulties with motor performance and motor learning. However, the multiple factors that contribute to the motor difficulties are still debated. The clearest marker of the difficulties with our assessment tools is the variability in the reported incidence of DCD. Depending on the assessment procedure and the background and experience of the assessor, the incidence can range from 3% to 22% (Gubbay, 1975; Kadesjo & Gillberg, 1999; Keogh, Sugden, Reynard, & Calkins, 1979; Mæland, 1992; Revie & Larkin, 1993). Current assessment tools provide us with relatively coarse-grained assessments for the identification of DCD, and the links between formal assessments and intervention are limited. The lack of precision in assessments can be a source of frustration for the practitioner. In turn, this contributes to limited use of reliable assessment tools for the identification of children with DCD and associated problems with the evaluation of intervention. In this chapter, we discuss some of the issues that professionals and researchers need to address in order to increase the validity of DCD assessment and evaluation. We explore historical influences that underscore some of the limitations of current tests. We discuss difficulties with the construct of DCD that constrain the development of better assessments and we investigate the influence of different theoretical frameworks on task selection and classification. We look at how the purpose of the assessment, initial screening, identification, diagnosis for intervention, and evaluation of intervention influences the tasks selected. Measurement issues particularly relevant to DCD are addressed. We also discuss future directions for development of assessment procedures that are context and culturally sensitive.

HISTORICAL INFLUENCES ON ASSESSMENT

The history of assessment in the area of mild motor impairment, dyspraxia, and clumsiness has provided a wide variety of instruments based on different definitions of the construct, with different purposes, as well as measurements with varying levels of sensitivity. Assumptions about motor ability, as well as deficit models of motor impairment, minimal brain damage, and perceptual-motor dysfunction have contributed to the development of a component approach to the assessment of motor proficiency. These components vary and overlap according to the level of analysis and/or the theoretical framework. At a behavioral level of description, the components include fine motor tests, gross motor tests, static and dynamic balance, and locomotion. At other levels of description, the components assessed include motor planning or motor execution or ideational and ideomotor dyspraxia. Exploring historical influences on test development can help us understand some of the current problems with testing. More importantly, our understanding of these influences can inform future development of methods for the identification and evaluation of children with DCD. How should we proceed? How useful are these approaches? Should we discard some and focus on the development of others?

Motor Ability

Two very early tests of motor performance (Brace, 1927; Ozeretzky, 1923, cited by Kemal, 1928) were precursors to tests that are still used to identify children with movement difficulties (Bruininks, 1978; Henderson & Sugden, 1992; Stott, Moyes, & Henderson, 1972; Stott, Moyes, & Henderson, 1984). These tests emerged at a time when a general construct of motor ability, somewhat paralleling a general construct of intelligence, was fashionable. The construct of motor ability, which is still contentious, has included overlapping classification systems. For example, Oseretsky in his 1923 test of motor proficiency measured the components of static coordination, dynamic manual coordination, general dynamic coordination, motor speed, simultaneous voluntary movements, and synkinesia (Lassner, 1948; Sloan, 1955). Brace (1927) in his test classified components of motor ability as agility, balance, control, flexibility, and strength, as well as more complex tasks measuring combinations of these components. Attempts to support these classifications have met with limited success. For example Vandenburg's (1964) study of the Oseretsky categories provided little support with more tasks loading off the predicted factors.

Scoring of these early tests was similar to some of the tests currently in use; the overall test score was a composite from all the test items. The Oseretsky (Lassner, 1948; Sloan, 1955) was scored on the basis of motor age with a score more than 1 year below expected motor age interpreted as a motor deficiency, with severity increasing as the discrepancy between chronological age and motor age increased.

Using the Brace test, a performer's motor ability could be ranked as excellent, above average, average, below average, or poor.

The construct of motor ability has had one of the strongest influences on test development. Brace (1927) in discussing the difficulty of defining the construct suggested use of three criteria to help judge motor ability:

1. Ease and proficiency in learning new coordinations
2. Proficiency in a wide variety of motor activities
3. Performing activities with easy and graceful form (p. 13)

A rating of poor motor ability, which Brace used to describe the lowest 10%, would adequately describe the motor performance of a child with DCD: difficulty and incompetence learning new coordinations; inefficiency in a variety of motor activities; performing activities with difficulty and labored form. Although there is still debate about the existence of motor ability, many current measurement tools reflect this general construct, using terms such as the Test of Motor Proficiency (Bruininks, 1978), and composite scores such as "a neuromuscular development index" (McCarron, 1982) and a "total motor impairment score" (Henderson & Sugden, 1992). There remain considerable difficulties with the construct of motor ability, the linking of different or overlapping components, and the selection of test items to represent these components. Nevertheless, the results of tests and the success of research with children identified with DCD or movement impairment lend some validity to the construct (Tan, Parker, & Larkin, 2001). More systematic research is needed to explore the usefulness of this construct with a view to future clarification of components that are clearly linked to suitable test items.

Perceptual Motor Influences

The perceptual motor framework continues to influence testing and intervention strategies. Tests based on this framework focused on perceptual-motor behavior rather than skills, but test components and test items overlapped with test items based on motor ability or neurological deficit frameworks. For example, the Purdue Perceptual-Motor Survey (Roach & Kephart, 1966) included activities to evaluate balance, identification of body parts, imitation of movements, and ocular motor pursuits. Other research-practitioners such as Ayres (1965, 1989) and Cratty (1969) included similar tests in their efforts to identify and understand perceptual-motor dysfunction. The perceptual motor assessments were generally linked with intervention of the processes considered to require remediation. While there was linking between construct, test items, and intervention, the link from perceptual motor processes to activities of daily living, sport, and leisure was relatively indirect. This issue has plagued theoretical constructs in the motor domain. The relationship between perceptual motor constructs and specific task performance is yet to be resolved. Other attempts have been made to link assessments of visual, tactile, vestibular, and kinesthetic processes (Ayres, 1965, 1989; Laszlo & Bairstow, 1985a, 1985b) to perceptual-motor dysfunction or clumsiness. A limitation of the model underlying the perceptual-motor framework is that it is based on a relatively simple unidirectional input-output model influenced by the information processing framework. Difficulties with this model arise from the complexity of multidirectional interactions between action and perception. Nevertheless, process-based assessments for identifying perceptual motor dysfunction continue to influence the development of assessment procedures for DCD and might be useful in the identification of subtypes (Hoare, 1994).

Neurobehavioral Influences

The assessment of motor difficulties in the neurobehavioral domain has been closely linked with the belief that the motor deficit was caused by minor brain damage or dysfunction. Two approaches to assessment, the pediatric neurological assessment and neuropsychological assessment, are driven by a focus on brain dysfunction. Touwen and Prechtl (1970) developed a neurological examination, designed to identify children with minor nervous dysfunction, later referred to as "minor neurological dysfunction" (Touwen, 1979). The items, explicitly targeted toward identification of motor functions, included "posture, spontaneous movement, resistance against passive movements, muscle power, reflexes and locomotion" (p. 8). Touwen and Prechtl (1970) distinguished the following components (aspects) of coordination: "the maintenance of balance, the ability to anticipate shifts in the center of gravity before making voluntary movements, the coordination of rapid rhythmical movements and of fine manipulations, and complex skilled motor performances" (p. 88). Tests for coordination and associated movements include mouth-opening finger spreading; diadokinesis; finger-nose test; finger-touching test; finger opposition test; and standing with eyes closed (Touwen & Prechtl, 1970). This type of testing has been used for identification and neurological evaluation of children with coordination disorder and related symptoms such as neurological soft signs. Gubbay (1975) used a different categorization in the development of his test specifically designed to identify clumsiness. Initially, items were selected to represent facial and lingual praxis, manual praxis, and trunk and leg praxis and further refined in terms of their success in identifying clumsiness.

The overlap in items across levels of testing provides evidence of the difficulties associated with the constructs that drive our assessments. Touwen (1979) also recognized other limitations of the neurological approach. He emphasized the difficulty of assuming a direct relationship between brain dysfunction and behavior, and the difficulty of distinguishing between impaired coordination and a retardation of coordination capabilities (Touwen & Prechtl, 1970, p. 88).

Functional Assessments

Although functional assessment has different nuances for different professionals, our definition is broad and includes motor skills that are part of everyday living, ranging from home to school, from the bathroom to the playground. Some of the earliest qualitative tests of motor development were constructed around the theme of motor skills that children do. These tests could be considered as precursors to the current ecological approach. For example, Gutteridge's (1939) Rating Scale to estimate motor skill focused on the process of motor skill development with the four main categories encompassing "no attempt made," "habit in process of formation," "basic habit achieved," and "skillful execution with variations in use." Within each category there were more specific categorizations. For instance, in the category "habit in process of formation," there were the following subcategories:

a. Attempts skill, seeking help or support
b. Tries when not helped or supported but is inept
c. Still using unnecessary movements
d. Practicing basic movements—no obvious effort directed to refining
e. In the process of refining movements

This assessment procedure was designed so that it could generalize to any motor skill, for example, catching a ball or riding a bike, or extended to manipulative skills such as writing or teeth brushing. This rating procedure was among the earliest efforts to directly link assessment and intervention.

Over the last 25 years, there has been a shift toward viewing motor development from a systems perspective where multilevel coactive interactions contribute to skill development. Discontent, particularly among practitioners, has led to a call for a change in approaches to assessment toward a more ecological approach (Davis, 1984). Limited progress has been made in the motor domain (Easly, 1996; Puderbaugh & Fisher, 1992). The ecological approach raises difficulties as it depends on qualitative assessment of motor tasks in complex contexts. Reliable field-based assessments require highly trained observers with appropriate pre-planned observational strategies (Knudson & Morrison, 1997). Consequently, many professionals continue to assess and evaluate with tools that provide sufficient information to make an informed identification. Few of these tools provide good guidance for intervention and evaluation of change.

ISSUES

One of the basic issues that still limits the development of better assessments for the identification of DCD is our difficulty with constructs and the motor tasks that we use to operationalize those constructs. For example, threading beads represents manual praxis (Gubbay, 1975), upper-limb speed and dexterity (Bruininks, 1978), and manual dexterity (Henderson & Sugden, 1992). It is also clear from the diverse terminology used to describe children with a range of mild motor problems (Barnett & Henderson, 1998; Polatajko, 1999) that clarification of terminology is important. Equally important is the relationship between constructs and test items, and test items and intervention.

Defining the Construct as a Basis for Assessment

Informative assessment of DCD is dependent on a well articulated understanding of the construct. What do we mean by developmental coordination disorder? What is motor coordination? Bernstein (1967) suggested that, "The co-ordination of a movement is the process of mastering redundant degrees of freedom of the moving organ, in other words its conversion to a controllable system" (p. 127). Observing at the movement level, we see many children with DCD who over constrain the degrees of freedom during the acquisition of a motor skill. Although this is considered an appropriate strategy during the early stages of skill development, many children with DCD do not seem to move beyond this point to develop more efficient and flexible strategies. As a consequence the motor skill is automated at a very inefficient level. We see other children with DCD who do not constrain the degrees of freedom in the early stages of learning. These children have very variable performances from trial to trial with little progress toward efficient skill development. Some of these children can articulate their movement plan but cannot implement it. With some of these children, the task is intermittently performed in a relatively coordinated or well-timed manner. If DCD represents a construct that we plan to use as a basis for assessment, then we have to establish a deeper understanding of coordination and how it relates to test items that we propose as a basis for assessment and the evaluation of performance changes.

When we talk about coordination, we assume a level of competence manifest by fluid and efficient performance of a motor task. There is appropriate application of forces resulting in topological and temporal contiguities in action. The motor task is successfully performed, and although the construct of coordination is difficult to define verbally, it is clearly observable at the behavioral level. Whether we view coordination as an emergent property of the multiple subsystems involved in the production of a motor task, or we take a more hierarchical view and see it as the manifestation of a motor plan, will alter how we interpret coordination and consequently how it should be assessed.

We need to clarify the subsystems that contribute to coordination of different task groupings. A further difficulty arises from the changing contributions of sensory and perceptual subsystems to the development of coordination and the production of a coordinated motor task. The contribution of each subsystem can vary according to the task and the point of learning. Learning to type provides a clear example of this shift, a task that initially relies heavily on vision for the development of spatial relationships, and changes to a more feedforward mode involving other subsystems as skill is acquired. How does DCD affect the dynamic reciprocal interaction between motor and perceptual subsystems involved with coordination? In order to address the complexity of motor coordination and the varying subsystems that contribute to the emergence or disturbance of coordinated movement, we must pose workable models of the development of motor coordination that link across levels of analysis.

Current assessments are not only limited by our understanding of coordination, but also by the meanings that we attach to the term "developmental." The developmental aspect can have many implications. Although DCD is identified during childhood and can continue to persist into adulthood, there appear to be no clear indications of the meaning attributed to developmental. In this chapter, we take the position that development implies not simply that the coordination disorder occurs during the childhood years, but it can continue to manifest at different stages of the life span contingent on the motor coordination needs at that time. The multiple influences during development can ameliorate or exacerbate the difficulties with coordination so we propose that developmental should be viewed broadly so that biological, behavioral, and social contributions are considered across the life span. Assessment and intervention might lead to more positive outcomes by influencing the developmental pathway at any level.

Given our emerging understanding of DCD, approaches to assessment will continue to develop and change. The interpretation of development as a life span issue dictates that we address the issue of assessment from infancy through adulthood. It is important that we remain open to change. Currently, many frameworks (functional, motor development, neurobehavioral) are used by different groups to guide assessment of DCD. Approaching assessment from a client-centered contextual perspective would result in assessments configured differently for different groups, children, adolescents, and adults, based on their cultural and movement needs and experiences.

Task Classification Issues

Classification of tasks has a strong influence on testing and intervention. Here we will deal with issues that need to be addressed when selecting and interpreting tests. What classification system are we using? Why are we using it? How does it relate to our overall purpose for assessment? Four levels of analysis are addressed here to demonstrate the variety in the classification of test components that approximate the general construct of coordination. These classifications include tasks considered representative of neurodevelopmental function, tasks grouped as fine and gross motor by the underlying neuromuscular contribution, tasks grouped on the basis of similarity of action, and tasks classified on the basis of action and their interaction with the environment.

Neurobehavioral Classifications

How successful are the neurobehavioral assessments for identification, and what do they contribute to specific diagnosis for intervention and future evaluation of intervention? Neurodevelopmental tests involving movement have been categorized on the basis of normal motor development expectations (e.g., hopping, finger touching; (Denckla, 1974) and observation of movements and motor activities that manifest motor dysfunction (choreiform movements, diadokinesia). Terms such as "posture," "spontaneous motility," "involuntary movements," "associated movement," "muscle power," "resistance against passive movements," "range of passive movements" and "reflexes" are used in a classificatory sense. Nichols and Chen (1981) identified 10 soft neurological symptoms: poor coordination (abnormalities on test of finger to nose, heel to knee, finger pursuit, rapid individual finger movements, or rapid alternating movements), abnormal gait (awkwardness when walking, running, walking on toes or heels, or hopping), impaired position sense, nystagmus, strabismus, astereognosis, abnormal reflexes, mirror movements, other abnormal movements, and abnormal tactile finger recognition.

Rassmussen, Gillberg, Waldenstrom, and Svenson (1983) organized their motor-related tests under the headings of muscular tone and reflexes, motor functions of the eye and face, gross motor coordination, fine motor, and visuomotor coordination. These tests are part of a tradition that grew at a time when hierarchical unidimensional approaches prevailed and pediatric neurologists were attempting to localize function. For DCD, these tests provide some guidance on neurodevelopmental levels and can be useful in terms of ruling out more serious neuromotor and neuromuscular disorders. Although the relationship between neurological soft signs and DCD is difficult to ascertain without more systematic research, research validating the COMPS (Wilson, Pollock, Kaplan, & Law, 1994) shows that children with DCD receive lower scores on these tests. Like the motor ability tests, they are signposts that intervention may be needed but provide limited information for intervention planning.

Fine and Gross Motor Tasks

There has been a tradition embedded into many motor tests and intervention protocols that DCD includes a problem with gross or fine motor coordination, or both. It is time for a reconsideration of this broad dichotomy so that DCD assessments provide more specific information and more direction for intervention. Although there were not definitive distinctions at the movement level between what constitutes a gross motor vs. a fine motor deficit, it is generally agreed that gross motor behaviors included activities such as running, hopping, throwing, and catching. Fine motor coordination included motor behaviors such as reaching, manipulation, discrete finger movements, eye-hand coordination (Case-Smith, 1994), and orofacial movements (Gubbay, 1975). Tasks from this classification are included in typical test batteries; for examples, see Table 6.1. Factor analysis of tasks considered representative of fine and gross motor skills fail to support a breakdown based on this broad classification system (Larkin & Rose, 1999; Tabatabainia, Ziviani, & Maas, 1995) and are in keeping with the extensive work done earlier by Fleishman and colleagues (Fleishman & Ellison, 1962; Hempel & Fleishman, 1955). For example, Bruininks (1978) reported that the factor analysis of the 46 items "gave some support to the grouping of items into the various subtests" (p. 30). Inspection of the analysis indicated that some items traditionally regarded as gross motor (e.g., running speed and agility, jumping up and clapping hands) loaded on the same factor as items traditionally regarded as fine motor activities (e.g., stringing beads and drawing vertical lines). In factor analysis of 32 gross and fine motor items, involving kinesthetically and visually loaded tasks, based on data from 80 children with coordination difficulties, nine factors emerged (Hoare, 1991). The fine motor factor included items involving object manipulation and transport. Copying shapes loaded on a separate factor as did finger opposition. One gross motor factor included bounce and catch, catch, throw, jump and run, while another gross motor or balance factor included hopping in place, walking a line, and balancing on one foot with eyes open and eyes closed. Again, there were indications that some gross motor items and some fine motor items loaded together but more specifically than implied by the very loose use of the terms found in some tests.

Since dynamic neurofunctional subsystems of the brain interact according to the specific nature of the task and the anatomical contributions, there is the possibility that a general dysfunction could arise effecting tasks predominantly dependent on

Table 6.1   Examples of Standardized Tests to Assess Aspects of Motor Performance

Test	Reference	Age (years)
Tests of motor proficiency		
Bruininks Oseretsky Test of Motor Proficiency	Bruininks, 1978	4.5–14.5
Movement Assessment Battery for Children (MABC)	Henderson & Sugden, 1992	4–12
Peabody Developmental Motor Skills–2	Folio & Fewell, 2000	Birth to 7
McCarron Assessment of Neuromuscular Development (MAND)	McCarron, 1982	$3\frac{1}{2}$–18
Test of Motor Proficiency	Gubbay, 1975	8–12
Test of Gross Motor Development (TGMD-2)	Ulrich, 2000	3–10.11
Fundamental Motor Skills Test	Victoria Education Department, 1996	5–12
Purdue Pegboard	Tiffin, 1960	4 to adult
Grooved Pegboard	Layfayette Instrument	4 to adult
Neurobehavioral tests		
Quick Neurological Screening Test–Revised	Mutti, Sterling, & Spaulding, 1993	5 to adult
Miller Assessment for Preschoolers	Miller, 1988	2.9–6.2
The Toddler and Infant Motor Evaluation (TIME)	Miller & Roid, 1992	Birth to $3\frac{1}{2}$
Clinical Observations of Motor and Postural Skills (COMPS)	Wilson, Pollock, Kaplan, & Law, 1994	5–9
Sensory Integration and Praxis Tests	Ayres, 1989	4–8.11
Visual-motor tests		
Bender Gestalt Test for Young Children	Koppitz, 1963	5–17
Developmental Test of Visual-Motor Integration, 4th ed.	Beery, 1997	2–17
Test of Visual Motor Skills–Revised	Gardner, 1995	3–13.11
Developmental Test of Visual Perception II	Hammill, Pearson, & Voress, 1993	4–10
Screening tests with a motor component		
First STEP (Screening Test for Evaluating Preschoolers)	Miller, 1993	2.9–6.2
Pediatric Examination at Three (PEET)	Blackman, Levine, & Markowitz, 1986	3
Pediatric Examination of Educational Readiness (PEER)	Levine & Schneider, 1982	4–6
Pediatric Early Elementary Examination 2 (PEEX 2)	Levine, 1996	7–9
Pediatric Examination of Educational Readiness at Middle Childhood 2 (PEERAMID 2)	Levine, 1996	9–15

manipulative or locomotor subsystems. The issue of deciding how we should classify tasks is ongoing, but finer grained classifications will provide us with more precise assessments (Case-Smith, 1994).

Locomotor and Object Control

In the physical education domain, tasks are classified by locomotion (e.g., running, hopping, and skipping) and object control (e.g., catching, throwing, and kicking). The later classification is demonstrated by the Test of Gross Motor Development (Ulrich, 2000). This qualitative test is based on specific tasks that are considered representative of either locomotion or object control. Each task is scored according to specific task components that are either present or absent.

Linking the Movement and the Environment

More extensive classification systems that emphasize the complexity of motor task and the environmental constraints have been developed (Gentile, 1987; Gentile, Higgins, Miller, & Rosen, 1975; Higgins, 1977). This taxonomy provides a means for task analysis within the environmental context and makes a useful start to moving the field to a multidimensional movement classification system. This classification system is currently used in the MABC parent/teacher questionnaire (Henderson & Sugden, 1992) and could provide a useful framework for classifying the heterogeneous movement difficulties manifest by children with DCD (Wright & Sugden, 1996).

Assessment for What?

Probably, the most important questions that the tester will start with are as follows: What is the purpose of the assessment? Is there a problem? How severe is the problem? What is the nature of the child's deficit? How modifiable is the child's performance? How will this assessment help the child? How will we use the assessment? Once these issues are addressed, the assessments selected are limited by our philosophical framework, our knowledge, and our ignorance. The practice of assessment of DCD is still strongly influenced by professional boundaries [e.g., medical vs. educational orientation vs. skill (ADL)]. What do we look for? What clientele do we assess? How do issues of funding influence our approach?

Screening and Identification

Tests for screening and initial identification of DCD or motor impairment include checklists (Henderson & Sugden, 1992; Keogh et al., 1979; van Dellen, 1986; Wilson, Dewey, & Campbell, 1998; Wilson, Kaplan, Crawford, Campbell, & Dewey, 2000) short gross motor tests (Johnston, Short, Crawford, Smyth, & Moller, 1987; Larkin & Revie, 1994) to longer batteries with a combination of perceptual motor items that include manipulative and whole body skills, and body awareness (Ayres, 1989).

Checklists

Checklists are designed to promote a simple and efficient means of identification of children at risk in the movement domain. They provide a means whereby the child can be assessed in context. However many classroom teachers may need further exposure to movement education to successfully use checklists for identification of DCD. Research studies with checklists have provided equivocal results. Henderson and Hall (1982) reported that classroom teachers who had received additional information successfully identified children with motor impairment. By contrast Keogh et al. (1979) reported a lack of agreement and difficulty with identification of kindergarten and first graders by teachers using checklists. Van Dellen (1986) initially used classroom teachers with a checklist to target children with suspected motor problems. Using the 20-item GMOS checklist, which included fine motor, gross motor, and general motor items, the teachers identified 111 from a sample of 1,443 primary school children. From this 111, 25 children were identified using the TOMI (Stott et al., 1984). There was a clear discrepancy in the numbers identified by the different procedures. Revie and Larkin (1993) reported a similar discrepancy where only 31 out of 75 children identified with movement problems using a classroom teacher checklist of movement behaviors were identified with the BMAT (Arnheim & Sinclair, 1979). The overall number of children identified with movement problems by teachers, 2.8%, was of further concern with this study. If a conservative population estimate of 6% is anticipated, then many children were missed using the checklist.

Studies with the MCC checklist (Sugden & Sugden, 1991), subsequently the MABC checklist, (Henderson & Sugden, 1992) also provide equivocal results. Wright, Sugden, Ng, and Tan (1994) reported retest reliabilities ranging from 0.33 to 0.86. The reliable identification of movement difficulties using any method requires individual observations over a number of tasks and that it is time consuming. Pless and colleagues (1999) raise another issue: performance variability in different contexts created difficulty when they assessed rater reliability in their study of 5- to 6-year-old children using the MABC checklist. Although checklists are an attempt to ease the burden of testing, unless teachers are specifically educated to observe movement better, the checklists cannot serve their purpose. Some of the foregoing issues need addressing before we can confidently use checklists as an identification procedure; one clear advantage of the checklist is that it serves an educative function in raising the awareness of teachers and parents to DCD.

Motor Tests

There are many screening tests to address difficulties in movement (AAHPERD, 1980; Burton & Miller, 1998; Henderson, 1987). A benefit of these tests is that they are inexpensive and have the potential to educate the public about motor difficulties. What we will address here are issues that arise with short screen tests used for preliminary identification of children who are struggling with their movement. These tests are simple and quick to administer and are intended to provide sufficient information about developmentally appropriate motor performance to indicate whether a more comprehensive test is required as a basis for intervention. What types of test items are appropriate in these short screens? Should we be using motor skills with contextual relevance, such as running and writing, or constructs such as balance and coordination with limited contextual and social relevance? Over the last 30 years, screening tests have focused on the 5–12-year age group with the intent that the movement problem should be identified in the early school years (Gubbay, 1975; Johnston et al., 1987; Larkin & Revie, 1994). Some of these screening tests are based on discriminant function analysis of manipulative and whole body activities. The items that best identified children with movement impairment were whole body activities, such as hopping and balancing, and some had relevance to the type of activities that children do in the playground (Johnston et al., 1987; Larkin & Revie, 1994). In other instances, a selection of tasks considered to cover fine and gross motor skills or a range of perceptual motor tasks were included. This approach may have face validity in terms of covering a range of tasks but may lack discriminative power.

A possible shortcoming of screening tests is that parents and teachers or others with a limited background in movement may administer them. This is particularly the case where qualitative judgements are required as it is well acknowledged that qualitative assessment of movement requires considerable training (Davis, 1984; Knudson & Morrison, 1997). It is important that good guidelines are provided to overcome the possibility that children with DCD may be overlooked.

Longer screens for use by movement professionals or trained nonprofessionals (for a review, see Burton & Miller, 1998) generally are adequate for identification of children with DCD. Most motor proficiency tests assume a construct of general motor ability. Although the preceding discussion of subtypes of DCD might suggest that there is no support for a general construct, this is still open to question (Hands, Sheridan, & Larkin, 1999). The motor proficiency tests are generally structured around manipulative and whole body tasks of varying complexity. For example, the widely used MABC includes skills under four categories: manipulation, ball handling, static balance, and dynamic balance. Another widely used test, the Bruininks-Oseretsky (Bruininks, 1978) has tests items organized into eight subtests or categories (running speed and agility, balance, bilateral coordination strength, upper-limb coordination, response speed, visual-motor control, upper-limb speed, and dexterity). Despite the focus on the individual performance during these types of test batteries and the somewhat arbitrary nature of the categories, they have proved useful for generations of teachers, therapists, and researchers for the initial identification of children with motor impairments. A weakness of these tests is that they provide a limited basis for intervention, particularly if the intervention is to take advantage of the child's development and context.

Assessment for Intervention and Change

Assessment of change following intervention has been plagued by a number of problems. The initial problem relates to what we believe we should change, a motor skill, handwriting, or an underlying process such as kinesthesis. The assumptions about a construct and the transfer of that construct to other tasks have created different problems (Case-Smith, 1994). How do treatment protocols affect our approach to assessment? Treatment categories make a difference. Recent reviews of remedial approaches used with DCD indicate a diversity of approaches (Miyahara, 1996; Sigmundsson, Pedersen, Whiting, & Ingvaldsen, 1998; Sugden & Chambers, 1998). Morris (1997) categorized treatment approaches to DCD as

1. Treatment of the motor deficit directly through drill or practice
2. Development of compensatory techniques or circumvention of a deficit
3. Correction/remediation of the hypothesized cause of the problem

When it comes to selecting the type of assessment to measure change, the assessment must clearly reflect the type of intervention, or risk failing to measure change when change is really occurring.

Assessment for motor skill intervention is developing along qualitative lines as well as quantitative assessments. Examples of motor skill tests that rely on qualitative assessment of motor skills include the TGMD (Ulrich, 2000) and an Australian fundamental motor skills test (Department of Education, Victoria, 1996). These tests include motor skills that children use in play and sport. The performance criteria assessed are considered to be important elements for the performance of that skill. For example, three performance criteria from the TGMD for the hop item include the following:

1. Nonsupport leg swings forward in pendular fashion to produce force
2. Foot of nonsupport leg remains behind the body
3. Arms flexed and swing forward to produce force (p. 21)

Normative values are provided indicating ages at which the criteria or components are generally achieved. In order to use this type of assessment well, it is important to have substantial training in movement observation. These types of assessments are particularly useful as precursors to task specific interventions. Children with DCD score poorly on these tests and are at serious risk of being socially isolated in the playground. A limitation of this type of assessment is the assumption that there is an optimal movement pattern for task performance.

Assessment of Subtypes

The issue of heterogeneity in the profiles of children with DCD is ignored in most assessment procedures currently in use. One approach for dealing with the heterogeneity is through the identification of subtypes of DCD. A number of researchers have identified subtypes using cluster analysis techniques (see Chapter 3). Additionally, subgroups of children have emerged from studies of postural control (Wann, Mon-Williams, & Rushton, 1998) and rhythmic coordination patterns (Volman & Geuze, 1998). By focusing at the level of motor behavior, hypothesized causal perturbations ranging from motor planning to sensory perceptual deficits, from timing to force control difficulties, can be explored as the basis for subtype differentiation. Despite the difficulties associated with the construct and identification of subtypes (see Chapter 3), we can view this as one direction to fine-tune our initial evaluation that might lead to better targeted intervention. For example if we identify that a child has difficulty with activities that involve visuomotor processes, then the focus of the intervention program can be directed toward remediation in that domain and also directed toward improving coordination through tasks that do not rely predominantly on visuomotor strategies. Identification of a subtype depends on increased understanding of DCD and has the potential to increase the specificity of motor interventions. However it is a difficult issue limited by the constraints of our knowledge and the theoretical frameworks we currently rely on. Already we have assessment tools that implicitly suggest subtypes of DCD. From a perceptual-motor framework, the assessment of kinesthetic sensitivity and awareness (Laszlo & Bairstow, 1985a, 1985b), although problematic (Hoare & Larkin, 1991), draws on the assumption that "dyskinesthesis" contributes to difficulties in the organization of movement. By contrast, there could be subtypes with deficits in the visuomotor domain, or in the planning or execution of movement. Difficulties in these different areas would contribute to different motor profiles for children with DCD (Pryde & Roy, 1999).

Assessment of subtypes also raises the possibility of counseling a child, adolescent, or adult with a specific motor impairment as to the type of physical activity that may be more suitable. For example, ball games in an open environment would be extremely difficult for a child with a visuomotor disorder, particularly if it involved dynamic vision. Swimming would be more appropriate given the identification of the subsystems that are contributing to the development of that coordinative structure and the repetitive nature of the movement.

It is clear from Chapters 3, 4, 6, 7, and 8 that there are many possible problems, matching the constructs that we have identified to date. What neural processes are involved in the development of coordination? How are these processes tuned by experience? Can we identify different developmental pathways within the DCD domain that provide a useful framework for assessment and intervention? Descriptions of DCD are still very loose and it is clear from attempts to find subtypes that researchers and practitioners are still struggling to refine the description of DCD, both for understanding, for better assessment, and for more finely tuned intervention.

MEASUREMENT ISSUES

Validity

Consistency of Identification

Research exploring the issue of consistency in identification of DCD or motor impairment shows that different tests vary in their agreement. For example, the MABC (Henderson & Sugden, 1992) and the Touwen test battery (Touwen, 1979) were both used in a study designed to identify timing difficulties in children with DCD. The results indicated that the two tests were not significantly correlated (Volman & Geuze, 1998). What is more troubling is the lack of agreement between tests based on relatively similar frameworks. In a study of two tests influenced by the earlier test by Oseretsky, the TOMI-H and the BOT-SF, 9 of 41 children were identified with motor impairment based on testing with the TOMI-H, while 4 of 41 were identified with the BOT-SF (Riggen, Ulrich & Ozman, 1990). In a recent study carried out in Australia, 21 of 26 children identified with motor impairment using the MABC were identified using the MAND while only 9 of the 26 children with DCD were identified using the BOT-SF (Tan, Parker, & Larkin, 2001).

Cut Scores

Another measurement issue contributes to the difficulty of identification of DCD. Inferences made on the basis of cut scores are fraught with difficulties (Dwyer,

1996). Cut scores, the score that is arbitrarily designated as the point of motor impairment (e.g., the 5th, 10th, and 15th percentiles), are based on the judgment of the test constructor (for examples, see Bruininks, 1978; Henderson & Sugden, 1992; Wilson et al., 2000). As Dwyer (1996) points out, "Cut scores almost always impose external differentiations on a continuous distribution. Very few tests can distinguish reliably between examinees with adjacent scores, yet applying a cut score in effect forces such a distinction" (pp. 360–361). Dwyer also emphasizes the importance of the context within which a test is used. For example, a cut score at the 5th percentile may be appropriate in a medical context, whereas a cut score at the 20th percentile might be more appropriate in an educational context. Dwyer emphasizes, "there is not one true cut score" (1996, p. 362).

Another difficulty when we use the recommended cut score for a standardized test such as the MABC, or the MAND as the basis for identification of DCD, we view only a small aspect of a child's movement behavior devoid of context. It is for this reason that additional criteria are needed to clarify interpretation of the score from the motor battery. A rigid adherence to a cut score as a basis for identification of motor problems is naïve. According to the ICD-10 (WHO, 1996), DCD (they use the term "specific developmental disorders of motor function") "is best assessed on the basis of an individually administered, standardized test of fine and gross motor coordination" (p. 194). Wisely, they do not identify the "cut-off" level that should be used to make the diagnosis.

Reliability

Probably one of the most difficult issues centers on rater reliability. Although some of the tests based on outcome scores, such as counts in 30 sec and distance jumped, provide relatively reliable results, the ability of the examiner to observe movement is still an issue. It is clear that this is the case with tests that involve quantitative and particularly qualitative measures. Underestimation of the importance of training in the observation of movement (Knudson & Morrison, 1997) has contributed to difficulties with reliability. A recent study of rater reliability using the Bruininks-Oseretsky Test (Wilson, Kaplan, Crawford, & Dewey, 2000) clearly emphasizes the difficulties involved in obtaining reliable measures across raters despite specific training with the test. If we are to have reliable estimates of motor performance for the identification of DCD and evaluation of intervention, we need to address the issue of competence in movement observation.

Recent technology including kinematic analysis has enabled a more systematic study of the differences in quality of movement and movement control parameters between children with coordination difficulties and those without (Larkin & Parker, 1998). While these methods of assessment are useful for understanding the nature of the disorder and have tremendous implications for remediation, they are not easily accessible to the clinician and have therefore been used primarily for research. There are also some limitations to consider. The movement analysis is based on biomechanical models that assume certain rigid segments that we often do not see in the DCD child. This can limit the reliability and validity of the information obtained from the analysis. Additionally the methods are extremely time consuming and until they are further automated have a limited contribution to make on a day to day basis.

Cross-Cultural Issues

Most tests developed for assessment of motor development were developed within specific cultures. Difficulties can arise when these tests are used outside their cultural context (Zhu, 2000). For example, the MABC, which was recently standardized in the United States, does not perform in the same way with a Japanese sample (Miyahara et al., 1998). Another test developed in the United States, the MAND (McCarron, 1982), translates well to the Australian sample when the composite score is compared but normative values for individual items show some marked variation. For example, the Australian sample do particularly well on the standing broad jump and very poorly on grip strength by comparison with the American norms (Larkin & Rose, 1999). The current practice of using tests developed in other countries leads to difficulties in the interpretation of the test results (Miyahara et al., 1998; Rosblad & Gard, 1998; Smits-Engelsman, Henderson, & Michels, 1998). From a contextual perspective, the cross-cultural issue raises a number of problems. Can we have tests independent of culture that are valid? Of particular interest is influence of different cultures on the motor development pathway (for a review, see Cintas, 1995). Future test development should plan for tests that cross cultures, in other words, tests that are relatively independent of local influences. In parallel, the development of multilevel tests (for a model of this type, see the AMPS; Puderbaugh & Fisher, 1992) that incorporate culture-free and culture-dependent elements into the item construction could provide a basis for cross-cultural research.

Gender Issues

By the early 1930s, it was well documented that gender differences were apparent in the motor profiles of children (Kemal, 1928; Yarmolenko, 1933). Testing motor ability and motor capacity in the physical education domain had established different tests or different weightings for boys and girls (Carpenter, 1942; McCloy, 1934). In general, the data indicated that girls excel in activities that require the use of finer coordination, while boys excel in those which require grosser movements and/or strength. During the assessment of the motor system, Touwen (1979) cautioned about differences in ranges of movement based on gender and body type. For example, a combination of physiological and morphological differences contributes to gender differences in locomotor tasks such as running and jumping. At the present time, gender differences have had limited consideration in motor assessment of children with DCD, despite the understanding of gender differences in the movement domain (Thomas & French, 1985) and many tests do not have separate norms for girls and boys.

Sociocultural differences in developmental pathways that link to being a girl or a boy will contribute to understanding differences in identification. It may be that sociocultural expectations contributed in part to differences in the identification of boys and girls with motor difficulties by teachers using checklists (Revie & Larkin, 1993). Only girls with particularly poor movement competence were selected, while boys with a wide range of movement competence were identified as having movement difficulties. This mirrors our observations of referrals to movement programs. Perhaps differences in social demands for motor skill proficiency and the higher social value for males has contributed to the general disregard for gender-based norms in motor tests for children and contributed to a gender bias in the identification of children with DCD (Larkin & Rose, 1999).

SUMMARY AND CONCLUSIONS

The assessment of DCD has been influenced by a number of broad theoretical frameworks. Although these frameworks have provided direction for some assessments, intervention, and the consequent evaluation of change, these frameworks were and still are limited by available knowledge of motor development and dysfunction. Most frameworks are also limited by the level of analysis or dimension (neural, sensory or perceptual motor, cognitive, information processing, motor ability) that influences the theorizing. Just how these different approaches facilitate or limit assessment needs to be addressed so that we can emerge with a multidimensional framework that can encompass a variety of approaches and developmental pathways. In turn, this will ensure that we address the movement difficulties within the context of the client's needs and culture.

PART

IV

Mechanisms Underlying DCD:
Sensory and Motor Issues

CHAPTER

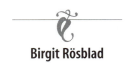

7

Visual Perception in Children with Developmental Coordination Disorder

Birgit Rösblad

Do the visual perceptual problems often reported in children with developmental coordination disorder (DCD) contribute to, or even cause, their movement problems? What is known about the nature of the visual-motor problems frequently reported? The aim of this chapter is to present findings from studies dealing with these questions and to discuss them in relation to the body of knowledge that exists on the role of visual information for movement control. Since the term "visual perception" will have different meanings for us depending on our educational background, I will start by defining how the term will be used in this chapter.

VISUAL PERCEPTION FOR APPREHENSION AND ACTION

Our sensory systems receive information from the environment through receptors at the periphery of the body and transmit this information to the central nervous system. Within the central nervous system, the information is being processed into meaningful information enabling us to apprehend the world and to act upon it. Traditionally, the term "perception" has been used for the process in which sensory information is transformed into conscious recognition of objects, events, individuals and scenes. This is for example how the term was used by the Gestalt psychologists at the beginning of this century. However, in the research tradition of Perception and Action, which has been heavily influenced by the work of James Gibson, the meaning of the term has been extended to include sensory information processed and utilized for the control of actions. One example of "perception for action" is how we can use visual information to catch moving objects. When a ball is thrown towards us, the image of the ball will expand on the retina as it approaches. The rate at which this expansion changes provides information for time to contact. The visual system is able to use this information for getting the hand to the right position at the right time to catch the object (Lee, 1980). Yet another example is that, when we reach out for an object, we perceive its properties and unconsciously preshape the hand in order to fit the object and the task we wish to perform (Jeannerod, 1984).

In this chapter, the term "perception" will be used to define the process in which we pick up and utilize sensory information to apprehend the world as well as to act upon it.

Perception and Action Are Coupled

Perception is necessary for action. Most of the motor activities we engage in involve interaction with the world. When we walk, reach out for a glass of water, catch a ball, or type on the computer keyboard, our acting body is interacting with the environment. Developing motor skills requires that there is development of the child's ability to perceive and utilize information about the outer world as well as of the properties of its own body. The functioning of the motor system is thus intimately linked to that of the sensory systems. Sensory and motor systems contribute collectively to the outcome, which explains why they are best conceptualized as a single functional unit or action system. "We must perceive in order to move, but we must also move in order to perceive" (Gibson, 1979, p. 223). Several sensory systems are important for movement control. Proprioceptors in the muscles, joints, skin, and vestibular apparatus will provide information about the length and tensions of muscles, joint angles, and the orientation of our body in space. The visual system enables us to recognize and detect the features of persons and objects, and informs us of their location in space in relation to our own body.

VISION PLAYS A CRITICAL ROLE IN MOVEMENT CONTROL

Vision plays a highly important role in the control of actions in humans. Unlike any other sensory system, it can provide us with detailed information about the world beyond our body surface. Seeing the environment gives us an opportunity to anticipate upcoming events and to plan our actions in an anticipatory fashion. One example of this is how we shape our hand prior to contact with an object. A blind person reaching for an object will have to touch the object first and then, guided by haptic information, shape the hand to fit the properties of the object. If we cannot foresee upcoming events and plan our movements ahead of time, those movements will of necessity be uncoordinated (von Hofsten, 1993).

Given the importance of the visual system for movement control, it is of interest to scrutinize the research carried out on the visual system in children with

DCD. In doing this, research on basic visual processing will be discussed first, after which higher order processing will be addressed.

PRIMARY PROCESSING OF VISUAL INFORMATION

The visual system is the most complex and highly developed of all our sensory systems. The auditory nerve contains about 30,000 fibers, but the optic nerve contains 1 million, which is more than all the dorsal root fibers entering the entire spinal cord (Mason & Kandel, 1991). Visual information is continually being processed on multiple levels and locations within the central nervous system, and as the information reaches higher levels the complexity of the processing increases.

A primary processing of visual information takes place in the retina. After this, information is sent via central visual pathways to three subcortical regions in the brain. Of these three subcortical regions, only one, the lateral geniculate nucleus, processes visual information that results in conscious visual perception. The other two process information involved in the control of pupillary reflexes, and information important for control of saccadic eye movements and control of eye and head movements. Information that has been processed in the lateral geniculate nucleus flows to the primary visual cortex in the occipital lobe. On this level in the nervous system, the cells are sensitive to stimuli of low complexity. Cells in the retina are sensitive to spots of light, while cells in the primary visual cortex respond to such stimuli as bars and lines (Mason & Kandel, 1991).

VISUAL STATUS AND THE CONTROL OF EYE MOVEMENTS IN CHILDREN WITH DCD

Basic Visual Processing in Children with DCD

A prerequisite for a functioning perception action system is that the involved sensory systems are intact. How then is the integrity of the low-level visual system in children with DCD? Lord and Hulme (1987) who tested near and far visual acuity and contrast sensitivity found no indications of impairments on this level of visual processing in "clumsy children."

These questions were investigated in greater depth by Mon-Williams and colleagues in a series of studies. In a first investigation, children diagnosed as having DCD were tested with a battery of ophthalmic tests, namely visual acuity, visual fields, refractive errors, strabismus, amblyopia, and binocular vision (Mon-Williams, Pascal, & Wann, 1994). No significant differences in visual status were found between the children with DCD and a tested control group.

The group additionally studied visually evoked potentials in children diagnosed as having DCD (Mon-Williams, Mackie, McCulloch, & Pascal, 1996). The aim of this study was to evaluate the integrity of the afferent visual pathways and to rule out the presence of neurological lesions affecting visual input. Does the visual information reach the primary visual cortex without disturbances? To assess this question, children were presented with visual stimuli consisting of black and white gratings with different bar widths. Recordings of evoked potentials in response to stimuli were made on the occipital scalp. No evidence of lesions in the afferent visual pathways was found.

Taken together these studies gave no indications of deficits in primary processing of visual information in children with DCD. It is, however, important to bear in mind that the sample sizes were small, and consequently generalizations to the entire population of "clumsy" children are unwarranted.

Coordination of Eye Movements in Children with DCD

To successfully stabilize the gaze on a target, we must be able track the target with smooth pursuit movements. Compensatory eye movements must also be initiated in response to head and body movements unrelated to the looking task. These abilities start to develop very early during infancy (von Hofsten & Rosander, 1996) and are functioning well by about 7 years (Ross, Radant, & Hommer, 1993).

The core symptom in the diagnosis of DCD is incoordination. It seems therefore reasonable to assume that the coordination of eye movements will be disturbed in ways similar to that of the other action systems. Evidence for a disturbed or delayed ability in children with DCD to coordinate the movements of the eyes with that of a moving target was also given in a study carried out by Langaas and colleagues (Langaas, Mon-Williams, Wann, Pascal, & Thompson, 1998). They recorded horizontal eye movements in children aged 5–7 years. The performance of a group of children diagnosed as having DCD and a group of prematurely born children was compared to that of a control group. Children with DCD as well as those prematurely born exhibited less proficient eye coordination compared to the control group, with the DCD children showing most pronounced problems. Both the DCD children and the prematurely born children were able to follow a target with pursuit eye movements but with a general problem of synchronizing the movements of the eyes with that of the moving target.

Higher Order Processing of Visual Information

What are the principles for higher order processing of visual information and where in the cortex does the processing take place? Ungerleider and Mishkin published an influential paper in 1982 in which they suggested that we have two cortical visual systems, a "what" and a "where" system. The "where" system was considered to be responsible for perception of an object's spatial location and located in the posterior parietal lobe. The "what" system was considered to be responsible for perception of objects' intrinsic qualities and located in the inferior temporal lobe. This functional and anatomical distinction between one visual system specialized for object vision and one for spatial vision has been widely accepted and has formed the framework for clinical reasoning. Damage in the posterior parietal cortex has been considered to cause disturbances in spatial perception, while damage in the inferior temporal lobe has been considered to disturb face and object recognition and discrimination.

Evidence for a "What" Versus a "How" System

This distinction between a "what" and a "where" system has been challenged by Goodale and Milner (1992). They have put forward an interesting proposal that is highly relevant for the topic of this chapter. They propose that the distinction between the two cortical visual systems should instead be between a "how" and a "what" system. According to their view, we have two visual streams originating in the primary visual cortex: the dorsal stream (the "how" system) projects to the posterior parietal cortex, while the ventral stream (the "what" system) projects to the inferior temporal lobe. Given their existence, what then are the functional roles of the two systems? Goodale and Milner propose that the "how" system is primarily concerned with perceptual control of guidance of actions while the "what" system is concerned with the recognition of objects, scenes and individuals. This is an important distinction between this model and the more traditional view of perceptual processing. In the model proposed by Goodale and Milner, both cortical streams process information about objects' intrinsic properties as well as their spatial locations, but the transformations they carry out reflect the different purposes for which they have evolved. The emphasis is now not on the input side of visual processing but on the output requirements (Figure 7.1).

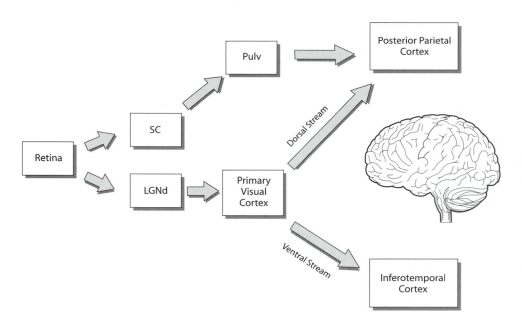

Figure 7.1 Schematic illustration of the flow of visual information through the dorsal and ventral streams. The dorsal stream carries visual information primarily used for the control of actions, whereas the ventral stream is concerned with object recognition. LGNd, lateral geniculate nucleus, pars dorsalis; Pulv, pulvinar; SC, Superior colliculus. (Adapted by permission from Goodale, Jakobson, & Servos, 1996.)

Most evidence for this dissociation is based on neurophysiological findings with monkeys and neurological findings with human adults. The proposed model has attracted much attention and inspired research within a variety of disciplines, among them infant development. Recent research on infant development adds support for the model and suggests that different factors contribute to the developmental changes within the two systems (Bertenthal, 1996).

Case Studies of Damage to the "What" Versus the "How" System

Milner and Goodale presented an extensive case study of patient D.F. who suffers from visual form agnosia after damage to the ventral stream. Her ability to recognize and differentiate between geometric forms is severely impaired and she has great difficulty in recognizing and copying line drawings. Despite this, she can reach out and grasp objects with accuracy, and she can catch objects thrown towards her. When instructed to make judgments on the orientation of slots, she erred markedly. When instead asked to insert her hand into the slots, she could correctly orient the hand. In this patient, there accordingly seems to be little correspondence between the ability to apprehend objects perceptually and the ability to guide actions perceptually. An example of a patient with damage to the dorsal stream is patient R.V. (Milner & Goodale, 1995). Despite good ability to recognize and distinguish objects, this patient shows an impaired capacity to shape the fingers in order to fit the properties of an object. Jeannerod, Decety, and Michel (1994) described a patient with similar problems who could not properly orient and scale the grip when reaching for an object but had no problems in recognizing and differentiating between objects. Evidence from brain-damaged patients also suggests that these two pathways are differentiated with respect to consciousness. One patient, D.F., appeared to have no conscious perception of the orientation or dimensions of objects, but in spite of this she could pick them up with precision (Milner & Goodale, 1995).

Incidence of Visual Perception Disorders in Children with DCD

How common is it that children with DCD have visual perceptual problems in addition to their motor problems? To answer this question, extensive epidemiological studies are needed. In a number of such studies, Gillberg and his colleagues investigated the incidence of clumsiness in childhood and its comorbidity with other neurodevelopmental disorders (e.g., Gillberg, Carlström, & Rasmusson, 1983; Gillberg & Rasmusson, 1982; Kadesjö & Gillberg, 1998). These studies clearly show that a high number of children who are clumsy suffer in addition from other disorders. There is, for example, a considerable overlap between ADHD and DCD, with about half of each diagnostic group also meeting the criteria for the other diagnosis (Kadesjö & Gillberg, 1998). Although the children in these studies were given visual perceptual tests such as the perceptual subtests from Wechsler Intelligence Scale for Children (WISC–III), findings regarding perceptual dysfunctions were not presented separately. Children were denoted as having motor-perceptual dysfunction if they showed marked (a) gross motor dysfunction *or* (b) fine motor dysfunction *or* (c) perceptual dysfunctions (Landgren, Pettersson, Kjellman, & Gillberg, 1996). No information was given on the degree to which perceptual and motor problems co-occurred. However, the fact that Gillberg introduced the diagnostic term "Dysfunction of Attention, Motor and Perception" (DAMP; Gillberg, Winnergard, & Gillberg, 1993) implies that perceptual and motor dysfunctions frequently did co-occur.

The information available on the occurrence of visual perceptual disorders in the population of children with DCD comes instead from a number of studies in which the performance on visual perceptual tasks was tested in groups of children with DCD and compared to that of age-matched peers (e.g., Dwyer & McKenzie, 1994; Henderson, Barnett, & Henderson, 1994; Hulme, Biggerstaff, Moran, & McKinlay, 1982; Hulme, Smart, & Moran, 1982; Hulme, Smart, Moran, & Raine, 1983; Hulme & McKinlay, 1984; Lord & Hulme, 1987, 1988; Mæland, 1992; Murray, Cermak, & O'Brien, 1990; Parush, Yochman, Cohen, & Gershon, 1998). The results from these studies vary to some degree. Although a majority of the studies indicate that visual perceptual problems are more common in children with DCD compared to typically developed children, this was only partly confirmed in some studies.

In a series of studies, Hulme and colleagues (1982, 1984, 1987, 1988) tested children with DCD on a battery of visual perceptual tasks such as discrimination of shape, area, slope, pattern, line length and size constancy. The groups of children with DCD were significantly less proficient than tested control groups of children on these measures of visual perception. That children with DCD perform poorly on tests of visual perceptual discrimination was also confirmed in a study by Henderson and colleagues (1994).

Some studies have shown that the performance components of WISC-R, which includes Block Design and Object Assembly items, differentiate between children with DCD and non-DCD children (e.g., Lord & Hulme, 1987; Barnett & Henderson, 1992), but this was not confirmed by Henderson and Hall (1982). Murray and colleagues (1990) tested children with DCD on the form and space subtests of the Sensory Integration and Praxis Test (SIPT) (Ayres, 1989). Results showed that the children with DCD performed significantly more poorly than a control group on four of the six SIPT subtests.

"Non motor visual perception" in children with DCD was tested with the Test of Visual Perceptual Skills by Parush and colleagues (1998), who also tested the children on the Developmental Test of Visual Motor Integration. Significant differences were found between the children with DCD and those without DCD on both tests.

Dwyer and McKenzie (1994) reported on a visual memory deficit in children with DCD. Children with and without DCD were to reproduce geometrical patterns immediately or after a 15-sec delay. While there was no difference between groups in the ability to reproduce the pattern immediately, the children with DCD were markedly less accurate after the time delay. In a subsequent study, Skorji and McKenzie (1997) tested the ability in children with DCD to reproduce a short sequence of simple movement directly after presentation and after a 15-sec time delay. Findings from this study were in agreement with those from Dwyer and McKenzie (1994) in that there were no differences between groups immediately after presentation, but children with DCD were significantly more affected by the time delay. Henderson et al. (1994), however, found the ability for graphic reproduction to be impaired in children with DCD, even when no time delay was introduced.

Considering that the sample sizes in these studies are relatively small and that children with DCD are a heterogeneous group, the difference in results between studies is not surprising. Accumulation of data from different studies can be one means of visualizing patterns otherwise obscured by high variability. This is also what Wilson and McKenzie (1998) did in a study aimed at identifying information-processing factors that characterize children with DCD. They conducted a meta-analysis in which a total of 50 studies were included. The results showed that children with DCD were inferior on almost all measures of information processing. The greatest deficits however were found in the area of visual-spatial processing. These deficits were found to be more pronounced for visual perceptual tasks that required a motor response of the child, but were significantly high also on visuo-perceptual tasks without motor response.

In conclusion, one can say that these studies strongly suggest that the DCD population performs poorly on visual perceptual tasks. There is, however, no knowledge available on the degree to which visual perceptual and motor disorders co-occur. Within the group of children with DCD there are probably visually competent individuals and not all children with visuo-perceptual disorders have coordination disorders.

On the Causality Between Visual Perceptual and Motor Disorders in Children with DCD

Do the visual perceptual problems often reported in children with DCD contribute to, or even cause, their movement problems? Given the fact that visual information plays a critical role in movement control and that disorders in visual perception commonly occur in children with DCD, this is a most relevant question. However, as discussed earlier in this chapter, there is evidence for a functional dissociation between a perceptual system for apprehension and a perceptual system for action (Goodale & Milner, 1992) and generalizations from one system to the other might be flawed.

Two lines of research emerge from the literature on visual information and movement control in children with DCD. One, which has been dominant, has focused on the relationship between performance on visual perceptual and motor tests. The perceptual tasks used in these studies are often traditional tests for visual perception, such as figure-ground tests, shape, and line discrimination, visual memory for shape and reproduction of geometrical patterns—tests that require the ability to recognize and distinguish between objects and geometrical patterns. These studies can be described as studies of perception for apprehension and its relationship with movement control.

In the other line of research, the ability to use perceptual information for movement planning and control is being tested, and movement outcome is often measured directly with various motion analysis systems. These studies can be described as studies of perception for action.

Perception for Apprehension and Its Relation with Movement Control in Children with DCD

Hulme and his colleagues carried out a series of studies in which they focused on the relationship between perceptual and motor ability in children with DCD (Hulme et al., 1982; Hulme, Smart, & Moran, 1982; Hulme et al., 1983; Lord & Hulme, 1987, 1988). In an early study (Hulme et al., 1982), the ability to match the lengths of lines within and between the modalities of vision and kinesthesis was studied in a group of children with motor impairment and compared to that of a control group. Results showed that the motor-impaired children performed less proficiently than the control group on all of these judgments. As a next step, the authors correlated the performance on a test of motor ability with the performance on the perceptual tasks. They found that only performance on the visual perceptual task correlated substantially with the performance on the motor ability test. This led the authors to conclude that "difficulties in the visual perception of distance and spatial relationships may be an important determinant of the clumsy child's poor motor co-ordination" (p. 468). In the next study, the same testing procedure was repeated but now in typically developed children aged 5 and 10 years (Hulme et al., 1983). As in the previous study, performance on the perceptual abilities was correlated with that on the motor test, but in this study, visual as well as kinesthetic judgments were substantially correlated with motor performance.

In a study in 1988, Lord and Hulme focused on drawing ability and its relationship with visual perception. Again, a group of motor-impaired children were tested on a visual discrimination test. Additionally, they performed a drawing task in which they were to copy the size and shape of a triangle, with and without visual feedback. The study confirmed earlier results that children with DCD perform poorly on visual discrimination tests. Drawing ability was less developed in the children with DCD compared to that of a control group of children, but both groups were equally affected by the withdrawal of vision. Again, the authors calculated correlations between performance on the perceptual and the motor tasks (in this case the copying task) and found correlations between performance only for the DCD group of children and only for the visual feedback copying task. This led the authors to the conclusions that "an adequate level of perceptual functioning is essential for adequate motor performance and beyond that level variability in motor performance is mediated by other factors" (p. 7).

The studies by Hulme and colleagues reviewed above are often cited and have inspired other researchers to investigate the causality between visual perceptual deficits and motor impairments. The conclusion drawn by the authors about a causal relationship between visual perceptual and motor disorders has however also been the target for criticism. Henderson et al. (1994) argue that one of the weaknesses of these studies is that they only tested an inconclusive dysfunction. Moreover, when attempting to replicate the findings by Lord and Hulme (1987, 1988), they failed to do so. Although they found the group of children with DCD to perform more poorly on visual perceptual discrimination tasks compared to a control group, these abilities were uncorrelated with motor ability even when restricted to the less proficient children. When aggregating across the studies by

Hulme and colleagues and their own, Henderson and colleagues found only 1 out of 10 correlations calculated to attain significance in each group. Considering that the claim made by Hulme and colleagues on causality between visual perceptual and motor deficits was based on the significant correlations obtained, it is clear that their claim must be questioned.

Subsequently, a number of other papers have been published in which performance on visual perceptual tests has been correlated with performance on motor tests (Mæland, 1992; Murray et al., 1990; O'Brien, Cermak, & Murray, 1988; Parush et al., 1998). Although a common finding in these studies is that children with DCD perform more poorly than matched control groups on tests of visual perception, the results regarding relationships between performance on visual perceptual tests and motor performance are inconclusive. In most of these studies, only a few of the tested correlations are substantial. Moreover, the result between studies varies when it comes to which of the tested perceptual abilities correlates significantly with motor performance.

PERCEPTION FOR ACTION IN CHILDREN WITH DCD
Visual Control of Goal-Directed Arm Movements in Children with DCD

A reaching movement can be divided into two functional components (Jeannerod, 1984). The first component is a transport phase, which brings the hand to the target. The second is a grasp phase, in which the hand is shaped in anticipation of contact with the object. For the transport phase of the movement, visual information on the position of the object is needed (the object's extrinsic properties). This information enables us to program the direction and extent of the movement. For the grasp phase, perception of the size and shape of the object is needed (the object's intrinsic properties). Thus, visual information is needed for planning and programming of the movement, and enables us to make corrections during the course of the movement. During development, children change from a probing strategy where they rely on feedback control to an anticipatory strategy (Forssberg, 1998). Accordingly, as the child becomes more skilled at controlling the movements of the arm and hands, the dependency on visual feedback during the course of the movement will decrease.

What do we know of the ability in children with DCD to use visual information for control of precise arm movements? Are they more dependent on visual feedback for movement control than typically developed children are?

Van der Meulen and colleagues (1991a, 1991b) tested the ability in children with DCD to make precise arm movements. In a first study, the task for the child was to reach to a target as fast and precisely as possible. In a second study, the ability to track a target that moved in an unpredictable way was assessed. In both studies, the children were tested in situations where they did or did not receive visual feedback of the moving arm. The results suggested that the less efficient movements performed by the children with DCD compared to those of a control group of children could be explained by a less developed ability for anticipatory control, and not by differences in the ability to use visual information for feedback control.

Another study, which addressed the question of whether children with DCD are relatively dependent on visual information for feedback control, was one by Rösblad and von Hofsten (1994). The task for the child was to pick beads from one cup and carry them to another cup. With the aid of a mirror arrangement and a curtain, visual information about the performing hand and the cups and beads was manipulated. The movements were monitored with an optoelectronic device. Results showed that both the children with DCD and the age-matched peers tested were similarly affected by the withdrawal of vision. However, in all conditions, the time taken for the children with DCD to move from one cup to the other was slower. That children with DCD exhibit a generally decreased movement speed is well in agreement with other studies (Forsström & von Hofsten, 1982; Henderson, Rose, & Henderson, 1992; van der Meulen et al., 1991a, 1991b). Why should children with DCD move consistently more slowly? One possibility is that anticipatory control strategies are less developed in children with DCD than in typically developed children and that they instead rely on feedback control. This is also in agreement with other studies pointing to the possibility that impaired capacity for anticipatory control is a limiting factor for children with motor impairments (Eliasson, 1995; Wann, 1986).

Catching Moving Objects

Anyone who has tested children with DCD knows that the task of catching a ball is something that is likely to give these children great problems. To reach for a moving object, the brain must process visual information about the object and its motion, as well as proprioceptive information about the current state of the body parts involved in the reach. A goal-directed plan must be constructed and the hand transported to the meeting point with the object. This requires that the visual, proprioceptive, and motor systems are well functioning and integrated. Moreover, the child must have acquired a necessary level of anticipatory or predictive control.

How can children with DCD utilize visual information for prediction of a ball's trajectory? To study this question, Lefebvre and Reid (1998) set up a task in which children watched a video of a person throwing a ball towards a target. The child was to predict the trajectory of the ball. Since the focus in this study was the ability to make predictions based on visual information, the viewing time of the ball flight was varied. The only motor response required of the child was to indicate if the ball would hit a target or go to the right or left. Children with DCD predicted more poorly at most viewing times, compared to a control group of children. One possible explanation for these results is that visual perceptual problems account for the poor predictive ability. However, it could also be accounted for by a more general problem with predictions that is not specific to the visual system. Yet another possibility is simply lack of experience with balls.

In the study by Lefebvre and Reid (1998), only the ability to predict the trajectory of a ball was investigated, not the child's ability to actually intercept and catch it. This was instead the focus of a study by Forsström and von Hofsten (1982), who investigated visually directed reaching in children who were clumsy and diagnosed as having MBD. The task was to catch a moving object that passed in front of the child. The movement parameters evaluated—speed, number of movement units, and length of the movement—revealed a less efficient movement performance in the children with DCD compared to a control group of typically developed children. When reaching for a moving object, a successful strategy is to reach for the meeting point with the object, and this was also the strategy adopted by both groups of children. The two groups mainly differed in that the children diagnosed as having MBD aimed their movements at a point further ahead of the target than the typically developed children did. This gave the children with MBD more time and compensated for their less efficient movements.

Influence of Visual Information on the Control of Stance

This chapter has mainly focused on the role of visual perceptual information for the control of arm and hand movements. Perceptual information is however also important for postural control, and three sensory systems contribute to upright stance: proprioception, vision, and vestibular information. Lishman and Lee (1973), who constructed a room with stable floor but with walls and ceilings that could move back and forth, investigated the role of visual information for stance. The motion in the visual field, induced by the swinging room, is perceived by the subjects as if they themselves are swaying and so they compensate with postural reactions. In a subsequent study, it was shown (Lee & Aronsson, 1974) that visual flow fields have a strong effect on postural control in young infants. Children who have just learned to stand will fall, stagger, or sway in the direction of the room to compensate for the perceived but nonexistent sway. Wann, Mon-Williams, and Rushton (1998) tested children with DCD in the "swinging room." They found that one subgroup of children with DCD had postural control problems and tended to use visual information in a similar way to nursery children. Yet another subgroup did not differ from age-matched controls in their response to the swinging room.

SUMMARY AND CONCLUSIONS

Results from a number of studies strongly suggest that visual perceptual and motor disorders co-occur in children. Tasks such as shape and size discrimination, reproduction of geometrical patterns, figure-ground discrimination, block design, and object assembly are among those reported to distinguish between children with DCD and non-DCD children. The degree to which visual perceptual and motor disorders overlap however remains unknown.

Perception and action are coupled. "We must perceive in order to move, but we must also move in order to perceive" as Gibson (1979, p. 223) put it. It is therefore a likely assumption that disorders in one system will affect the other. It has also been suggested that visual perceptual problems contribute to, or even cause, the motor problems in children with DCD. Studies aimed at testing this relationship have adopted traditional tests of visual perception, such as figure-ground tests, shape and size discrimination, visual memory for shape, reproduction of geometrical patterns or block design, or object assembly tasks. Results from these studies are to some extent inconclusive, and several studies have failed to find significant correlations between perceptual and motor abilities.

This failure to find substantial correlations between performance on traditional perceptual tests and motor performance could be explained by a proposed dissociation between two visual systems. Goodale and Milner (1992) suggest a distinction between two cortical visual systems. The dorsal stream (the "how" system) projects to the posterior parietal cortex, while the ventral stream (the "what" system) projects to the inferior temporal lobe. The "how" system is primarily concerned with perceptual control of guidance of actions, while the "what" system is concerned with the recognition of objects, scenes, and individuals. This dissociation between a perceptual system for apprehension and a perceptual system for action does not imply that these systems are completely independent. The message is however that it is difficult to generalise from one system to the other. That a child has problems when asked to discriminate between objects of various shapes or to differentiate between lines of different lengths does not necessarily imply that the child will have problems when acting upon these objects.

Tasks traditionally used to test visual perception are of interest in that they can provide us with information about the child's capacity for perceptual apprehension. These abilities are probably of great importance for school performance and everyday activities. However, if the interest is in the child's ability to use visual information for movement control, one might question the relevance of these tasks. So far only a few studies have focused on the ability of children with DCD to use visual perceptual information for the control of movements. Results from these studies do not indicate the use of visual information to be a main problem in movement control for children with DCD. Instead, the results indicate that one problem may be a lack of progression from a visual feedback probing strategy towards a more mature anticipatory control strategy. It is however important to point out that we still lack basic understanding of the motor problems in children with DCD. Moreover, the population of children with DCD is heterogeneous and we cannot expect to find one underlying cause of the movement problems exhibited by these children.

CHAPTER
8

Motor Control in Children with Developmental Coordination Disorder

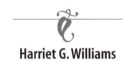

Harriet G. Williams

The study of motor control in children with DCD has involved a wide range of tasks. Some have focused on the sensory components that contribute to motor control and have examined, in particular, the use of visual and proprioceptive information. Others have focused on intersensory integration or cross-modal matching. A large number of studies have examined the motor aspects of control and have focused on temporal and timing aspects of control, and force generation/production; a few have examined potential underlying neuromuscular processes. Most studies suggest that children with DCD exhibit poorer performance on all of these tasks than do children without DCD. The review that follows discusses selected research on a variety of characteristics of motor control in children with DCD; this includes research on reaction time, movement time, timing control, unimanual and bimanual coordination, balance and postural control, and other related motor control issues.

REACTION TIME, MOVEMENT TIME, AND MOTOR CONTROL IN CHILDREN WITH DCD

Reaction Time

Reaction time provides important information about the speed and accuracy of sensory information processing, the translation of that processing into a plan of action, and the initiation of an overt response. Several studies have investigated reaction time in children with DCD and have indicated that children with DCD have significantly longer reaction times than do children without DCD. This is true for tasks involving the processing of both proprioceptive and visual information (Henderson, Rose, & Henderson, 1992; Smyth & Glencross, 1986). Smyth and Glencross (1986) used simple and two-choice reaction time key-press tasks to examine reaction time to simple visual and proprioceptive information in children with DCD. They reported that 5-year-old children diagnosed with DCD had significantly longer reaction times than did control children when they processed proprioceptive information. There was little or no difference between the two groups when they responded to a visual stimulus. Data on this issue, however, are far from clearcut.

Henderson et al. (1992) used a visual stimulus and studied reaction times of older children with DCD, aged 7.8–11.6 years. They found that older children with DCD also had significantly slower reaction times than age-matched controls. Children with DCD took an average of 367 msec to process a simple visual stimulus (a green arrow pointing toward a target) and then initiate a simple reaching response to depress a key. In contrast, reaction times of control children were, on average, 326 msec, a 41-msec difference. Thus, it appears that, at least in older children with DCD, there is some slowness in processing visual information that is not reported for younger children.

Williams, Huh, and Burke (1998) studied children with and without DCD and examined the time required to initiate unimanual and bimanual reaching movements toward end targets located at near and far distances. Some reaching movements were symmetrical; that is, the two hands moved to targets located at the same distance. Other movements were asymmetrical; that is, the two hands moved to targets located at different distances. There was little or no difference in the time required to initiate one- versus two-hand movements for children without DCD; children with DCD, however, took significantly longer to initiate bimanual than unimanual reaching movements. For both symmetrical and asymmetrical bimanual reaching movements, Williams et al. (1998) reported that children with DCD had significantly slower reaction times than control children (DCD symmetry = 315 msec; asymmetry = 312 msec; without DCD symmetry = 269 msec; asymmetry = 274 msec). If one views reaction time as an indirect indicator of the nature of the planning process involved in reaching movements, it would appear that planning two-hand movements is more problematic for children with DCD than for control children. Based on the foregoing observations, it seems there is a potential explanation for some of the differences between the two groups of children. For children with DCD, the two hands may be treated as independent, unrelated units, while for control children, the two hands may be treated as a single or coupled unit of movement.

Along with the slowness of reaction time, it is also frequently observed that children with DCD are much less consistent in the time taken to process information and plan a response (Henderson et al., 1992). With regard to consistency of reaction time in bimanual movements, Williams et al. (1998) indicated that children with and without DCD were equally consistent in the time taken to initiate symmetrical reaching movements. In contrast, children with DCD were significantly more variable than control children in the time taken to initiate movements toward asymmetrical end targets. Thus, under one circumstance, the reaction time of these children may be fairly rapid; on other occasions or under different conditions, it may be quite slow. Variability or inconsistency of function, whatever system may be involved, has often been associated with young children with immature systems or with individuals or systems that are weak or vulnerable (e.g., have some underlying dysfunction in one or more systems involved in task performance). What if anything does this mean in terms of motor control of children with DCD? Clearly, if processing information related to planning and initiating a behavioral response is slow, unstable, or both slow and unstable, then overt responses based on these processes will, by necessity, also be variable or inconsistent. Thus, the rather commonly observed variability and inconsistency of performances of children with DCD on a wide variety of reaction time and other movement tasks may have their origin, in part, in the slowness and inconsistency that characterizes underlying central nervous system processes involved in organizing the upcoming movement.

Coincidence Anticipation Timing

Response synchronization and interception tasks that involve moving stimuli may be particularly sensitive to movement planning problems as they rely on the ability to estimate accurately when to initiate a movement in response to external events. A simple keypress synchronization task was employed by Henderson et al. (1992) to examine coincident anticipation timing in children with and without DCD. Their data clearly indicated that all children tended to respond late to the moving target (mean time = 129 msec). Still, both the magnitude of the timing error and the variability of response initiation were greater in children with DCD than in control children. Overall, children with DCD were significantly less accurate and less consistent in timing responses to moving external stimuli. These authors also reported that slowing down the movement rate of the target had equally deleterious effects on both groups of children, and, therefore, suggested that cognitive processes involved in time estimation were not a major factor contributing to differences in the coincidence timing abilities of these children. It seems more likely that it is an inability to generate responses with consistent timing that differentiates these two groups of children.

Movement Time

Movement time is a measure of the speed of movement execution and can be viewed as an indirect indicator of the efficiency of motor system function. Movement time data, reported by Henderson et al. (1992), clearly indicate that children with DCD move more slowly in executing simple arm movements than do children without DCD. In fact, children in this study moved almost twice as slowly as control children; the mean movement time for children with DCD was 641 msec and that of control children 338 msec. When children moved their hands to a smaller end target, the difference in movement times nearly doubled. These data suggest that children with DCD are much more vulnerable to increased accuracy and/or control demands than are control children and thus are more likely to show deficits in performance under conditions which place added demands on speed and accuracy of movement responses. Henderson et al. (1992) also reported that children with DCD moved slowly and inconsistently even when accuracy was not a critical factor in carrying out reaching actions. These data indicate that precision of control and end point accuracy differentially affect responses of control children but have minimal effect on responses of children with DCD. One might speculate that this is due to some underlying inefficiency or immaturity of their motor control.

Huh, Williams, and Burke (1998) used a simple discrete reaching task to examine movement times of children with and without DCD (6–7 years and 9–10 years). Children were asked to perform simple unilateral reaching movements to either near or far targets; both movement time and underlying neuromuscular processes (electromyographic activity) were studied. As with other investigations, these authors found that discrete unilateral aiming responses were significantly slower and more variable in children with DCD. Importantly, the slowness of these discrete unilateral aiming movements in children with DCD were characterized by slower onset latencies of antagonist muscle activity and increased duration of agonist muscle activity. The interaction of these two neuromuscular parameters (longer duration of agonist burst and delayed activation of antagonist activity) determines to a large extent the speed of movement. Agonist activity generally provides the muscular force to move the hand/limb through space; activation of the braking action of the antagonist muscle is needed to stop the movement. Since antagonist muscle activity is delayed in children with DCD, agonist muscle activity continues for a longer period of time. As a result movement times are generally longer (slower). These underlying neuromuscular responses were also more variable in children with DCD; this of course may help to explain the more variable movement times in these children.

Several studies (Forsstrom & von Hofsten, 1982; Schellekens, Scholten, & Kalverboer, 1983) have reported that children with coordination difficulties tend to "require multiple steps," reminiscent of Parkinson's patients, when they have to generate fast movements. Therapists working with children in clinical settings often report that movements of children with DCD are "jerky" and "staccato," a description that suggests that their movements may indeed be carried out in a series of short, segmented steps. Short jerky movements could also be a factor contributing to the slowness and variability of movements often seen in children with DCD.

Huh et al. (1998) reported an interesting laterality effect in children with DCD. Movement times and underlying neuromuscular parameters of limb movements to both near and far targets were similar for right and left limbs of control children. In contrast for children with DCD, movement times of the right limb to a far target were slower than those for the left limb. In all instances, durations of agonist and antagonist muscle contractions were longer and the onset latency of antagonist muscle activity delayed in these slower right-limb movements. Although evidence for laterality effects in children with DCD is at best equivocal, left hemisphere dysfunction has been associated with deficiencies in selected temporal aspects of skilled unimanual movements (Geuze & Kalverboer, 1994). A potential left-hemisphere dysfunction in some children with DCD could manifest itself in the observed slower right hand movements involved in more complex aiming tasks (e.g., in reaching movements to distant targets).

TIMING CONTROL AND DCD

Rhythmic coordination or timing of movements is universally recognized as a common deficit in DCD. During development, children typically improve in a variety of aspects of timing or rhythmic actions and thus become more skilled at intercepting balls, skipping to a beat, tapping rhythms with one or both hands, and playing games that involve timing actions with moving objects on a computer screen. This improvement or change in timing ability during development is often not observed in children with DCD. What is the nature of the difference between these children and those who show the expected change or improvement in timing? What is the origin of these difficulties? What factors contribute to this difference? I will first summarize studies on unimanual coordination followed by studies that have focused on bimanual or two-hand coordination processes in children with and without DCD.

Unimanual Coordination

A common approach to the study of unimanual coordination and repetitive rhythmic control in children and adults is one that falls within an "information processing" paradigm. These studies typically use tapping tasks of various kinds to examine rhythmic control in children who are asked to tap under a variety of different conditions. The universal instruction to the child is to try to establish a given rate of tapping to an external stimulus (visual or auditory) and then to continue that rate of tapping when the external stimulus is no longer present. In general, data from studies that have looked at timing or rhythmic control from this perspective have consistently reported that children with DCD have great difficulty in consistently "tapping" or reproducing time intervals (e.g., they are much more variable than age-matched controls). Lord and Hulme (1988) examined performances of children with and without DCD on a task that required the synchronization of rhythmic limb movements with a periodic visual signal. The children with DCD were extremely poor at rhythmically tracking the visual signal and consequently spent significantly less time on target than did control children. Others have reported similar differences between children with and without DCD in tracking an unpredictable visual signal (Van der Meulen, Denier van der Gon, Gielen, Gooskens, & Willemse, 1991). Data from Van der Meulen et al. (1991) suggested that the tracking delay was significantly longer in children with DCD. These observations point to a deficiency in children with DCD in detecting a change in the visual environment and in initiating an appropriate corrective response. This, in a sense, may be viewed as a type of reaction time to a changing, unpredictable environment.

Other studies have used tapping tasks that involve a temporally spaced auditory tone. Typically, the child listens to the tone for a period of time and, when ready, begins to tap in time with the tone. After a set time period, the tone ceases and the child continues to tap and attempts to maintain the original rate of tapping. Using this type of task, Williams, Woollacott, and Ivry (1992) studied 6–7-year-olds and 9–10-year-olds and reported that children with DCD were significantly more variable than control children in maintaining a given rate of tapping. For most children with DCD, time lags in tracking the tone ranged from early, anticipatory responses to very late responses. In contrast, control children were much more consistent in keeping time with their rhythmic tapping action. If a consistent rate is not established with the tone present, it is unlikely that the tapping response will improve when the tone is removed. Although not often commented on, even when the tone was present, children with DCD exhibited greater variability in maintaining a close synchronization between the tapping action and the auditory tone. Thus, it is not surprising that children with DCD were more variable in their tapping responses without the tone.

Another consideration in this research is that, more often than not, only successful attempts (responses that fall within certain set parameters) are analyzed and reported. However, in the Williams et al. (1992) study, for example, children with DCD had twice as many unsuccessful trials as control children, suggesting that their timing control may be even more inconsistent than reported in the past. Performances of these children may be especially vulnerable to failure when tasks require consistent, repetitive actions or involve complex timing of movements in relationship to stimulus events in the external environment.

Important age-developmental effects are also frequently present. Young children with DCD have been reported to be the most variable in tapping rate with young control children the next most variable. Older children with DCD are more variable than older control children who are the least variable. This suggests that difficulty with timing control (as represented by variability of tapping performance) is present in young children with DCD and that although it improves to some degree with age, rhythmic timing of motor responses continues to be problematical in older children with DCD.

What are the potential underlying factors or mechanisms involved in timing control? Williams et al. (1992) used the Wing-Kristofferson model (Wing & Kristofferson, 1973) to examine the possible locus of timing control difficulties in children with DCD. Their data suggested that timing control deficits of children with DCD were more related to problems with "central timing mechanisms" than to peripheral mechanisms involved in response implementation. Thus, the observed rhythmic coordination deficits in children with DCD were attributed to an inability to organize temporal aspects of movement by central motor control systems. These authors also reported that children with DCD were significantly less accurate than control children in making perceptual judgments about time intervals. This lead the authors to speculate (1) that both sensory and motor processes involved in time functions are affected in these children and (2) that this may be a manifestation of a general "time-based" disorder in the central mechanisms involved in movement control. There are converging data that suggest that this may, in fact, be a real possibility. For example, Ivry and Keele (1989) have shown that individuals with cerebellar lesions exhibit greater variability in producing timed, rhythmic movements and in judging time intervals than do "normal" individuals. Although individuals with other types of central nervous system dysfunction (e.g., Parkinsonism, etc.) also frequently show increased variability in timed, rhythmic responses, they do not exhibit deficits in perception of timed intervals. In the Williams et al. (1992) study, children with DCD showed a pattern of "perceptual and motor timing deficits" similar to those seen in cerebellar patients. Thus, the authors speculated that a potential underlying cause of inefficient timing control in children with DCD may be a manifestation of subtle cerebellar dysfunction. The observation that timing control difficulties persist in older children with DCD suggests that such difficulties are less likely to be due to a "delay" in development and/or to maturational differences between the two groups.

Using a tapping task similar to that of Williams et al. (1992), Lundy-Ekman, Ivry, Keele, and Woollacott (1991) examined subgroups of children with DCD and control children. Children with DCD were categorized into two groups: those with soft neurological signs associated with cerebellar dysfunction (e.g., dysmetria, inability to perform rapid, alternating movements, intention tremor); and those with soft neurological signs associated with basal ganglia dysfunction (e.g., choreiform or jerky, irregular movements; athetotiform or small, slow, writhing movements, and synkinesis). These authors reported that although there were no differences in the mean rate of tapping between the two groups of children, the groups were significantly different in consistency of tapping rate. Children in the cerebellar subgroup were significantly more variable than both control children and children with basal ganglia soft signs in maintaining steady, repetitive rhythmic tapping responses. Data indicated that the inability of children with cerebellar signs to maintain a steady tapping rate was of central origin. That is, it was due to a deficit in a "central clock or timing mechanism." Importantly, the authors found a similar pattern of differences in the perception of time intervals in children with cerebellar signs. These differences in motor and perceptual timing were identical to those reported by Williams et al. (1992). Again, subgroups of children with cerebellar signs were the only children to exhibit both motor and perceptual timing deficits.

To address possible force control differences in these same children, Lundy-Ekman et al. (1991) asked children to perform a force control task that required the child to produce a series of isotonic movements to reach a given target force level on a computer screen. Both the consistency with which children could reproduce a given amount of force and the duration of force pulses were evaluated. All children produced, on the average, similar mean amounts of force. More importantly, children with basal ganglia signs were significantly more variable than both the control group and children with cerebellar signs in producing specified target forces. The authors suggest that there may be a double dissociation between timing and force control deficits in children with DCD; certain children exhibit timing control deficits, while others exhibit force control deficits. Thus, the nature of motor control deficits in children with DCD may be in part a function of deficits in different underlying neurological systems. This may contribute to the heterogeneity of characteristics of motor control displayed by children with DCD.

Interestingly, Lundy-Ekman et al. (1991) reported that children with cerebellar signs produced smaller amounts of force than control children or children with basal ganglia signs. Since there is a strong positive relationship between the amount of force produced and the variability of force responses (e.g., as force is increased, variability decreases), one might expect children with soft cerebellar signs to be more variable than either of the other two groups of children. When the variability of the force response was examined in relationship to mean force produced (using a coefficient of variation), children with cerebellar signs were significantly more variable than control children in producing specific target forces. Thus, it would appear that children classified as DCD with soft cerebellar signs in this study exhibited both timing and force control deficits.

Temporal features of force pulses also support this observation; children with cerebellar signs had longer force pulse durations and longer times to peak force than control children. Lundy-Ekman et al. (1991) suggest that children with cerebellar signs may show some deficit in force production because timing control may be involved at a different level in this type of response. In other words, timing control may be important in the force control task because of the need to regulate the temporal relationship between onset of activity in agonist and antagonist muscle groups involved in producing the force pulse. If the onset of antagonist muscle activity is delayed, force production may exceed the specified target force. In contrast, if the onset of antagonist muscle activity is early, it is more likely to lead to an underproduction of target force. Thus, increased variability in timing of agonist and antagonist muscle activity could indirectly lead to increased variability in force production. Since deficits in timing control were not present in children with basal ganglia signs, one might speculate that timing control deficits lead to more pervasive deficits in movement control than do force control deficits. More evidence is clearly needed to clarify the nature and extent of potential differences in timing/force control in children diagnosed with DCD.

Geuze and Kalverboer (1994) studied timing control in children with DCD and compared them with age-matched controls and with children with dyslexia. Although dyslexia is typically defined as a failure to acquire normal reading skills, these children have frequently been shown to have difficulty with tasks that involve timing of limb movements (e.g., tapping tasks). Results indicated that all children tended to increase the rate of tapping when the auditory tone was removed. However, three times as many children with DCD and four times as many children diagnosed with dyslexia increased the rate of tapping as compared to control children. These authors also reported that, although children with DCD were more variable than control children on all tapping tasks, the differences were not statistically significant. Children with dyslexia were significantly more variable than control children but were not different from children with DCD. The Test of Motor Impairment (TOMI) scores indicated that children with dyslexia had motor performance scores comparable to those of control children, while scores of children with DCD were much poorer than either of the other two groups.

How is it that children with dyslexia failed to exhibit the motor control deficits seen in children with DCD and yet were as variable as these children in maintaining a repetitive rhythmic response of the upper extremities? Wolff, Michel, Ovrut, and Drake (1990) have suggested there may be a common underlying deficiency in children with DCD and those with dyslexia, and that this deficit is a reflection of inadequate temporal "resolution." Some have theorized that speech and skilled movements share common neural mechanisms that regulate timing and serial order control and thus timing control deficits are manifested in different ways in each of the two diagnoses. The exact origins of such timing related problems, however, is still unclear.

A Dynamic Systems Analysis of Timing

Volman and Geuze (1998) used a dynamic pattern approach to examine the stability of rhythmic coordination patterns in children with DCD. This approach is concerned with studying spatial-temporal invariance (i.e., dynamic stability) of movement patterns and how transitions from one stable behavior pattern to another occur. The theory proposes that stable coordinated movement patterns seen at a behavioral or macroscopic level emerge in an autonomous fashion (i.e., are self-organized) as a result of appropriate coupling among different systems or components that contribute to the movement pattern. For example, movement patterns at the behavioral level are the result of contributions from the postural control system, the muscular system, the sensory systems, the bony skeletal framework as well as other biomechanical, physical, and physiological factors. Thus, the action patterns we observe and examine are a manifestation of the "intrinsic dynamics" of the body, its systems, and the information constraints placed upon them as a result of past experience and the task environment.

Unimanual Control

Children (7–12 years) with DCD ($n = 24$) and those without DCD ($n = 24$) were asked to perform a visuo-manual coordination task (Volman & Geuze, 1998). The task involved executing smooth flexion-extension movements of the left or right index fingers in time with a visual signal that oscillated at a specified frequency between two light emitting diodes (LEDs). In one condition, the "in-phase" condition, finger movements were made in concert with the oscillation of the light; in another condition, the "anti-phase condition," finger movements were made in a direction opposite to the oscillation of the light. In the first task, the visual signal oscillation was set at 0.8 Hz and children simply moved the right or left index finger (in-phase or anti-phase as designated) with the visual signal. Data from this task provided a basis for describing the stability of a coordination pattern when the pattern was known, predictable, and not interfered with by unexpected perturbations. In another condition, children were asked to perform a task similar to the one just described; in this task, however, the movement itself was unexpectedly disturbed by the insertion of a braking action at two different points in the action cycle. This allowed the authors to examine the adaptability characteristics of the system. Children also performed a third task that involved a gradual change in the frequency of the oscillating light. The oscillation frequency began at 0.8 Hz and was increased by 0.05 Hz after each four stimuli to a maximum of 1.8 Hz. Performances on this task provided insight into conditions (e.g., rate-limiting factors) that affect the stability of coordinative patterns. All children were given opportunities to practice all tasks prior to data collection.

Actions that involve visuo-manual or visuo-motor coordination have an inherently important person–environment interaction. Thus, it is important to note that four children with DCD could not perform the simple finger flexion-extension task when the finger movements had to be made in the opposite direction to the oscillating visual signal (anti-phase pattern). For those who could perform the tasks, there were no differences between children with and without DCD in terms of the absolute deviation between finger action and the visual signal (e.g., relative phase differences). Both groups of children were equally accurate and thus capable of producing a small relative phase difference. However, children with DCD were more variable in sustaining a simple, repetitive visuo-manual coordinative pattern than control children. When the coordinative pattern was disrupted by an unexpected braking action, children with DCD also took a much longer time to return to the initial level of stability than did children without DCD.

When children moved the fingers in concert with the visual signal and the frequency of the oscillation of the light was increased, some phase drifting eventually occurred and was similar for all children (i.e., differences between the timing of the finger actions and the oscillation of the light increased). When children moved the fingers opposite to the direction of the visual signal (anti-phase condition), there was a switch to the in-phase pattern for all children. Importantly, however, the switch from the anti-phase pattern to the in-phase pattern occurred at a significantly lower frequency for children with DCD. Thus, children with DCD were less able to meet increasing movement demands as represented by increased rate or frequency of movement. Since phase transitions involve proprioceptive, visual, and auditory information, transitions from anti-phase to in-phase patterns may be the result of the system reaching a ceiling for handling sensory information. The outcome is a change to a different, more stable pattern, the in-phase pattern which has reduced information demands. The fact that children with DCD required more time to return to the initial level of stability after a disturbance to the movement and that the coordination pattern was "stable" across a smaller range of frequencies, points to a potential lack of capacity of the system. This, of course, makes the child with DCD extremely vulnerable to a changing environment and to increasingly greater movement demands.

Bimanual Coordination

Relatively few studies have examined the repetitive timing of bimanual movements in children with DCD. The study by Volman and Geuze (1998) used a dynamic pattern approach to examine the timing of the two hands in a simple finger flexion and extension task. Children (7–12 years old) were asked to execute movements of the index fingers of right and left hands under two conditions. In one condition, children produced self-paced rhythmic movements of the index fingers in in-phase (in this action homologous muscles are used) and anti-phase (in this action nonhomologous muscles are used) patterns. In the other condition, children produced self-paced rhythmic movements of the index fingers but with unpredictable perturbations applied to the movement. In general, children with and without DCD produced self-paced movements of approximately the same frequency (DCD = 1.15 Hz; control = 1.23 Hz). However, the timing of the bimanual movements were significantly more variable in children with DCD; this was true for both in-phase and anti-phase conditions. As with unimanual movements, children with DCD had greater difficulty sustaining a steady, repetitive pattern of bimanual movements and at least one child with DCD was unable to maintain a steady enough pattern to allow perturbations to be applied. As before children with DCD were more variable, took longer to reestablish the original rhythmic pattern following a perturbation, and shifted from an anti-phase to an in-phase pattern at a lower critical frequency than controls. These observations all point to a system that is more affected by even small environmental perturbations and less able to adapt to increased movement demands. The fact that children with DCD shifted to an in-phase pattern at a lower critical frequency than controls may help to explain the slower limb movements characteristic of these children and may be a reflection of the system's attempt to maintain stability of action.

An interesting observation reported by Volman and Geuze (1998) is that although both unimanual and bimanual rhythmic coordination patterns were less stable in children with DCD than in control children, one-hand visuo-manual coordination patterns were even more unstable in children with DCD than were bimanual or interlimb coordination patterns. The authors suggest that this is due in part to the fact that coupling in visuo-manual and interlimb coordination systems is functionally different. In bimanual coordination tasks, coupling is bidirectional; in unimanual coordination tasks, it is unidirectional. Control of bimanual coordination also relies more on proprioceptive information while visual information is critical to the control of visuo-manual actions. The authors propose that bimanual coordination patterns are more stable in general because the "rhythmic units" involved in these two-hand patterns have a tighter coupling (e.g., a more stringent frequency relationship) than is the case for visuo-manual coordination patterns (i.e., the coupling between vision and the hand is looser). Importantly, in their study Volman and Geuze (1998) identified children with DCD who had very poor bimanual coordination patterns but stable visuo-manual coordination actions and vice versa. A third group of children was also identified; these had poor bimanual and visuo-manual coordination patterns. This suggests again that the motor control difficulties of children labeled as having DCD are quite diverse. Overall, control of bimanual and unimanual actions in children with DCD seems to be characterized by unstable spatial-temporal organization of movement. The potential locus of dysfunction at the neural level is still unclear.

In a different approach, Geuze and Kalverboer (1994) examined performances of children with and without DCD in two different bimanual tasks. In one task, children tapped the two hands alternately to each beep of an auditory tone; in the second task, one hand was used to respond to every tone or beep, the other tapped to every other beep. In general, although children with DCD were slightly more variable on both tasks than controls, the difference between the two groups was not significant for either bimanual task. The authors do not provide any detail about children in the control group, but they do indicate that control children "had some problems." This might account for the lack of differences between the two groups of children.

Bimanual Coordination: Discrete Actions

Huh et al. (1998) used a discrete bimanual aiming task to study the development of bilateral motor control in children with DCD. Children (6–7 years and 9–10 years with and without DCD) moved the two hands to targets of either (1) the same amplitude or distance (symmetrical or synchronous bilateral movements) or (2) different amplitudes or distances (asymmetrical bilateral movements). In one instance in the asymmetrical bimanual aiming task, the right hand moved a longer distance than the left; in the other instance, the left hand moved a longer distance than the right. We also examined neuromuscular processes underlying these movements in the form of duration of agonist and antagonist activity and latency of onset of antagonist activity. Overall, children with DCD were significantly slower in executing bimanual aiming movements than controls (control: short distance = 163 msec; long distance = 204 msec; children with DCD: short distance = 198 msec; long distance = 240 msec). Movement times of children with DCD were also almost twice as variable as those of controls (control SD = 33 msec; children with DCD SD = 59 msec).

At a behavioral level, both groups of children showed evidence of bimanual coupling in two-hand symmetrical movements (e.g., the two hands moved synchronously to and arrived at near/far targets in similar amounts of time). With regard to underlying neuromuscular processes, there were clear differences between the two groups of children in how this coupling was achieved. For control children, there were changes (from single limb movements) in the duration of agonist and antagonist muscle activity and in the onset latency of antagonist muscle activity; these changes occurred in parallel in both limbs. The neuromuscular activity exhibited by children with DCD was quite different. Along with slower and more variable latencies in onset of antagonist muscle activity [near target-control: 294 msec (49 msec); children with DCD: 358 msec (65 msec); far target-control: 300 msec (51 msec); children with DCD: 382 msec (74 msec)], these children also exhibited nonparallel modifications of duration of agonist muscle activity in the two limbs. Although at a behavioral level, children with and without DCD tended to couple the two hands in symmetrical bilateral aiming movements, the speed with which these aiming movements were executed, and the way in which the motor control system regulated the muscle activity involved in these actions, was quite different.

When asymmetrical movements were performed, both groups of children tended again to couple the movements of the two hands so that they arrived at appropriate end targets in similar amounts of time. Both groups of children showed evidence of slowing the movement of the hand moving to the near target (left hand)

and increasing the speed of the movement of the hand moving to the far target (right hand). However, as with symmetrical movements, the underlying neuromuscular responses were quite different in the two groups of children. Control children achieved coupling in the asymmetrical two-hand coordination task by modifying the duration of antagonist muscle activity. Thus, in relationship to activity observed in unilateral aiming movements, duration of the left antagonist activity increased and duration of right antagonist activity decreased. Consequently, movement times and duration of antagonist activity were temporally consistent in control children.

For children with DCD, coupling was achieved in a very different way. Coupling was achieved through changes in duration and onset latency parameters of agonist *and* antagonist muscle activity. Generally, duration of right agonist muscle activity increased, while that of the left decreased. Onset latency of right antagonist activity also decreased. These data suggest that children with DCD have difficulty programming agonist and antagonist muscle activity in producing fast, accurate movements. The observation that agonist muscle activity is prolonged and onset of antagonist muscle activity is delayed is important as these neuromuscular parameters directly affect speed of movement in motor tasks that have speed-accuracy constraints (Gottlieb, Corcos, & Agarwal, 1989, 1990, 1992). Prolonged agonist burst duration and delayed antagonist electromyographic activity have also been observed in patients with cerebellar lesions during execution of fast, accurate movements (Diener, Hore, Ivry, & Dichgans, 1993).

Overall data from Huh et al. (1998) suggest that, for control children, regulation of antagonist activity (burst duration) is the underlying motor control strategy used to achieve bilateral motor coordination in asymmetrical aiming movements. For children with DCD, the strategy for regulating muscle activity is much less uniform and consistent. There is some evidence to suggest that motor control strategies that involve regulation of antagonist muscle activity represent an advanced stage of motor learning and/or hierarchical motor development (Jaric, Corcos, Agarwal, & Gottlieb, 1993). Thus, the bilateral motor coordination deficits often observed in children with DCD may, in part, be a result of a less advanced motor control system and lack of capacity to organize and employ appropriate motor control strategies.

DCD: ISSUES IN BALANCE AND POSTURAL CONTROL

Skilled movement performance, regardless of its end goal, is believed to be a product of two interrelated phases of action: a positioning, postural or preparatory phase, and an executory or manipulative one. To balance effectively, the individual must process visual information about the body and external environment, proprioceptive information about limb and body position, and then initiate an appropriate corrective response. The integration or mapping of these two sources of sensory information is also a critical ingredient in balance control.

One of the common features of the child with DCD is poor balance and/or postural control. It is possible that the poor balance of these children is a major source of the problem underlying the pervasive and diverse incoordination that characterizes many of their movement patterns. The following section focuses on research that has examined the nature and extent of differences in balance and postural control in children with and without DCD.

Sway Characteristics

Sway is considered by many to be a general indicator of the integrity of the postural control system. Frequency and amplitude of sway are known to change with age and are influenced by a number of other factors (e.g., gender, vision). Amplitude of adult sway is, on the average, reported to range from 2.7 cm to approximately 4 cm and is characterized by low- and high-frequency components. The low-frequency component is at approximately 0.2 Hz and accounts for the major portion of the sway. The high-frequency component is a tremor component and is thought to account for a smaller proportion of the sway observed in adults. Wann, Mon-Williams, and Rushton (1998) have reported data on children with and without DCD who were asked to stand in a simple, upright position with eyes open. Children with DCD swayed significantly more than control children and other groups to which they were compared. For example, in the normal standing position, on average, children with DCD swayed 7.37 cm, control children 3.5 cm, nursery school children 4.89, and adults 4.86 cm. There were no differences among these latter three groups. When children with DCD balanced without vision, the mean amplitude of sway increased; in contrast, sway amplitude did not change for control children, nursery school children or adults. Together, the data suggest that some children with DCD sway more under typical, everyday balance conditions than do age-matched and younger control children and that they may have a greater dependence on vision for regulation of balance than other children.

Wann et al. (1998) also studied postural control of these groups using the moving room paradigm. The room was moved at approximately 0.17 Hz and was displaced 40%, 80%, and 120% of the base of support of the individual. Under these conditions, sway was synchronized with the movement of the room to some degree for all individuals. Synchronization occurred on 76% of exposures for children with DCD, on 72% of exposures for control children, on 80% of exposures for nursery children, but on only 35% of exposures for adults. Regardless of age and developmental level, the dominant frequency of postural sway was approximately that of the movement of the room.

Mean changes in sway are an indication of the degree to which postural sway is driven by the motion of the visual surround, in this case, the moving room. Wann et al. (1998) reported that adults and control children reached their sway limit (i.e., the mean gain in sway) when the room was displaced at approximately 40% of the base of support and did not exceed this limit when greater displacements of the room occurred. Although children with DCD exhibited higher mean gains than adults in response to the moving room, their mean gain was not different from that of control children. Importantly, children with DCD had significantly higher peak sway than controls. Wann et al. interpret these data to mean that children with DCD exhibited significant sway components at frequencies other than those associated with room movement. That is, a significant proportion of the sway response of these children was outside the frequency band of the room motion. Thus, in terms of peak frequency of sway, children with DCD seem to be more vulnerable to disruption of posture by optical flow than age-matched peers. In this respect they are more like children 4–5 years their junior. Young children are much more affected by perturbations of the optical flow, exhibit responses that are directly coupled to the visual motion of the room, and are more reliant on visual input and less on proprioceptive information in regulating balance. Wann et al. (1998) propose that, in general, children with DCD tend to show a strong reliance on vision in maintaining balance and suggest that this tendency to rely on visual information for balance control may be an indication that children with DCD are slow in developing the capacity to process proprioceptive input and to effectively integrate visual and proprioceptive information.

Both visual and vestibular/proprioceptive systems play a major role in regulating sway. Vestibular and proprioceptive systems are important in the execution of rapid adjustments to postural disturbances and sway. Visual information is believed to contribute to slower postural adjustments (Nashner & Berthoz, 1978). Visual information may also play a role in helping to calibrate proprioception and may at times be the dominant source of information in regulating balance control (Lee & Lishman, 1975). This appears to be the case for children with DCD. Primary reliance on visual information to regulate posture may handicap these children in responding to disturbances to balance since vision may mediate slower postural adjustments.

Postural Synergies

In general, evidence indicates that healthy, young individuals (children and adults) respond to external perturbations to balance by activating stereotyped muscle responses. These responses are referred to as postural synergies and involve activation of the muscles of the legs and trunk. Although postural synergies are present in children as young as 15 months, they are not refined until 7–10 years of age at which time they appear to be adult-like in both latency and variability characteristics. There is a dramatic period of change in latency and variability of postural responses between 4 to 6 years. This change is important to keep in mind since reduction in response variability may reflect important changes in the development of the young nervous system and has been shown to characterize other central nervous system functions.

Williams and Woollacott (1997) examined postural responses of children with and without DCD. Children, 6–7 and 9–10 years of age, stood on a force platform with eyes open and feet shoulder width apart. The platform was unexpectedly perturbed in either a forward or backward direction; this movement created posterior and anterior sway, respectively. The speed with which the postural synergy was activated (latency) and the pattern or sequence of muscle activation were the primary characteristics of interest. In general, the average onset latency of muscle activation, that is the speed with which the postural synergy was initiated, was similar in the two groups of children. For example, in backward sway, ankle flexor muscles were activated in approximately 88 msec in control children and in 89 msec in children with DCD. Thus, children with DCD initiated responses to perturbations to balance as quickly as children without DCD.

When intraindividual variability of onset latencies was examined, children with DCD were found to be significantly more variable than children without DCD in activating postural synergies to counteract anterior sway. There was no difference in variability between the two groups in initiating postural responses to backward sway. These data on anterior sway suggest that the postural control system of the child with DCD tends to activate responses quickly on one occasion and extremely slowly on others. Importantly, this inconsistency in onset latency is present in both younger and older children with DCD. Williams and Woollacott (1997) argued that, if motor control difficulties of children with DCD were due to a developmental delay, they should not only be more variable than control children but should also show a decrease in variability with age, a phenomenon commonly seen in children without DCD. This was not the case for children in this study as older children with DCD were only slightly less variable in response latencies than younger children with DCD. However, this interpretation is based on cross-sectional data and some caution is warranted.

Williams and Woollacott (1997) also suggest that if motor control problems are due, in part, to a motor dysfunction, not only should there be little or no decrease in variability with age (as was observed) but there should also be other evidence of dysfunction. In support of this hypothesis, the authors provide evidence that children with DCD are significantly different from control children in the pattern of muscle activation used in responding to disturbances of balance. Overall, control children consistently exhibited the characteristic distal-proximal pattern of leg muscle activation seen in response to these types of perturbations to balance. This pattern was present on 100% of perturbation trials. Children with DCD were less consistent and often exhibited a less efficient proximal-distal pattern of activation. Thus, on 28% of trials, young children with DCD activated the upper leg muscles prior to activating stretched ankle muscles. Older children with DCD exhibited this proximal-distal pattern of activation on 17% of trials. Approximately two-thirds of young children with DCD and one-third of older children with DCD showed a proximal-distal pattern of muscle activation on at least 40% of trials on which perturbations to balance occurred.

When trunk and neck muscles were examined as a part of the pattern of muscle activation, Williams (1999, personal communication) indicated that control children tended to exhibit two patterns of muscle activation in responding to perturbations of balance. Both were equally common. One pattern involved the activation of stretched ankle muscles first, followed by activation of the upper leg muscles and then simultaneous activation of trunk and neck muscles. The other pattern involved activation of stretched ankle muscles first followed by simultaneous activation of upper leg, trunk, and neck muscles. These patterns were observed in response to sway in both anterior and posterior directions. Thus, control children counteracted the initial displacement of the center of gravity through the action of leg muscles; they then immediately stabilized the trunk and upper body to bring the total body back into a more stable state.

In contrast, children with DCD exhibited different and varied patterns of leg, trunk, and neck muscle activation. A common pattern that was used primarily to counteract posterior sway was activation of upper leg muscles initially, followed by activation of stretched ankle muscles, then trunk and finally neck muscles. When perturbations to balance created anterior sway, children with DCD tended to activate the stretched leg muscles first (either ankle and then upper leg or vice versa); this was followed by activation of neck muscles (presumably to stabilize the head) and then trunk muscles. These patterns of muscle activation point to a different and potentially less efficient organization of postural responses in children with DCD.

Data on variability and sequencing of muscle responses in children with DCD reported by Williams and Woollacott (1997) support the notion that the motor control difficulties of children with DCD are, at least in part, the result of some motor dysfunction. Nashner and Grimm (1977) have reported increased variability of postural responses in patients with cerebellar lesions, even though absolute muscle response onset latencies were "normal." Nashner et al. (1983) also have reported reversals in distal-proximal muscle activation patterns in the involved leg in children with spastic hemiplegia. Other data indicate that it is possible that the inconsistent timing and sequencing of muscle activity and thus the difficulty with postural control observed in children with DCD may be a symptom of a more general problem of timing; this is also the case for patients with cerebellar dysfunction.

Neuromuscular (Electromyographic) Aspects of Postural Control

Wilson and Trombly (1984) studied children with and without sensory integration dysfunction ($n = 8$ per group) and examined integrated eleectromyographic activity in the upper and middle fibers of the trapezius and the pectoralis major during performance of two fine motor tasks. The tasks included a line drawing task and a motor accuracy task. Children with sensory integration dysfunction (SID) exhibited significantly greater eleectromyographic activity than children without SID in all muscle groups and under all task conditions. Interestingly there were high correlations between scores on the two fine motor tasks for control children ($r = 0.958$) but little or no correlation for children with SID ($r = 0.299$). Similarly, there were stronger correlations between the amount of muscle activity and performance on fine motor tasks for control children ($r = 0.731$) than for children with SID ($r = -0.119$). The authors suggest that (1) there is a deficiency in the use of proximal muscles by these children in providing appropriate stability for performing fine motor tasks and (2) there is a tendency for children with SID to overuse muscles to fixate the joints for stability. This latter characteristic is reminiscent of early stages of motor development. The authors point out that there is a difference between the coordinated cocontraction of muscles for stability at a joint and the tiring and rarely needed stiff and rigid fixation of joints that does not allow for more flexible adjustments to posture or joint position. Thus, instability in these children may be a manifestation of both inappropriate amount and application of muscle force.

Williams, Fisher, and Tritschler (1983) investigated static postural control in 4-, 6-, and 8-year-old children who were described as either being motorically awkward or as having developmentally appropriate levels of motor coordination. Children were asked to assume six different positions that included balancing in the extensor prone position, on all fours, in full and half-kneel positions, and standing upright. Amplitude of electromyographic activity in lower leg (gastrocnemius and tibialis anterior), upper leg (quadriceps and hamstrings), and trunk muscles (abdominals and paraspinals) was significantly greater in children who were motorically awkward than in control children. This was true for all positions assumed by the children. In addition, control children showed a pattern of diminishing amplitude with increasing age; 4-year-olds exhibited significantly greater muscle activity than 8-year-olds in maintaining the same position. In contrast there were no differences in levels of muscle activity involved in static postural control in 4- and 8-year-old children classified as motorically awkward. Equally important, Williams et al. (1983) reported that children identified as motorically awkward were characterized by patterns of muscle activity that involved greater levels of activity in *both* leg and trunk muscles when maintaining upright posture. These data suggest that in maintaining a simple upright stance, children with motor coordination difficulties seemed not to establish adequate trunk stability initially, and, thus, trunk muscles were active throughout the period of upright stance. For control children, maintenance of upright posture was achieved primarily through leg muscle activity.

In a more recent study, Williams and Castro (1997) investigated timing and force parameters of muscle activity in children with and without DCD during standing. They examined amplitude, duration, and sequencing of muscle activity in tibialis anterior (distal muscle) and quadriceps muscles (proximal muscle) when children stood in an upright position on a moveable platform under three conditions: with vision, without vision, and with the head tilted backward. The platform was moved forward and created backward sway. Children with DCD exhibited significantly greater amplitude of muscle activity (e.g., produced more force) than control children in all balance conditions. Interestingly, control children increased amplitude of both distal and proximal muscle activity when they balanced without vision or with the head tilted backward. Children with DCD did not show any increase in amplitude under these perturbation conditions. Thus, control children tended to respond to potentially destabilizing postural conditions with an increase in neural drive to both upper and lower leg muscles. Williams and Castro hypothesized that a similar increase in neural drive to leg muscles may not have occurred in children with DCD in part because the force output was already high and an increase in muscle activity may have been outside the capacity of the system.

When ratios of distal to proximal muscle activity were examined, it was clear that for control children the force output of the distal muscle was greater than that of the proximal muscle. In contrast, the distal/proximal ratios of children with DCD indicated that a disproportionate amount of force was produced by the proximal muscle. This relationship between forces produced in proximal and distal muscles was present in all balance conditions. Williams and Castro (1997) also examined duration of muscle activity in these same children and reported that control children exhibited a pattern of activity in which the distal muscle was active one and one-half times longer than the proximal muscle. Characteristic of children with DCD was a pattern in which the duration of distal muscle activity was either equivalent to or less than that of the proximal muscle. In terms of the sequence of muscle activation, children without DCD maintained a consistent distal-proximal pattern of activation with and without vision. For children with DCD, the incidence of proximal-distal activation of muscle activity when they balanced with vision was greater than for control children. When they balanced without vision, the incidence of proximal-distal muscle activation was increased even more; there was evidence of proximal-distal activation of muscles on one in every three trials.

Amplitude (force), duration, and sequence of muscle activation data all suggest that proximal muscle control may be a primary mode of regulating posture/balance in children with DCD. Proximal muscle control generally represents a cruder, less refined level of motor control. Distal muscles are used more often to produce finer gradations of force and involve finer control. Therefore, greater use of distal musculature to regulate balance may represent a more refined and advanced level of motor control and may be more characteristic of control children. Reliance on proximal muscle control in responding to changes in balance that require finely graded force production may present children with DCD with a difficult challenge.

OTHER ASPECTS OF MOTOR CONTROL IN CHILDREN WITH DCD

There is some scientific evidence that points to central nervous system involvement in motor control difficulties of children with DCD. However, there are many details that are unknown about potential differences in central nervous system function in these children. The following section considers research evidence from the "conditioned patellar tendon reflex paradigm."

Conditioned Patellar Tendon Reflex Paradigm

The planning and execution of skillful motor acts is clearly a complex process; one important aspect of that planning and execution is the precise regulation of input-output activity of the alpha motor neuron pool. Activity of the alpha motor neuron pool is influenced by a variety of inputs including crossed spinal inputs, descending inputs from various brain centers, and inputs from the periphery. The patellar tendon reflex response is a safe, noninvasive tool for studying input-output characteristics of the alpha motor neuron pool in humans. The nature and extent of the contributions of different sources of input to the motor neuron pool can be examined through the "conditioned patellar tendon reflex" paradigm. In this paradigm, for example, a tap is applied to the left patellar tendon (conditioning stimulus) prior to the application of a tap to the right patellar tendon (test stimulus). The conditioning stimulus is used to activate crossed spinal and supraspinal pathways that are known to influence the input-output activity of the alpha motor neuron pool. Which pathways, crossed spinal or supraspinal, are activated is related to the time between the application of the conditioning and the test stimulus. Thus, tendon taps are applied at different time intervals after the conditioning stimulus (e.g., 15–600 msec).

By comparing the force of the "test" patellar tendon reflex response at different time intervals after the "conditioning" patellar tendon reflex response, Williams and Burke (1995) examined the potential contributions of crossed spinal (i.e., force produced at intervals ≤ 75 msec) and supraspinal pathways (i.e., force produced at intervals ≥ 90 msec) to activity of the motor neuron pool. The authors studied input-output properties of the alpha motor neuron pool of children with and without DCD. It is important to understand how the motor neuron pool functions in these children since successful performance of voluntary movements depends upon the capacity of the central nervous system to regulate the output of the alpha motor neuron pool. The authors hypothesized that motor neuron excitability via either a peripheral reflex loop, crossed spinal pathways, and/or supraspinal pathways might be impaired in children with DCD.

Williams and Burke (1995) reported that, in general, the force of the basic patellar tendon reflex was greater by 105% in children with DCD. With regard to conditioned patellar tendon reflexes, peripheral reflex effects (e.g., short latency responses at 15 and 60 msec) were often present in children with DCD but were never seen in control children. These data imply that the sensitivity of the peripheral reflex loop may be increased in children with DCD. Thus, at least in some children with DCD, there is stronger peripheral input from the Ia afferents for a given stimulus intensity. Perhaps one characteristic of children with DCD is that a greater percentage of the alpha motor neuron pool is recruited through peripheral reflex loops than for control children. What might explain this increase in tendon reflex force in children with DCD? The authors suggest that this could be a result of an increase in muscle spindle gain via central mechanisms (e.g., the gamma motor system) or of an increase in muscle tendon stiffness via peripheral mechanisms. Since there is little or no evidence to suggest that increases in muscle tendon stiffness are characteristic of children with DCD, one is inclined to point to the possibility of central involvement.

An increase in muscle spindle gain in the resting muscle might also contribute to reduced capacity for processing proprioceptive feedback during movement. Precision processing of proprioceptive feedback is maintained during performance of voluntary movements, in part, by alpha-gamma coactivation (cf. Hagbarth, 1993). A high background level of activation of the gamma motor neuron pool could adversely affect the capacity of the central nervous system to set appropriate muscle spindle gain during voluntary movement (Hulliger, 1993; Llewellyn, Yang, & Prochazka, 1990). Thus, the ability to maintain precision of proprioceptive feedback during movement control could be compromised in DCD. It is also interesting to note that the cerebellum has been shown to influence the background activity of the gamma motor neuron pool (cf. Gorassini, Prochazka, & Taylor, 1993) and that exaggerated tendon reflexes have been observed in patients (2–14 years) who were diagnosed with cerebellar disorders and no concomitant peripheral neuropathy. These data point to a possible central nervous system dysfunction in children with DCD.

An increase in the excitability of alpha motoneuron pool in children with DCD could also help to explain their apparent inability to regulate muscle force (Lundy-Ekman et al., 1991). It is well known that Ia afferent input influences the recruitment of alpha motor neurons for the production of voluntary movements in walking (Capaday & Stein, 1986; 1987) and in running (Capaday & Stein, 1987;

Dietz, Schmidtbleicher, & Noth, 1979). Thus, increased proprioceptive feedback during voluntary movement via peripheral reflex loops may act to impair the capacity of the central nervous system to regulate appropriate recruitment of alpha motor neurons and, consequently, muscle force gradation in children with DCD. It is important to note that children with DCD also varied considerably in terms of the effect of the conditioning stimulus on motor neuron activity. Some children with DCD showed evidence of fluctuating but strong inhibitory influences of both crossed spinal and supraspinal pathways. Others showed consistent and very strong facilitatory crossed spinal and supraspinal influences on the alpha motor neuron pool. This is another indication of heterogeneity in children with DCD.

SUMMARY AND CONCLUSIONS

What then do we know about motor control in children with DCD? Although the amount of research available on motor control characteristics of children with DCD is limited, there is some consistent evidence to suggest that the following are frequently observed in children diagnosed as DCD:

- Significantly slower reaction, movement, and response times
- Universal difficulty with timing control
- Frequent difficulty with force control
- Increased variability of performances on a wide variety of motor tasks
- Greater vulnerability to perturbations of movement
- Inability to adapt quickly to changes in movement demands
- Tendency to rely on vision for maintaining balance/postural control
- Tendency to rely on proximal muscle control to regulate balance
- Poorer intersensory integration than peers of similar chronological age especially with regard to mapping visual and proprioceptive information
- Use of different neuromuscular/motor control strategies to regulate bimanual coordination
- Tendency for deficiencies in motor control to persist with age and to be more related to central nervous system dysfunction than to developmental delay

Overall evidence clearly indicates that there is extensive heterogeneity in motor control characteristics of children with DCD and that no one set of characteristics can be associated with individual children with DCD.

PART
V

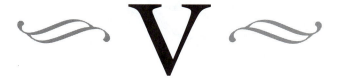

Functional Implications

CHAPTER

9

Daily Living Skills and Developmental Coordination Disorder

Teresa May-Benson, Peg Ingolia, and Jane Koomar

"Her life is a challenge, from the minute she wakes up, all through her day!" This is how Julia's mother describes her first grade daughter's difficulty in the tasks most children perform easily and most parents take for granted.

Developmental coordination disorder (DCD) affects the most basic and familiar tasks children attempt. These basic and familiar tasks are frequently referred to as functional skills, activities of daily living (ADLs), and instrumental activities of daily living (IADLs) (Shepherd, Proctor, & Coley, 1996). DCD is characterized by motor coordination problems that interfere with a person's ability to perform functional activities of daily living (American Psychiatric Association, 1994). De Ajuria-guerra and Stambak (1969) note that, in the child with poor praxis, "movements are jerky, badly integrated and poorly coordinated, as can be seen in every day activities like dressing, writing, drawing and playing, in the form of clumsy movements which make it difficult for any of these activities to become automatic" (p. 454).

What constitutes activities of daily living or functional skills is not well defined among all professions, however. Difficulties in the ability to perform everyday tasks and activities often subsequently results in an inability to fully participate in appropriate social roles (World Health Organization, 1997). The International Classification of Impairments, Activities and Participation (ICIDH-2) identifies activities as being associated with the daily tasks of everyday life that a person is expected or needs to perform and participation as being the societal phenomena of the person's ability to be actively and fully involved in those life situations. These two concepts form the foundation of activities of daily living.

Taber (1997) defines "activities of daily living" as tasks that enable individuals to meet basic needs. Five task areas of personal care, family responsibilities, work or school, recreation, and socialization are identified. The field of occupational therapy, which specializes in facilitating people's ability to independently participate in activities of daily living at both the personal and societal levels, refers to participation in these daily life activities as occupational performance (Moyers, 1999). "Activities of daily living" have been specified in the uniform terminology of the field of occupational therapy as those purposeful tasks necessary for self-maintenance, for example, grooming, hygiene, dressing, feeding, and socialization. However, work and purposeful activities, productive activities that are necessary for self-development, social contribution, and livelihood (e.g., home management, chores, meal preparation, vocational activities, or school), and play or leisure activities (e.g., activities for amusement, relaxation, enjoyment, or self-expression such as games, sports, or crafts), are also considered occupational performance areas (American Occupational Therapy Association, 1994). Within the rehabilitation literature, daily living skills are separated into self-care skills and IADLs. While self-care skills encompass tasks such as eating, grooming and dressing, IADLs are considered to be more complex ADL skills needed to function independently in home, school, community, and work environments and include those performance areas of work and productive activities such as preparing meals (Shepard et al., 1996).

Therefore, "activities of daily living" is a term that may refer to a narrow range of skills and abilities affecting only performance of self-maintenance activities, or a broad range of functional life skills necessary for successfully completing routine activities. ADLs involve the ability to perform as well as the ability to participate in self-care tasks, vocational and home maintenance activities, play/leisure skills and social situations. This chapter takes the broad view of daily living skills and occupational performance. The infant, toddler, child, and adolescent with DCD may demonstrate difficulties with any number of these skills which can range from performance of self-care activities, to performance of chores around the house, to success in school, to participation in sports and social activities. What these specific tasks are and the importance they have vary throughout childhood, adolescence, and adulthood. For the child with DCD, motor coordination difficulties become apparent in the home, school, and community settings in which the child functions.

HISTORY OF DCD AND DAILY LIVING SKILLS

Historically, children with motor coordination problems have been referred to as "clumsy children" with other terms used such as developmental dyspraxia (Ayres, 1973, 1979; De Ajuriaguerra & Stambak, 1969; Wall, Reid, & Paton, 1990), developmental apraxia (Gubbay, 1978; Reuben & Bakwin, 1968), physically or motorically awkward (Gubbay, 1979, 1985), and minimal cerebral dysfunction (Paine, 1968). Different disciplines and different researchers tend to favor one descriptor over another in describing and classifying the child demonstrating motor clumsiness, and the terminology used to describe different subgroups is highly variable (Missiuna & Polatajko, 1995).

The term "clumsiness" may be seen as a clinical descriptor identifying a large population of children exhibiting motor coordination problems, which impacts on the child's ability to perform daily life tasks. However, the term does not reflect a diagnostic label, connote causality, nor does it reflect a specific set of clinical symptoms beyond general delays in the development of motor coordination skills. The term "developmental coordination disorder" (American Psychiatric Association, 1994) has been increasingly used among researchers and clinicians since 1994 (Polatajko, Fox, & Missiuna, 1995). This diagnostic label encompasses a broad category of motor coordination problems, with the primary characteristics being motor coordination problems that are below age and IQ level and that significantly interfere with school or activity of daily living performance. Among researchers this classification has been the most frequently used term in recent years, however, clinicians and other professionals often still refer to these children as "clumsy" or dyspraxic.

In 1937, Orton identified a group of children with movement difficulties that manifested as problems with functional developmental skills such as walking and running, use of the hands, copying motions, and daily living skills such as climbing stairs, spilling food, dressing, buttoning, shoe tying, and spoon use. Little attention was paid to this group of children until the 1960s, when Walton, Ellis, and Court (1962) presented a series of case studies. These children were described as having less efficient coordination and control of their muscles, their movements were performed with excessive expenditure of energy, and they had an inaccurate judgment of required force, tempo and amplitude of their movements. These authors identified problems in functional daily life tasks as a primary characteristic of the disorder, citing the inability to write, draw, or make block designs. They also identified problems with dressing, ball skills, play skills, feeding and handling utensils, manipulating objects, and traversing stairs.

Reuben and Bakwin (1968) subsequently presented a case study of a child with developmental clumsiness and provided a list of symptoms that they felt represented a syndrome of developmental apraxia. The symptoms were (1) clumsiness severe enough to interfere with everyday activities such as dressing, eating, and playing games; (2) dysgraphia or deficits in handwriting; (3) impaired ability to draw a person and/or ability to reproduce geometric forms; (4) a pattern of low performance and high verbal scores on intelligence tests such as the Weschler; (5) frequent co-occurrence with articulation deficits; and (6) frequent occurrence of a family history of developmental motor or language disorders.

Shortly following the publications of Reuben and Bakwin, Dare and Gordon (1970) presented 35 case studies providing a framework for differential diagnosis of the clumsy child from other movement or developmental delays. They described the cases as falling within three distinct categories: (1) a specific developmental disability "apparently affecting only the acquisition of skills movement"; (2) minimal cerebral palsy; and (3) overall developmental delay including mental retardation. For the developmental disability group (whose primary characteristic was motor clumsiness) individuals were reported to have particular problems with handwriting, completing puzzles, tying shoes, being untidy in appearance, difficulty throwing and catching balls, difficulties with buttons, and problems chewing.

Following these early case studies, ADLs, as they related to the clumsy child syndrome, received limited attention. Then, in a series of papers, Gubbay (1975, 1978, 1979, 1985) provided a clear picture of the functional challenges faced by these children. He noted problems with manipulation skills such as opening doorknobs and door handles; self care skills such as dressing, manipulating fasteners, hair combing, tooth brushing, and washing; and feeding skills such as using cutlery, keeping food on the plate and avoiding knocking over glasses. In addition, he noted the impact of these motor difficulties on school performance in the areas of handwriting; limited playground motor skills; and decreased participation in gym class and sports.

In summary, early research in the area of clumsiness in children consistently identified deficits in performance of daily life tasks as a primary feature of the motor coordination disorder. This was in contrast to the motor execution or quality of movement problems seen with other motor disorders such as cerebral palsy, ataxia, or brain damage. Problems in daily life tasks were found to fall within three general areas: self-care, home- and school-related tasks, and leisure/play skills. Difficulties in these areas are routinely recognized by clinicians working with children with DCD and have been noted in numerous case reports and clinical summaries on children with DCD and motor coordination problems (Ayres, 1979; Cermak, 1985, 1991; Dawdy, 1981; Wall et al., 1990). Although research on specific aspects of functional daily living skills has been conducted on children with other motor impairments such as cerebral palsy, spina bifida, and head injury, empirical research in this area on children with motor coordination problems and DCD in particular is extremely limited.

DEVELOPMENTAL MANIFESTATIONS OF DAILY LIVING SKILLS IN DCD

Children with DCD often manifest different patterns of motor and functional skills at different ages and stages of development. Consistent across ages is a reported impairment in the quality and efficiency with which these children complete daily living tasks. A. Jean Ayres (1979, 1985) described the functional difficulties of children with dyspraxia. She reported that they often perform some skills later than peers do, and that even when tasks are accomplished at the expected age, they are often done so inefficiently. She aptly described the constant frustration that can occur from trying to master new daily living tasks and frequently encountering failure.

Coster and Haley (1992) stated that, in evaluating the performance of tasks, it was necessary to determine what qualities best represented function. They indicated that the ability to initiate activities at the correct time in the correct situation and with sufficient frequency was important. In addition, the ability to complete tasks in the required amount of time without interference from undesirable or inappropriate behaviors was important in determining a child's independence and success in completing daily living skills. Frequently, children with DCD not only are unable to complete some tasks, but more often have difficulties in quality of motor production and task completion as identified by Coster and Haley.

The Infant, Toddler, and Preschool Child

Michael was born two weeks early, but was considered to be a full-term birth. He was a docile baby whose milestones appeared to be within the expected range, with the exception of learning to walk at 18 months of age. In addition, he did not go through a period of putting his toes in his mouth, which is typical of children at 8–10 months of age. He was content to lie on his back, but he did not explore his body in this position. His parent's first concerns centered on his delayed walking and the limited repertoire of foods that he would eat as a toddler. He seemed to have a difficult time handling any mixture of textures and tended to avoid foods that he needed to chew. As he learned to walk, he tended to bump into things readily and would fall more often than his peers. When he was 2½, his mother noted that he did not seem to anticipate what to do with his body as other children in his playgroup did. If he desired help in jumping off of a bench, he might reach for his mother's hands, but would fall forward into her rather than truly jumping. When he was 3 years of age, she noted that, when she gave him a regular glass to drink from, instead of his usual cup with a spout, he did not know how to bring the cup to his lips or move his mouth to try and drink from it. Despite his lack of experience drinking from a cup, it was striking that he had such little awareness of how to approach this unfamiliar task.

Although motoric dysregulation has been noted in infancy and toddlerhood (Zero to Three, 1994), the DCD diagnosis is rarely used, as it is necessary to achieve an age where competency in motor tasks is expected before dysfunction is diagnosed. In addition, achievement of motor milestones and early functional skills are highly variable which can make assessments for this age group highly unreliable (Parham, 1986). In a longitudinal study of normal and mild neurologically dysfunctional infants, Touwen (1993) found that there was broad variation of ranges in functional development among both groups. No fixed time schedules for developmental phases were noted and, in the same child, the early development of one skill (e.g., sitting) might be followed by the late development of another (e.g., walking). It was noted, however, as described in the case at the beginning of this section, that the infants were typically clumsy and had decreased smoothness or accuracy of movements. Mild neurological signs that did not result in overt handicaps (e.g., cerebral palsy) primarily characterized these infants.

Ishpanovich-Radoikovich (1993) suggested that no diagnosis of dyspraxia be given until age 4 or 5, when the child enters school, because of the variability of emotional immaturity and psychomotor skills in this age group. Miller (1993), however, has developed a screening tool, The First Step, to assess praxis and ADLs in 2.9–6.2-year-olds. Miller developed this assessment because she believes that it is important to identify children as early as possible who may be at risk for DCD and other developmental problems, so that intervention may be offered to minimize the impact of the problems on later skill development. Infants and young children with motor coordination problems and suspected DCD may demonstrate problems in qualitative aspects of motor performance involving motoric interaction with the environment, exploration of objects, ease of manipulation of objects, and movements from one position to another (Jirgal & Bourna, 1989; Parham, 1986). These children, who may also master motor milestones more slowly and perform them less consistently than other children, may later be diagnosed as having DCD. For the infant, toddler and preschooler, motor coordination problems most often affect the development of self-care and play skills. In the next sections, problems that often are observed clinically will be described.

Self-Care Development

Jennifer's mother describes that she and her husband have always been "on duty" from when Jennifer awakens until she goes to sleep at night. Since she was an infant, Jennifer has required assistance in meeting her needs. Due to Jennifer's limited stamina and endurance for motor activities, her parents pushed Jennifer in the stroller for a much longer period than other children. As her mother describes it, "Everything was more of an effort." The parents continued to perform tasks for Jennifer or to support her for longer than they had expected, "to do things that with a regular kid you would give up earlier."

In infancy, self-care skills involve both the child's ability to make his or her needs known, and to begin to actively engage in activities that will help meet those needs. It may be difficult for an infant to coordinate the movements required to suck his/her thumb for self-calming and soothing. Reaching for a pacifier, a stuffed animal, or a toy for comfort may be similarly problematic. Early feeding skills may be compromised in the infant with motor coordination problems, as it may be difficult for the infant to master the suck, swallow, and breathing patterns required for bottle drinking or nursing for both nutrition and calming (Oetter, Richter, & Frick, 1988).

As the child matures into toddlerhood, the task of feeding becomes more complex as the child actively tries to grasp and place food in the mouth, reach for and drink from a bottle or cup, and begin to use a spoon to scoop food. Children with DCD experience a great deal of difficulty not only in using utensils but also in expressing their needs to figure out what to do and how to begin to get what they want. The child may tend to eat all foods with his or her hands rather than attempt the use of utensils. The child may rely on use of a cup with a spout rather than mastering an open cup. The child may have difficulty eating a mixture of textures and may also have difficulty chewing foods. As increased independence occurs in eating, the child may be reluctant to try and pour liquids from a pitcher or milk carton into a cup and, in addition, may have difficulty with the preschool task of clearing his or her plate and cup from the table.

The young child may also have difficulty with dressing and pre-dressing skills. The toddler with DCD may not assist in dressing by lifting the arms up or extending the foot and leg. A typically developing toddler will frequently voice that he or she would like to "do it all by myself" and will attempt dressing and manipulation of fasteners that are somewhat beyond the child's capabilities. A child with DCD will often prefer to be helped and, when required to dress independently, will have more difficulty with what clothes to put on first, the placement of clothes on the body, and the appropriate body awareness for the adjustment of socks and shoes. Learning to use fasteners can be particularly difficult. Buttoning, zipping, snapping, and shoe tying can all be delayed. In some cases, the child may lack the physical strength needed for these tasks; in other cases, the sequence of movements needed to complete the task (e.g., buttoning and tying) is difficult to master.

In the preschooler, there may be signs of DCD when the child is learning to bathe and brush teeth, although these tasks aren't expected to be independent until the child reaches school age. They may also experience difficulty with becoming independent in toileting, having difficulty with wiping and with clothing management associated with toileting. Any task that relies heavily on a sound awareness of body scheme, such as wiping after toileting, hair combing, and tooth brushing, are frequently delayed. Many self-care skills emerge during the toddler and preschool age; consequently, it is an important time to compare children with suspected DCD to those of typically developing peers (Shepherd et al., 1996).

Research on the impact of motor coordination problems, and DCD specifically, on self-care skills in young children is very limited, although this area is well studied in populations of more frank motor impairment such as cerebral palsy. Only a few studies have looked at children with predominately mild motor coordination problems. Case-Smith (1995) examined the relationship of foundational fine motor coordination skills to functional self-care skills in motor delayed children (which included primarily developmental delays but also some children with cerebral palsy, mental retardation, and Fragile X). She found no relationship between children's performance on foundational fine motor skills and self-care skills such as eating, although there was a relationship with social function and play.

Play Skills Development

Nisha was "floppy," and she reached developmental milestones more slowly than did her older brother. She did not reach for objects from the supported sitting position, and she did not explore her surroundings without help from others. As she got older, Nisha did not experiment with toys and objects around her, as is typical of infants and toddlers, and she did not develop age-appropriate skill and competency in playing with these toys. When she was old enough to go to the playground, Nisha required constant supervision to remain safe. Her mother relates that, while other parents sat on benches and chatted among themselves, she and her husband needed to be right next to Nisha so that Nisha did not fall, walk into the path of swings, or otherwise become injured. Nisha's mother felt that Nisha wanted to do things and could plan the steps, but she could not "get it going." Her mother felt that Nisha had trouble initiating the task in order to accomplish the desired activity.

Competency in play skills reflects an important daily living skill achievement for the developing child. Development of play skills in typical children has been well-documented (American Occupational Therapy Association, 1986; Chandler, 1997; Hughes, 1995; Leipold & Bundy, 2000; Piaget 1963; Reilly, 1974). Play skills for toddlers and preschoolers involve imitation, exploration of objects and the environment, as well as manipulation and combining of objects using both gross and fine motor activities (Morrison, Metzger, & Pratt, 1996). Motor coordination problems in the developing child can significantly impact on the development of play skills. Frequently, toddlers and preschoolers are noted to have delays in riding a push toy, peddling a bike, and pumping a swing.

As was reported to be true for Nisha, young children with motor coordination difficulties or DCD are often less precise in their body movements, resulting in an awkward appearance (Jirgal & Bourna, 1989; Parham, 1986). As they begin to use their arms, they are often observed to reach ineffectively into their environments, if they even reach for objects. They may request adult assistance, verbally or by pulling the adult's hand, in order to hold and play with toys. They may not readily understand how to navigate around the environment; for example, they may crawl over an adult's legs to secure a toy, instead of going around the adult's legs. They may not have the sensory awareness of their own body scheme to draw upon in planning such actions. Consequently, their own exploration of toys, objects, and people is less independent and they receive less feedback from their actions. Since this feedback, which is thought to be important to motor learning, is diminished, the development of mature and consistent motor patterns leading to skill is also delayed.

Infants and toddlers with suspected DCD often prefer to be held and carried, remaining visual observers of their world in situations where peers would actively explore. When they do explore, it may be more random and with less focus. Spangler (1984 cited in Losche, 1990) describes a sequence of development for four types of action differing in complexity: (1) the action-effect contingency, for example, banging and hitting; (2) the action with continuous effect, for example, pulling a toy, pushing a chair; (3) the separation of action and effect, for example, throwing or kicking a ball, throwing a toy; (4) action aimed at a goal (multiple steps to a goal), for example, building a tower, placing puzzle pieces in a puzzle. For toddlers and preschoolers with suspected DCD, they are often observed to have difficulty moving to the last stage, remaining at the stage of throwing objects, often with too much force due to poor sensory awareness from their muscles and joints, causing social difficulties in play groups and preschool.

Preschool age children often rely on adults to structure play situations, as the children have problems either conceptualizing the activity they wish to play or actually initiating and following through on the steps involved in their chosen game. For example, they may pull the adult to hold and manipulate a toy they want or, as is often observed, they may choose to line up toys, rather than to engage in creative games of pretend. When they do master an activity they often repeat that very same activity, with little variation in the themes. As older preschool children enter group situations, their lack of flexibility becomes even more apparent, with the child often requiring or demanding control of the game or withdrawing to the sidelines, while the other children give and take more freely. Sharing and turn taking often are more difficult than is expected at this age. A frequent result is anxiety when group situations are imminent, as when friends and families arrive for playgroup.

Although play skills have been examined among many groups of children with overt motor or cognitive deficits, little research has been conducted regarding the impact of impaired motor coordination skills on the development of play skills in young children. One study by Puderbaugh and Fisher (1992) examined the play skills of children with developmental dyspraxia between the ages of 12 and 54 months. They examined the qualitative aspects of play and found that the children with motor coordination delays had poorer play skills than typical peers in the areas of motor skills (including skills such as reaching, moving, and manipulating objects) and in process skills (including skills such as sequencing, organizing, and investigating objects and actions).

As children begin to participate in more structured academic programs, their parents frequently mention social skills as a major area of concern (Cohn, Miller, & Tickle-Degnen, 2000). The children often have trouble with "personal space," that is, stepping on other children in their games and on materials with which they are working. They may be a safety risk to themselves and to others. Many parents of children with DCD remark that their children are less frequently sought out for play dates outside of school. They feel this is due to the difficulty their children have with the "give and take" of play activities and with the fact that they often inadvertently hurt other children or destroy their projects due to clumsiness, less predictable movements, and inappropriate use of force.

The School-Aged Child

As a third grader, Pedro stated he did not like school. When questioned further, he said that he hated handwriting and gym class, but that he liked recess and lunch. His classroom teacher found him to have slow, labored, often illegible handwriting, and she noted that he often fell into the role of class clown. He was clumsy by nature, but would exaggerate this and make it into a joke in front of the other children. His physical education teacher noted that he had more difficulty learning new motor skills and games than other children, and that his peers saw him as less competent, often choosing him last for team sports. His parents noted that he was highly verbal and tended to have friends who were highly verbal but less coordinated than their peers. Their activity of choice was to play computer games for hours on end. Getting dressed in the morning was always a chore, with Pedro needing many reminders and a long time to get dressed. Pedro also had difficulty following through on his chores.

As the child with DCD reaches school age, his or her problems with motor coordination broaden to affect their performance of tasks in school and community environments. There are increased demands for independence at home and at school. Social interactions become more complex, and more refined motor skills are required for play and sports activities. Many clinical descriptors of this population of children with motor coordination problems are available, but empirical research on their performance of specific daily living skills is limited (Cermak, 1985; Dawdy, 1981; Fox & Lent, 1996; Hoare, 1994). These children are described as often falling down, bumping into things, knocking things over, being unable to "keep up" in physical play, and having problems with fine motor manipulations such as writing, buttoning, and tying shoes (Dawdy, 1981). Managing their bodies and cognitively planning many activities that others perform automatically consumes a great deal of energy. It can be difficult to have energy and focus left for attending to the increasing complexity of social interaction.

Problems in motor coordination, and the subsequent impact on daily life skills, take a toll on other aspects of the life of the child with DCD. O'Dwyer (1987) found that 11-year-old boys with motor coordination problems were less outgoing, less emotionally stable, less tough-minded and self-reliant, less shrewd and calculating, less self-assured, and more introverted, and had lower self esteem and poorer peer acceptance than their more coordinated peers. Similarly, Schoemaker and Kalverboer (1994) found that clumsy children were more anxious, had low self-concept, were more insecure and isolated, and were less competent in social and physical skills than their peers. Koomar (1996) also found that anxiety co-occurred with dyspraxia for 5- to 13-year-old children, with a greater degree of anxiety manifesting with more severe dyspraxia.

These problems have been reported to affect the child with DCD's skill performance across many areas of daily life functioning. Gubbay (1979) noted problems in school and the classroom, sports, and household chores. Cermak (1985) noted difficulties with self-care skills and sports. Dawdy (1981) indicated difficulties in the areas of eating, dressing, household and school tasks, and play. However, empirical research on the specific ages at which many of these specific tasks should be mastered and the percentages of typical children who have mastered these skills is limited, making identification of delays in these areas very subjective. Clinically, however, parents frequently report that the school-aged child with DCD demonstrates functional motor difficulties in four main areas: management of self-care skills, home activities and chores, school-related tasks, and play and sports-related activities.

Self-Care Skills

Ching Lee's mother noted her daughter's difficulty in dressing, shoe tying, and performing hygiene activities. Although she mastered these skills, it took her longer than most children and she required more teaching and practice. Her parents needed to help Ching Lee brush her teeth; no structure or routine seemed to adequately help her sequence the steps and actually perform the motor components of tooth brushing. While she improved in her ability to brush her teeth, Ching Lee continued to require parental involvement for this self-care activity. Toileting has also been a particular problem, especially cleansing after toileting.

At home, mealtime skills often present particular difficulties for the child with DCD. Using eating utensils, especially cutting meat into small pieces, is a troublesome and very persistent problem for children with DCD. Usually, merely picking up food on a spoon or fork is mastered by school age, although cutting food remains difficult for the children (Gubbay, 1985; Hoare, 1994). Similarly, putting salt on their food (in the right proportions), drinking milk without spilling, and serving food for themselves are daunting tasks that often result in failure or frustration for the children and their families (Gubbay, 1979). They also have difficulty with setting the table, assisting with measuring during cooking, coordinating switching from chewing to talking during meals, and noticing that food is on their faces after meals. Dressing issues often continue, particularly managing fasteners, and learning the several steps to tie shoes can be very difficult (Hoare, 1994). Overall, they often remain slow at dressing and eating even when skills appear to be adequate.

With increasing age, more is expected of the child in terms of independence with hygiene skills, for example, thoroughness in hair washing, toothbrushing, bathing, fingernail cutting, hair combing, and brushing. Children with DCD are often noted to have difficulty in these areas (Gubbay, 1985). While early development of many self-care skills is well documented and developmental scales are available for young children, ages of expected proficiency among older children for more independent performance of these tasks is not readily available. Specific empirical research on the performance of these life tasks by children with DCD in comparison with typical peers is almost nonexistent. In addition, although frequently clinically reported to be a problem for this population, the percentage of children with DCD who exhibit problems in specific areas has rarely been examined. In one study of school-aged children with dyspraxia, 71% of the population had problems with tying shoes and using utensils, 67% were reported by their parents to be messy eaters, and 46% had difficulty with dressing or fasteners (May-Benson, 1999). These results suggested that a substantial portion of school-aged children with dyspraxia continue to exhibit problems with self-care skills.

Home Management Skills

Alex's lack of independence necessitated his parents' constant vigilance. As they reported it, "we needed to think about everything." Commonplace tasks, including getting in and out of the car, required supervision to avoid injury and to minimize the frustration both Alex and his parents experienced as a result of his difficulty mastering and independently completing functional tasks. He also had difficulty with chores that had been expected of his older brother at the same age, such as setting the table, making his bed, hanging up his coat, putting dirty clothes in the hamper, and feeding the cat.

Many parents report that enforcing house rules about completing chores is abandoned with children who have DCD. It is just too hard to follow through with the supervision and reminders to finish the jobs. They realize that most tasks require more time and energy for the child with DCD, so that, although they want to have the same expectations as for siblings without DCD, it is not necessarily realistic to maintain the same expectations. Families often focus first on the most essential tasks, such as establishing routines for completing homework, and developing an organizational system for the child's room so that clothing and other objects can be located without extreme frustration. Development of a chore list often is done with a focus on completion of chores that best fit with the child's capabilities, such as taking out the trash, helping to load and unload the washer and dryer. It is often recommended to minimize chores that require more precise planning and skill for the child with more severe DCD.

Social, Leisure, and Play Skills

As a school-aged child, delayed development of Paul's play skills was especially frustrating to his father. While he did have coordination difficulties and he required help getting some activities started, his father felt that there were also times that Paul could perform a task or play a game by himself, but instead he requested help and would not play alone. He confided that, "Everything could be an ordeal." Teaching play skills and making up stories about play activities, however, was tremendously helpful in expanding Paul's repertoire of play themes and choices. He began to consult his special book of play stories for ideas and was eventually able to play alone at home.

When children enter school, their difficulties with motor coordination and planning appear in the area of academic performance, as well as in sports and organized group activities. These leisure and sports activities have received more notice from researchers than other areas of daily life skills, and restricted participation in sports is often one of the diagnostic criteria for DCD used by researchers. Poor performance of various gross motor skills such as balancing, throwing and catching a ball, skipping, hopping, or jumping are frequently examined and form the foundation for a DCD diagnosis. Many parents report that their children of school age "are just not sports people." The children do not enjoy physical activities or competition (Adler, 1982). They generally prefer individual sports to group sports, if they pursue them at all, and often seek out younger playmates (Clifford, 1985). For example, they may choose swimming or bike riding, while they avoid soccer, basketball, and baseball.

The most common problems that parents report their children experience during group sports include difficulty following the rules of the game and "spaciness" about where they should be at a given point in the game. For example, the child will often become confused as to which goal is his or her team's goal in soccer and he or she does not know which way to run or to kick the ball. Many children with DCD frequently have difficulty maintaining their own "personal body space" and as a result, they bump into other people and objects. Body movements in space, as in playing soccer, kickball or other running games are difficult to sustain and the children frequently have trouble figuring out where to be and anticipating what might happen next. Other children with DCD seem to anticipate difficulty and they will often sit on the sidelines and even provide excuses as to why they do not wish to play in games. Although there is little research in this area, it appears that the differences in participation could be related to severity of DCD. Koomar and May-Benson (1999) found that children with dyspraxia had less participation in and exhibited less skill in avocational activities, than would be expected of typical peers. They found that both parent and therapist ratings and objective measures of the children's praxis skills were strongly related to the children's participation in avocational activities.

The awkwardness described in sports is also apparent in physical education class. The organized nature of the activities is similarly problematic, and children report that they have to try very hard in order to keep up with their classmates. Gubbay (1975) notes that children with motor coordination problems tend to have repeated truancy from school on physical education day, and Clifford (1985) notes that they often have a history of quitting community-sponsored physical activity programs. Similarly, May-Benson (1999) found that 50% of children with dyspraxia had problems riding a bicycle, 67% had poor ball skills, and 71% had difficulty with sports.

School Skills

His teacher relates, "Billy attempted to paint with his friends, only to spill the paint (on the floor and on his friends) when he reached for it. In his subsequent attempts to wipe up the paint, he tore the paper towel and got the paint on himself, also knocking down the easel in the process. As he tried to right the easel, he pushed it onto another friend, who was understandably upset with this new development. All in all, the experience was an exercise in frustration for him—and his classmates."

Problems in school for the child with DCD manifest in numerous ways, from poor handwriting to poor organizational skills. When children with DCD attempt to complete activities with their peers, their difficulties become even more apparent, as they now have to comply with the structure and "agendas" imposed by other children. Experts who work with children who have DCD note their frequent resistance to change and their accompanying preference and need for structure, routine and predictability. When they work within specific schedules and predictable routines, the children experience more success than when they are required to accommodate unexpected changes or to "go with the flow" in unstructured settings. Their organizational skills are often reported to be problematic, and they require additional strategies to help maintain notebooks for assignments, records of their work, and drafts of their assignments. They frequently have difficulty getting assignments done on time, and homework often takes them longer.

Handling tools and objects used in school, as in manipulating materials for art projects and actually putting together constructional projects (fine motor and visual motor tasks), can be very hard, as many parents, teachers, and students report. Handling objects with the body requires a particular type of coordination and skill, and it can be performed differently than tasks that involve only body movements, separate from the body using tools. Within this category, clinical and empirical reports indicate that the most readily identifiable and most often discussed areas of difficulty for children with DCD are poor handwriting, pencil skills, and drawing skills. Children exert a great deal of effort in the mechanical aspects of writing, such as holding the pencil correctly and moving it in the correct directions to form letters and words. They often report fatigue in these paper/pencil and writing activities and their teacher's report that their work is much less detailed and rich than their verbal descriptions of the same material. A very real concern is that the children expend so much energy as they concentrate on the technical aspects of writing that they have little energy left for the conceptual content they are attempting to master (Cermak, 1991). In addition, case studies and clinical trials have shown that children with DCD have poorer handwriting than their typical peers (Gubbay, 1978, 1979, 1985; Henderson & Hall, 1982; Hoare, 1994). Gubbay found that over 60% of the children with clumsiness in his studies had handwriting problems and nearly half had problems completing homework. Similarly, May-Benson (1999) reported handwriting problems in 71% of a population of dyspraxic children.

Wright and Sugden (1996) found that children with DCD had difficulty with routine motor tasks in the classroom, from writing to passing out papers, to moving about the classroom. They concluded that these motor problems reduced the children's participation in school activities. Similarly, Piek and Edwards (1997) found that difficulties in daily life skills, as identified by classroom and physical education teachers, were an important indicator of motor coordination problems and a subsequent DCD diagnosis. In this study, 25% of children identified by their teacher as having functional problems in the classroom, and 47% of children identified by physical education teachers, were later identified with DCD.

The Adolescent and Young Adult

Despite his pediatrician's early prediction that Sam would outgrow his clumsiness, his parents and Sam noted that this did not occur by the time he graduated from high school. Sam often found ways to skip physical education class in middle school. In high school, where he had choices of physical education classes, he selected noncompetitive classes such as swimming and biking. Although his handwriting had improved some over the years, he took sparse notes in class, tape recording lectures he knew he would need to listen to again. He used a computer at home to word process all of his homework assignments that required written text. One of the greatest challenges for him was taking driver's training. He was highly motivated to learn to drive and gain the independence that would bring, but he had difficulty mastering certain skills such as backing up and parallel parking. It was difficult for him to judge exactly where the car was in space.

For adolescents who were diagnosed with DCD at younger ages, research indicates that those with mild DCD may not have many functional difficulties by adolescence, but those with moderate to severe DCD may continue to manifest functional difficulties later on (Cantell, Smyth, & Ahonen, 1994). Although evidence suggests that many children do not outgrow DCD (Cermak, Trimble, Coryell, & Drake, 1991; Geuze & Borger, 1993), there is also research that suggests that some adolescents may experience improvements in coordination following their growth spurt, perhaps due to enhanced maturation of some parts of the central nervous system (Visser, Geuze, & Kalverboer, 1998). In addition, it is possible that some adolescents with mild DCD may learn to compensate for their problems more effectively than those with more impairment.

When children reach middle school and high school age (roughly ages 11–17) they, and their parents and teachers, tend to report organizational problems in school, at home, and, later, in tasks such as driving. Teachers and parents report that frustration and discouragement are common when children reach middle and high school age. Their effort can diminish as they perceive that their efforts do not "pay off" for them. This frustration can take the form of aggression, anger, or withdrawal for different adolescents (Hay & Missiuna, 1998).

Self-Care Skills

Jack's mother reports that, "He just doesn't seem to care about how he looks. He wears rumpled clothes, his shirts are half-untucked and he never seems to comb his hair. At times, I am concerned that he hasn't bathed properly and may have forgotten to apply deodorant. I know he knows that these things are important, but some mornings it seems difficult for him to maintain his morning routines."

Self-care and leisure tasks, frequently involving tool use, are often reported to be challenging. These activities range from using dental floss, shaving, applying make-up, styling and combing hair to dealing cards, cooking from a recipe, and participating in wood shop or art classes, and a wide variety of other IADLs. Evidence suggests that the motor problems of adolescents with DCD may primarily remain in areas involving manual dexterity (Geuze & Borger, 1993). Parent's report concerns about their children's self-esteem, as a result of needing assistance with personal care activities, such as handling menstruation needs and shaving properly. In addition, they also have concerns about how their children will function when they no longer live at home. Parents have witnessed the difficult transition from grade school to middle school or high school, involving the use of lockers and combination locks, the change of classes and many books and assignments to organize. They are concerned that a move to college or out of the house into an apartment will be a further challenge without their parents there to guide and give assistance as needed.

Home Management Skills

"I know Sarah's a teenager, but can't she at least be responsible for some of the chores around the house without needing to be reminded over and over?" laments Sarah's mother. It has become a huge problem for the family that she requires so much attention and support to complete even the smallest tasks, from household chores to beginning and following through with her homework assignments.

Performing chores at home is a problem similar to others the children experience. They have difficulty following multi-step directions and completing multi-step tasks. They may require frequent reminders, and they tend to "get lost in the middle" of chores. Their parents report that the adolescents are often "daydreaming" or doing something completely different long after the parents expected the chore to be completed. Transitions and schedule changes can remain stressful, as they were in childhood, but the stress now often surfaces around managing time (like completing homework), work schedules, social appointments, and finding one's way around a new environment, which are the types of situations encountered in adolescence and adulthood. More is expected of adolescents, such as handling their own laundry, emptying and loading the dishwasher and washing dishes, mowing the lawn, raking, cooking, and handling small appliances and home office equipment.

School and Vocational Skills

One of Seth's middle school teachers states that Seth "is a good student who would get good grades if I could only get him to take the right books and papers home to do his homework. His in-school work and tests are good, but he's missing a big part of his grade—homework."

Geuze and Borger (1993) cite evidence to suggest that adolescents with DCD may have more frequently repeated a grade by the time they reach middle school, or that they have been placed in a lower level of secondary education than their peers. In addition, they may have more difficulty with concentration and attention, social contacts, and expected classroom behavior. Another study found that adolescents with stable motor problems had lower academic ambitions for their futures (Cantell et al., 1994).

With respect to school organizational skills, getting the right books to each class, as well as home from school, are frequently cited issues by parents. Keeping track of papers and assignments is also a challenge, and the subsequent loss of homework and pertinent class materials often results in poorer grades than would otherwise be achieved. Note taking is often demanding, as the child is attending to the mechanical aspects and may miss the content of the lecture. The organizational difficulties are compounded by unresolved handwriting problems, as is described by students, parents, and teachers. Even students who have mastered the mechanical aspects of writing (e.g., formation, size, and spacing of letters and words; copying from samples) can still have difficulty translating their ideas into written form and/or fatigue with longer assignments. Once again, handwritten assignments are performed with less enthusiasm, thoroughness, and complexity than if the material can be relayed verbally. There are concerns about using a copier, fax machine, or other machines in future jobs that require an understanding of several steps. Psychologists and occupational therapists report that they frequently work with adults in their twenties with repeated job loss who appear to have DCD. In reviewing the histories of these individuals, they find that they often have all of the cognitive skills needed for their vocational area, but they have difficulty in organizing and prioritizing their work. They are often much slower at completing tasks than the job demands, and they have difficulty in working independently.

Social Participation/Leisure/Play Skills

Michelle is a very hard worker in school. She gets very good grades, but most of her free time is spent on homework, giving her little time to participate in after school activities. When she was younger, she enjoyed gymnastics, but as she grew older, the skill level of her peers increased beyond hers, so she stopped taking classes, partly due to embarrassment. When she has time, she likes to hike with her family on the weekends, and her parents are encouraging her to join a local hiking group for teens. Her parents worry that she is somewhat isolated socially, with only one really good friend, but Michelle feels she really doesn't have time to make more friends due to schoolwork demands.

Cantell and colleagues (1994) found that adolescents with persistent motor problems had fewer social hobbies and pastimes than a comparison group of typical peers. There is evidence that adolescents with DCD continue to experience difficulty with sports and any new motor skill (Cermak et al., 1991; Haines, Brown, Grantham, Rajagopalan, & Sutcliffe, 1985; Losse et al., 1991). Further research needs to be done to assess whether or not the adolescent with DCD lacks the motor competence needed to compete at the adolescent level. It is suspected that poorer motor competence interacts with a lack of motivation to continue to engage and practice skills that are difficult (Johnston, Short, & Crawford, 1987; Wall, McClements, Bouffard, Findlay, & Taylor, 1985). Parents often report that, by the time their children with DCD reach high school, they tend to avoid group sports activities and have opted for other activities, such as individual endeavors like biking and swimming.

Safety issues associated with understanding spatial concepts both in the car and even on foot (as in crossing the street) are particular concerns for parents. It is interesting to note that the adolescent frequently perceives that he or she is competent to drive a car, the parents' concerns notwithstanding. Transitions and schedule changes can remain stressful, as they were in childhood, but the stress now often surfaces around managing social, medical, and after-school appointments and finding one's way around a new environment, which are the types of situations encountered in adolescence and adulthood.

ACCOMMODATIONS AND MANAGEMENT OF DAILY LIFE SKILLS IN DCD

As professionals work with persons who have DCD, the interventions they suggest often encompass both direct remediation and indirect adaptations to the environment. Direct intervention is generally provided in individual or group settings and a variety of approaches are employed, prominently among them, occupational or physical therapy, with an emphasis on sensory integration treatment principles as well as mastering specific ADLs and IADLs. Adaptations to the environment are suggested to increase the success children and adolescents with DCD experience in their daily activities. Many such accommodations and strategies have been suggested by researchers and experts in the field (Bissell, Fisher, Owens, & Polcyn, 1993; Levine, 1987; OTA–Watertown, P.C., 1998a, 1998b). A sampling of recommended accommodations and strategies can be found in the Appendix of this book.

SUMMARY AND CONCLUSIONS

It appears that across the age span from infancy to adolescence, individuals with DCD experience difficulties with daily living activities. In infancy, toddlerhood, and the early preschool years, determining whether or not a child differs significantly from peers in motor skill performance can be difficult. The problems may be more in the effectiveness and quality of movement rather than in whether or not the child can complete specific tasks and skills by a certain age. In the later preschool years and early school age years, the problems may become more evident in self-care, school, and play tasks. As the young child grows older, the expectations increase and frustration is experienced when attempting many ADLs. By adolescence, some individuals who experienced mild difficulties earlier in childhood may be able to perform fairly well on daily living tasks, but those with moderate to severe difficulties continue to have trouble with a wide variety of skills, including handwriting and other manual skills, sports, academics, and social activities. Further research is needed in all of the above areas to further delineate the types of problem individuals with DCD experience across the childhood spectrum in individualized ADLs.

C H A P T E R
10

Hand Function and Developmental Coordination Disorder

Jane Case-Smith and Naomi Weintraub

Development of hand function has traditionally been described in the literature according to performance components of hand skill, for example, reach, grasp, release, and bimanual coordination. Analysis of performance components helps to identify reasons for deficits in hand skills. We have approached this topic by identifying and describing the primary hand functions that relate to the occupations of childhood, including play, self-care, and school. The hand functions discussed in this chapter include (1) construction activities, (2) tool use, (3) action on a surface, (4) in-hand manipulation, and (5) handwriting. All of these functions which involve the hand's manipulation of objects may be difficult for the child with developmental coordination disorder (DCD). The first section of this chapter describes these categories of hand function, reviewing development, related performance components, and then associated occupations. The second section of this chapter describes performance problems documented in children with DCD and the implications of those problems for hand function.

CATEGORIES OF HAND FUNCTION

Construction Activities

The child first combines objects in simple ways by placing objects side by side or placing them in a container. The child learns to stack blocks around 12 months of age, and by 2 years, he or she can stack six cubes. The toddler fits simple puzzle pieces into their correct form spaces and places pegs in pegholes. These skills rapidly improve such that by preschool age, the child is building elaborate structures, can copy three dimensional designs made with blocks and can put together puzzles with interlocking pieces (Gesell et al., 1940).

The sensory-motor-perceptual performance components that define a child's ability to construct are listed in Tables 10.1 and 10.2. Construction activities require precision grasp, accurate placement of the object, and precision release. In most construction activities, the child carries objects, maintaining a stable grasp of the object while moving his or her shoulder and elbow. The object is generally released without stabilizing the proximal arm on a surface, for example a block is released on top of other blocks. Construction activities involve both hands moving reciprocally and/or simultaneously. Actions are planned and sequenced to create structures that match the child's goal.

Visual perception is a primary contributing component of construction. The integration of visual motor skills enables the child to create three-dimensional structures from a model or from memory. A good understanding of spatial orientation and spatial relations is matched to the motor skills to enable the child to position and place objects in containers or next to, on top of, behind, or in front of objects. Haptic perception is needed to identify shapes that fit together, on top of, or within each other. Accurate use of force is needed to stack or fit objects together. Cognition is also needed to plan or sequence movement so that the goal is achieved. In addition, construction play is pursued only when the child has a vision or image of the structure he or she is attempting to create.

A child needs construction skills in many play and school activities. Projects at school involve assembly; for example, completing puzzles and buildings are part of science and math. These skills are later important to adults in housekeeping, cooking, and vocations that include assembling, building, or maintaining work or living spaces. The preschool child with motor difficulties tends to avoid these fine motor skills and the limited experience can contribute to long-term difficulties with hand skill development (Cermak, 1991).

Tool Use

Tool use is a primary hand function that involves using a utensil or tool to act on self or the environment. Infants use tools at early ages (e.g., 10–12 months) to bang, make sounds, or cause other objects to move (Connolly & Dalgleish, 1989). In the child's first use of a tool, he or she holds the tool using a static palmer grasp and moves it from the shoulder. By 12 months, the infant hits a spoon on the surface of his or her high chair. By 1½–2 years, the child bangs with a hammer or a stick on a xylophone. Although striking continues, the child begins to use tools in more refined ways. Two-year-olds experiment with drawing by scribbling with crayons or markers (Folio & Fewell, 2000). By 3 years, the child may demonstrate a static tripod grasp with the marker and is making lines and circles on paper. He or she copies horizontal and vertical lines, and can copy a cross (Gesell et al., 1940).

The preschooler uses a tool for a much different purpose and with much greater precision than the infant and toddler. Now the tool is used in drawing or creating forms and shapes. The 3-year-old child also learns to use tools that move within the

Table 10.1 Motor Components of Hand Functions

Performance Components

Hand Functions	Proximal (Shoulder) Stability	Proximal (Shoulder) Mobility	Precision Grasp: Fingertip Prehension	Precision Release	Isolated Finger Use	Thumb Stability and Strength	Blended Grasp	Graded Force	Motor Planning	Motor Sequencing
Construction activities	Ranges from sometimes to often related	Appears to be essential to hand function	Appears to be essential to hand function	Appears to be essential to hand function	Ranges from sometimes to often related	Ranges from sometimes to often related	—	Appears to be essential to hand function	Appears to be essential to hand function	Appears to be essential to hand function
Tool use	Ranges from sometimes to often related	Appears to be essential to hand function	Appears to be essential to hand function	—	Appears to be essential to hand function	Appears to be essential to hand function	Appears to be essential to hand function	Appears to be essential to hand function	Appears to be essential to hand function	Ranges from sometimes to often related
Action on a surface	Ranges from sometimes to often related	—	Ranges from sometimes to often related	Open hand is needed	Appears to be essential to hand function	Appears to be essential to hand function	—	Appears to be essential to hand function	—	Appears to be essential to hand function
Gathering and holding: In-hand manipulation	Ranges from sometimes to often related	—	Ranges from sometimes to often related	—	Appears to be essential to hand function	Appears to be essential to hand function	Appears to be essential to hand function	Appears to be essential to hand function	—	Ranges from sometimes to often related
Handwriting	Ranges from sometimes to often related	—	Ranges from sometimes to often related	—	Appears to be essential to hand function	Appears to be essential to hand function	Ranges from sometimes to often related	Appears to be essential to hand function	Appears to be essential to hand function	Appears to be essential to hand function

Table 10.2 Sensory and Perceptual Components of Hand Functions

| Hand Functions | Performance Components | | | |
	Visual Perception	Tactile Discrimination	Kinesthesia/ Proprioception	Visual Motor Integration
Construction activities	Appears to be essential to hand function	Ranges from sometimes to often related	Appears to be essential to hand function	Appears to be essential to hand function
Tool use	Ranges from sometimes to often related	Ranges from sometimes to often related	Appears to be essential to hand function	Ranges from sometimes to often related
Action on a surface	—	Appears to be essential to hand function	Appears to be essential to hand function	Initially— when learning
In-hand manipulation	—	Appears to be essential to hand function	Appears to be essential to hand function	—
Handwriting	Appears to be essential to hand function	Ranges from sometimes to often related	Appears to be essential to hand function	Appears to be essential to hand function

hand (e.g., scissors). Cutting with scissors requires that one hand open and close the blades. The child demonstrates a blended grasp in which the ulnar fingers are stable and the radial fingers control the tool. As cutting skills develop, he or she uses this blended grasping pattern with appropriate force to open and close the blades while maintaining the paper within them. The child also develops the eye-hand coordination needed to guide the scissors along a line. By 4 years, the child moves the marker or pencil using intrinsic muscles. Intrinsic muscles are critical to precise pen or pencil use because they function to provide the finger stability and mobility necessary to apply appropriate force in writing and drawing. The sensory-motor-perceptual performance components that contribute to tool use are listed in Tables 10.1 and 10.2.

Tool use is an aspect of human performance that crosses the life span. Children and adults use tools that require coordination of arm and hand together (e.g., those for grooming and eating) and that require power with force applied through the shoulder (e.g., hammer and heavy tool use). Handwriting requires precise tool use with actions of the fingers sequenced and planned. Handwriting is learned through kinesthetic and visual systems. Feedback from both systems is essential for error correction and legible handwriting. The efficiency of these systems is also associated with speed. Because handwriting is associated with perceptual and cognitive performance, it is categorized as a unique hand function and is discussed in detail later. Given the complexity of the skill, it is not surprising that handwriting difficulties are experienced by some children with DCD (Mæland, 1992).

Action on a Surface

Keyboarding and use of a computer are important skills for children and adults. Actions on a surface refer to simple tapping finger movements or complex handling, such as buttoning or fastening, where the hand acts on a surface, pushing or moving an object without fully grasping or holding the object. The infant first demonstrates actions on a surface pushing and hitting the levers or buttons on busy boxes and interactive toys that produce music, sounds, or visual effects. Toys for 1- and 2-year-olds that require action on a surface are toy pianos or typewriters. Although little is known about the developmental sequence of action on a surface in children with DCD, observations of typical children show that initially children use their palms or fists to press objects. By one year, they use their fingertips, usually together as a unit. The 15–18-month-old toddler uses an isolated, extended index finger for pointing and pressing. Children vary in their preference for using one or several fingers to act on a surface. Use of isolated movements of all fingers to keyboard often does not develop until children are in 4th or 5th grade when they are formally exposed to these activities.

The components required for efficient keyboarding are listed in Tables 10.1 and 10.2. Action on a surface requires that the upper body and proximal arm remain relatively stable while the fingers are active. Because effective action on a surface involves isolated finger movements, the intrinsic muscles are used. The most efficient keyboarding skills involve movements initiated from the metacarpal-phalangeal joints (MCPs). Because the movement is rapid and often forceful, both stability and mobility at the MCPs are important.

Vision is instrumental to the initial learning to keyboard. Similar to handwriting, once learned, keyboarding appears to relate more to kinesthetic input and less to visual input. However, by observing young children use the keyboard, it is apparent that they use their eyes frequently (Rogers, 1999). Action on a surface when performed rapidly is planned ahead and relies on predictive feedback to refine or correct the movements. When the goal is word processing, cognitive components, including language and memory are important to performance. In efficient keyboarding, the hands move sequentially and simultaneously. These complex movement patterns may pose difficulty for children with DCD when learning to keyboard.

In-Hand Manipulation

The fourth hand activity, in-hand manipulation involves moving objects within the hand. Primary categories of in-hand manipulation are rotation of the object within the fingers and translation of objects in and out of the hand (e.g., moving from finger tips to palm and palm to finger tips). In-hand manipulation is observed first in the 1-year-old who simply adjusts a cracker or toy within his or her hand by pushing it outward or bringing it more into the palm. By 2 years, the simplest in-hand manipulation is observed, that is, bringing one or two objects into the palm. At this age, the child also exhibits simple rotation (i.e., turning the lid of a jar). These skills require isolated movements of the fingers. Between 3 and 4 years, the child demonstrates more complex patterns in which the fingers move sequentially to rotate the object (Pehoski, 1995). This sequential, isolated movement enables the child to rotate a pen or pick up multiple objects and hold them in his or her hand. Exner (1992, 2000) indicated that most of the complex in-hand manipulation patterns are performed by 4- and 5-year-olds. However, these skills continue to develop, becoming increasingly efficient until children reach preadolescence.

The sensory-motor-perceptual components of in-hand manipulation are listed in Tables 10.1 and 10.2. Wrist and palmar stability provide a base for the rapid isolated movement of fingers. Intrinsic muscles need to be well developed so that MCPs are stable and mobile and can simultaneously hold and move an object. The thumb is instrumental in most in-hand manipulation and must be stable when opposing the fingertips.

Pehoski (1995) indicated that appropriate application of force which can be difficult for children with DCD (Lundy-Ekman, Ivry, Keele, & Woollacott, 1991), is essential to in-hand manipulation. The object must be held with sufficient force so that it is not dropped but also light enough so that it can be moved within the hand. This just-right amount of force requires accurate perception of touch and kinesthesia; as these senses guide the hand's use of force. In-hand manipulation, when compared to the other hand activities described, involves minimal visual perception. At the same time, it is probably the hand activity most directly linked to somatosensory input and use of force.

In-hand manipulation is needed in most daily activities. Efficient handling of keys, coins, and other materials involves complex in-hand manipulation. In self-care activities, individuals open containers and manipulate small objects within the hand. Most vocational and avocational tasks include materials handling requiring these skills. It is important that problems in in-hand manipulation are identified and remediated early so that the child with DCD has positive experiences and develops movement confidence in these life-long motor skills.

Handwriting

Although handwriting builds on previously learned tool use and drawing skills, it is strongly associated with language and cognition. In addition to new levels of dexterity and visual motor integration, the child learns to write only if he or she is interested in letters and words and is learning to read. Even with these interests, children with DCD can become frustrated in their efforts to write.

Alston and Taylor (1987) documented the development of handwriting as a graphomotor skill. By 3 years, a child has learned to use a crayon or marker to scribble and make lines and circles. The 4-year-old copies a circle and the 5-year-old a square and triangle. Beery (1989) indicated that children who consistently copied diagonal lines correctly were ready to make simple printed letters. The 5-year-old draws a person with multiple parts. By 6 and 7 years, the figures drawn are contoured rather than constructed of multiple parts and are inclusive of all body parts known to the child (Ziviani, 1995). These drawing skills are an important foundation for handwriting skills.

A 5-year-old is very interested in copying and tracing printed letters. By 6 years, children can print their name and copy all letters. Many have learned to write the alphabet. As motor and perceptual abilities improve and enable the child to form letters with a crayon or marker, preliteracy skills, attention span, cognition, and memory enable him or her to attach letter forms (graphemes) to sounds.

Models of the handwriting process using an information processing framework reflect the complexity of this skill and imply that handwriting requires the orchestration of linguistic, cognitive, sensory, and motor skills (Ellis, 1982, 1988; Margolin, 1984; van Galen, 1991). When compared to the other hand activities, handwriting is unique in that it uses an orthographic system or the brain's graphic representation of letters or word. Writers need to have an intact representation of the alphabet letters relevant to their language, maintained in a long-term memory storage. In response to a visual or phonological cue, these codes are retrieved and stored in a working memory, while writers retrieve the appropriate allographs required for writing a specific word or letter. The allographs are a specification of letter forms, namely, upper- or lower-case letters, manuscript, or cursive form. Once an allograph is selected, the writer needs to generate or retrieve from a long-term memory an abstract motor plan for executing the specific allograph (Weintraub & Graham, 2000). This is followed by the recruitment of the movements used in writing. Handwriting requires high levels of motor control, including the smooth execution of a structured sequence of coordinated movements, working under precise temporal and spatial constraints (Thomassen & Teulings, 1983).

Sensory components that contribute to handwriting include visual and tactile/kinesthetic systems. The role of the visual and kinesthetic systems is to monitor the hand's movement when writing and to compare it with the sensory image of previous movement stored in memory. When a mismatch occurs between visual and kinesthetic systems, motor commands are generated to correct the movement (Copley & Ziviani, 1990; Meulenbroek & van Galen, 1988). The visual and kinesthetic systems each provide different types of information and have a different role in the feedback process; together they influence the quality and the fluency of handwriting. Difficulty with handwriting performance may be a result of a breakdown at one or more of these stages of handwriting.

HAND FUNCTION AND SENSORY AND PERCEPTUAL PROBLEMS IN CHILDREN WITH DCD

Specific performance components (kinesthesic, visual, cross-modal matching, and motor control) are associated with each of the hand functions, giving therapists a method for analyzing these hand functions in children with DCD. The following section describes the sensory-motor-perceptual problems that influence hand function in children with DCD. Each performance component is described using the research literature of children with DCD and then is related to the hand functions described above.

Hand Function and Kinesthetic Perception

Perceptual impairments have been associated with the fine motor difficulties of children with DCD (Laszlo & Bairstow, 1984, 1985a, 1989; Lord & Hulme, 1982; Piek & Coleman-Carman, 1995). Laszlo and her colleagues defined kinesthesis as the critical defining perceptual problem of DCD. Despite their strong belief in the importance of kinesthetic perception to movement and motor planning, the results of studies that have compared kinesthetic ability in children with and without DCD have been inconclusive.

Hulme, Smart, Moran, and Raine (1983) and Lord and Hulme (1987) did not find a difference in kinesthesis between groups of children with and without DCD. Smyth and Glencross (1986) found that children with DCD processed visual information at a normal rate, and processed kinesthesia slowly. In a more recent study, Piek and Coleman-Carman (1995) found differences in kinesthetic sensitivity (Laszlo & Bairstow, 1985b) in children with DCD. In their sample, kinesthetic sensitivity correlated with performance on the Movement ABC (Henderson & Sugden, 1992). Children with DCD made more errors on the perception and memory test (with stylus passively moved along a pattern), indicating that children with DCD may have difficulty in visual-kinesthetic integration or mental rotation as the test involves both these elements. Although studies regarding kinesthetic perception are equivocal, clinicians report problems that suggest kinesthetic difficulties in children with DCD (e.g., appropriate modulation of force).

Kinesthetic perception contributes to performance of most hand functions. Kinesthesis with touch provides the sensory information that guides the hand's movements when holding small objects or a tool. The hand functions that appear to be most associated with kinesthetic accuracy are tool use and in-hand manipulation.

When tool use involves precise and rapid movement, immediate feedback from kinesthesis appears to be primary, with error correction from vision as secondary. Specifically, the force used and the accuracy of movement patterns appear highly related to kinesthetic perception (Eliasson, 1995). When tools are used with precision (e.g., a pencil for handwriting) the kinesthetic system is active in providing feedback for error correction.

In-hand manipulation appears to use feedback from the fingers' movement to adjust force and motor patterns of the fingers. The accuracy of the fingers in rotating and moving small objects depends on the acuity of the kinesthetic system. Kinesthesis is believed to play an important role in legible handwriting (Alston & Taylor, 1987; Benbow, 1995). Kinesthetic perception is required for setting the correct overall force level to the writing implement and via the implement to the writing surface (Van Galen, Meulenbroek, & Hylkema, 1986). This system provides information regarding directionality and size of letters (Laszlo & Bairstow, 1984).

Kinesthesis appears to be related to pencil grip (Levine, 1987; Schneck, 1991). Levine, Oberklaid, and Meltzer (1981) found that 20 of 26 students with DCD had awkward grasping patterns. Half of these students showed evidence of finger agnosia, as measured by an imitative finger movement and a finger differentiation tasks. In a study that compared the pencil grip of first-grade students with good and poor handwriting skills, Schneck (1991) found that students with poor handwriting and poor kinesthetic awareness demonstrated immature pencil grip patterns.

Kinesthetic awareness appears to relate to qualitative aspects of handwriting. Berninger and Rutberg (1992) studied the performance of 300 students in grades 1–3 on various finger tasks that required kinesthetic perception. Finger tasks consistently related to handwriting fluency. Kinesthetic ability also related to handwriting accuracy in a study by Tseng and Murray (1994). These researchers compared kinesthesis (using the Imitative Finger Movement subtest of the PEERAMID and the Finger Position Imitation test) in children with good and poor handwriting. Students with good handwriting performed significantly better than students with poor handwriting on both tasks. A moderate, but significant correlation was found between the finger tests and handwriting legibility.

The relationship between handwriting performance and kinesthetic perception was examined in several other studies. Bairstow and Laszlo (1981) reported a significant correlation between their kinesthetic test and a writing task. Copley and Ziviani (1990) compared first-grade students with good and poor handwriting on the Test of Kinesthetic Sensitivity (Laszlo & Bairstow, 1985b) and the kinesthetic test of the Southern California Sensory Integration Tests (Ayres, 1972). Only the latter test differentiated between good and poor handwriters. Lord and Hulme (1987) compared children with and without DCD on handwriting performance, motor ability, and kinesthetic sensitivity. In students that were identified with coordination problems, kinesthetic acuity correlated with handwriting accuracy ($r = 0.50$).

In summary, the research to date suggests that kinesthesis is associated with hand functions that are complex in nature and require high levels of precision. In particular, in-hand manipulation, tool use and handwriting appear to be associated to kinesthetic accuracy and memory. However, the mixed findings indicate the need for more systematic research to verify these claims.

Hand Function and Haptic Perception

Haptic perception is the ability to discern and interpret an object's size, weight, shape, texture, and other physical features using tactile and kinesthetic systems. Also termed "active touch," individuals use haptic perception to gather information about an object's physical characteristics when grasping and manipulating the object. Lederman and Klatzky (1998) described the movement patterns that are associated with haptic perception of the various sensory qualities of an object. To detect the roughness or smoothness of an object, the hand scans the surface by moving fingers back and forth on the surface. To detect the weight of an object, the object is held in the palm. Judgment about weight is gathered primarily from the kinesthetic system and secondarily from mechanoreceptors of the skin. Hardness and softness appear to rely on both cutaneous and kinesthetic inputs to determine an object's compliance or rigidity (Lederman & Klatzky, 1998).

Active touch or haptic perception is likely to be diminished in children with DCD. Ayres (1965, 1977) consistently found a relationship between tactile perception and dyspraxia. Ayres, Mailloux, and Wendler (1987) found that both tactile and visual perception correlated highly with praxis. This relationship was confirmed through structural equation modeling that demonstrated a relationship between somatosensory deficit and generalized dyspraxia (Mulligan, 1998). Haron and Henderson (1985) found that children with dyspraxia had more difficulty matching geometric shapes explored in their hands. Although these children were more accurate in identifying shapes when active versus passive touch was used, differences in haptic perception acuity were not as great as expected. One possible reason for similar accuracy when passively holding the object versus actively touching may have been an inefficient manipulation of the object. The children may have had difficulty identifying the objects because their focus was on manipulating while maintaining grasp rather than perceiving the objects' sensory features.

Haptic perception is particularly important to in-hand manipulation and construction skills. In-hand manipulation is a key strategy for determining the sensory features of an object and by extension, possible functions of that object. With information about an object's size and shape, a child can complete a puzzle or play a game. With information regarding hardness and texture, the child constructs buildings and play structures or creates art projects. Haptic perception linked with in-hand manipulation is essential to handling fragile objects so that they are not broken and slippery objects so that they are not dropped. Although there is anecdotal evidence that children with DCD have difficulty with in-hand manipulation, further research is needed to extend our understanding of this relationship between hand function, haptic perception and DCD.

Hand Function and Visual Perception

Some children with DCD appear to have impairments in visual perception that affect hand function. Hulme, Biggerstaff, Moran, and McKinlay (1982) looked at children with and without DCD matching the length of lines using vision, kinesthesia or both of these modalities. Only the visual perceptual test correlated with motor performance, leading the authors to conclude that visual perceptual deficits were the basis of the motor problems. Lord and Hulme (1987) found a significant correlation ($r = 0.52$) in children with DCD between drawing ability and visual discrimination. This correlation between visual discrimination and drawing was not significant in typical children ($r = 0.10$).

Van der Meulen, Denier van der Gon, Gielen, Gooskens, and Willemse (1991) investigated whether children with DCD efficiently used vision to guide their movement patterns when reaching. The children with motor difficulties adopted slow movement strategies that allowed visual feedback to make a larger contribution to movement accuracy. It appears that they also have difficulty using visual information to guide their movement when reaching to a specific target. In the goal directed reaching movements, the children with DCD demonstrated more variability and less accuracy. Van der Meulen et al. (1991) expected these children to be more accurate when they were allowed visual feedback; however, the children with DCD demonstrated increased times to process when visual feedback was present.

Several aspects of visual perception appear to relate to handwriting. Some children with DCD have difficulty in accurate formation of letters and in spatial arrangement of letters on a page. In handwriting, a motor program consists of an abstract representation of a grapheme, symbolizing the number of strokes and their spatial relations (Meulenbroek & Van Galen, 1990). The formation of each of the letter-forms necessitates visual-constructive-perception of the various strokes to create a specific letter. Thus, in the handwriting process the child integrates visual images of letters or shapes with appropriate motor responses (Tseng & Cermak, 1993). The assumption that visual motor integration is related to handwriting performance gains support from several empirical studies. Weil and Cunningham Amundson (1994) examined the relationship between letter-form errors and the Visual Motor Integration Test (Beery, 1989) with 60 kindergarten students. The students' scores on the letter-form copying tasks and the VMI were significantly correlated ($r = 0.47$). Several studies found that students with poor handwriting scored significantly lower on design copying tests compared to students with good handwriting (Cornhill & Case-Smith, 1996; Tseng & Murray, 1994). This relationship is not strong in older students (i.e., students above 5th grade). Some children with DCD consistently make more errors in and take more time to complete visual motor tasks. Ayres (1989) believed that certain children had constructional dyspraxia. These were children who had concurrent problems in visual perception.

Hand Function and Cross-Modal Integration

Some researchers suggest that children with DCD have problems in the integration of visual and kinesthetic/proprioceptive information, rather than in perception of any single sense (Mon-Williams, Wann, & Pascal, 1999; Smyth & Mason, 1997, 1998; Wilson & McKenzie, 1998).

Mon-Williams and colleagues (1999) investigated differences between children with DCD and controls in replicating limb position based on visual-proprioceptive information or only proprioceptive information. The children with DCD made more errors than the controls in both the visual-proprioceptive and proprioceptive tasks, but they made significantly more errors when vision of the limb was available than when it was occluded. The authors speculated that the basis for increased errors when vision was available were difficulties in cross-modal matching.

Deuel (1995) described a type of developmental dysgraphia observed in children with spatial perception deficits. The handwriting of children with spatial dysgraphia is often found to be disorganized and illegible. These children display poor letter formation and have difficulty copying texts. They are not always able to discriminate between letters that are similar, such as b/d/p/q, resulting in reversal or transposition of letters (Cunningham Amundson, 1992). Due to deficits in spatial formation, they have difficulty writing on the lines and maintaining proper margins. In arithmetic, they may have problems aligning numbers. Visual and proprioceptive perception are combined to guide movements and if the processing of both systems takes longer or is less accurate, cross-modal maps may not be well established in children with DCD. Children with DCD may require a multisensory approach in which information about the action needed is provided through multiple channels, for example, auditory, visual, kinesthetic, and tactile.

HAND FUNCTION AND MOTOR CONTROL

Problems with hand function have also been related to difficulties with aspects of motor control, including control of force, timing, and motor planning. Children with DCD appear to have difficulty modulating force, and as a result they crush or break objects that need to be handled gently or they close containers or place objects with too much force. To apply appropriate grip force, the hand perceives the surface and weight qualities of the objects. Objects with lower surface friction (smooth or slippery surfaces) require a higher grip force and objects that are more textured require less grip force. When an object is moved slowly, less grip force is applied than if the object is moved quickly. Grip force when lifting an object upward tends to be higher than grip force when lowering an object. Hill and Wing (1998) completed a pilot study examining the difference in grip force and acceleration of movement in a child with DCD and a matched control. The child with DCD showed a large increase in grip strength at the end of his movement (i.e., when placing the object on the surface). This child also had greater acceleration in the downward direction. In general, the child with DCD used greater grip force than the typical child.

Force control has also been studied as a basis for the movement errors and motor control difficulties in children with DCD (Lundy-Ekman et al., 1991). These researchers identified two groups of children with DCD: those with neurological signs, indicating basal ganglia disorders and those with cerebellar signs. To measure force, the participants pressed a button to reach a targeted level of force. As predicted, the children with basal ganglia soft signs were more variable at producing force pulses. The children with cerebellar signs tended to produce smaller forces and make slower force pulses. The most salient characteristic of the children's use of force was increased variability. Difficulty in modulating force may relate to limitations in sensitivity to kinesthesis, although Hill and Wing (1998) hypothesized that modulation of force relates to limitations in planning, because individuals plan the degree of force to be used to grasp and lift based on visualizing the object. For example, picking up a china plate (i.e., a disk-shaped object) requires a different motor plan to picking up a glass of milk (i.e., cylinder); the hand orients in different directions, and different forces are applied.

Appropriate use of force is important to all hand functions. In construction activities, force is used to stack objects on each other. The research suggests that children with DCD lower objects more quickly and apply greater force when releasing the object. Force in placing of one object on another would create problems, for example stacking a number of small blocks may not be a functional activity or part of the play repertoire of a child with DCD.

In most actions with a tool, appropriate pressure is required so that the pencil lead is not broken, the paper torn, or the hammer too forcefully applied. Appropriate modulation of force is particularly important to the small midrange finger movements used when cutting, such that the scissors' blades move, but, at the same time, the paper is held in between the blades. Because tools are used successfully only when they are held dynamically (e.g., in a hand that provides both stability for holding and mobility for using the tool), appropriate force of fingers on the objects is essential.

Force is also used in action on a surface. The force applied is graded to the resistance of the keys or the object on a surface. In-hand manipulation of objects requires grading of force so that the objects can move within the hand without dropping. Clinical experience reveals that children with DCD drop small objects more frequently when manipulating them within the hand. They also use alternative strategies to stabilize the objects against other body parts to prevent them from being dropped. Tool use and in-hand manipulation are similar activities in that objects are held while manipulated; that is, an appropriate use of force is necessary to allow for the movement of the tool or small objects within the hand.

Force is an element of handwriting in determining the degree of pressure of pencil on paper and in creating letter forms. Children with difficulty modulating force may demonstrate poor letter formation. They may be unable to maintain uniform size of letters. These problems often result in written output that is illegible and messy. Children with DCD have difficulty regulating the amount of pressure they exert on the writing implement or on the paper. With poor regulation of force, they press too hard with their pencil and fatigue early. They may tear their paper or break the pencil lead due to excessive force. Inconsistent force results in combination of dark and light letters on the page.

Levine et al. (1981) found that 20 of 26 students in grades 5–9 who were described as having "developmental output failure" had awkward grasps. Awkward grasping patterns are often associated with application of too much force and poorly formed letters (Schneck, 1991). Both excessive force and variability in application of force appear to pose problems in handwriting of children with DCD.

A number of studies have demonstrated that children with DCD require more time to respond in fine motor activities (Lundy-Ekman et al., 1991; Smyth, 1994). In a recent study, Rosblad and von Hofsten (1994) investigated the differences in 10 children with DCD and matched controls in transferring beads from one cup to another with and without vision. The children with DCD demonstrated slower movement speeds and less consistent movement patterns. These researchers concluded that children with DCD use slower and more variable feedback monitoring rather than anticipatory monitoring in planning movement.

Timing of movement patterns is an important aspect of in-hand manipulation tasks as well as bimanual tasks. In-hand manipulation was found to be slower in children with mild fine motor delays and typical cognitive performance (Case-Smith, 1993). The children with delays in in-hand manipulation used less efficient movements to rotate small pegs in their hands, more often stabilizing them on another surface or dropping them.

Lundy-Ekman et al. (1991) referred to the timing error (as measured in a tapping task) as a computational disorder. They felt that the timing problem related to regulating the use of antagonist and agonist muscles together so that appropriate force and accurate movements were made. Smyth (1991) suggested that the longer time required related to difficulty with programming movements. His findings that complex movements, but not simple movements, are slower in children with DCD suggest that these children are more dependent on feedback for motor control. Others have found that movement patterns in children with DCD do not become automatic and that they particularly rely on vision to guide their movement (van der Meulen et al., 1991). One reason that children with DCD move slower may be to reduce their error. Timing may also be increased when an individual relies more on vision to guide movement because it requires more time to process (van der Meulen et al., 1991). Goodgold-Edwards and Cermak (1990) suggested that simplistic models cannot explain the basis of timing delays in movement patterns.

How do these motor control problems affect hand function in children with DCD? Motor planning is particularly important to construction, tool use, and handwriting. Taken together, the implications of these motor control difficulties are evidenced in all hand functions. In construction, children sequence motor actions to construct a design. Motor planning problems are evident when the child selects the correct puzzle piece to match the form space but has difficulty correctly turning and rotating the piece to fit it into that space.

The level of motor planning required in tool use varies according to the complexity of the task. To use a tool efficiently, the child postures his hand prior to reaching to a target, then moves to it with speed and precision varying according to the size and distance of the target. Studies have consistently found children with DCD are slower and less accurate in reaching a target.

Handwriting requires high levels of motor planning. When writing, a child forms a motor plan consisting of sequences of strokes. Difficulty in selecting or executing a motor program for forming a letter may result in poor letter formation or many erasures. In addition, due to poor motor control, these children may demonstrate handwriting that is illegible and messy. A number of studies have demonstrated that children with difficulty in handwriting have associated problems in motor planning.

SUMMARY AND CONCLUSIONS

Children with DCD can have visual, somatosensory, and motor problems that affect hand function. Consistently hand function activities are performed more slowly with greater error, when children with DCD are compared to children without DCD. Problems in use of force affect accuracy and speed in in-hand manipulation and tool use activities. Motor planning impairments negatively influence performance in construction, tool use, and handwriting. Understanding the links among perceptual processing, use of force, and motor planning appears essential to designing better interventions. Inconsistent findings in descriptive studies of children with DCD suggest that they differ in the relative degree of perceptual and motor problems and that intervention programs focus on the specific patterns of perceptual motor performance observed in the individual child.

CHAPTER
11

Physical Fitness and Developmental Coordination Disorder

Beth Hands and Dawne Larkin

The importance of fitness to our general health and well-being is well documented; however, health specialists, worldwide, are increasingly concerned that children, in general, are not sufficiently active on a daily basis to maintain a healthy level of fitness. What about children with developmental coordination disorder (DCD)? Are they physically fit? Although the evidence available is limited, it indicates that children with low motor competence are even less fit and less physically active on a daily basis than coordinated children. In turn, their low fitness levels can have a negative impact on motor performance compounding the effect of their coordination difficulties. The maintenance of physical fitness is particularly important for the child with DCD. In this chapter, we will draw on the limited research that has investigated fitness in children with DCD, poor coordination, and low motor proficiency and compare it with research from normative populations, and children with other disabilities particularly those that involve the motor system.

WHAT IS FITNESS?

Physical fitness is "a set of attributes that people have or achieve that relates to the ability to perform physical activity" (Casperson, Powell, & Christenson, 1985). A number of measurable components that contribute to overall physical fitness are categorized into two types: health-related and skill-related fitness. The health-related components of cardiorespiratory endurance, muscular strength, muscular endurance, flexibility, and body composition are important for general health and well-being, in particular, the prevention of diseases associated with a sedentary lifestyle. For example, poor abdominal muscle strength, endurance, and flexibility in the lower back and thigh, often found in children with DCD, have been linked to lower back pain. The skill-related components of agility, speed, and power contribute to improved athletic performance and are sometimes referred to as "measures of motor fitness." Health-related fitness is considered achievable by all, not only those with high motor ability. Most practitioners focus on the health-related components, although the skill-related components are very important for children with DCD and could be helpful in diagnosis and remediation.

PHYSICAL FITNESS AND DCD

Children with DCD are at greater risk of low levels of physical fitness. Most young children develop fitness through their daily activities while they perform fundamental movements such as running, walking, skipping, climbing, hanging, and rolling. Some skills are important to the development of fitness as they contribute to strength (jumping, hopping, hanging, climbing), power (hopping, kicking, throwing), or endurance (running, riding, swimming). Because movement is so hard for children with DCD, they are less likely to be physically active, and consequently, the development of physical fitness, as well as skill, is compromised.

There are a number of other factors that can influence the development of fitness in children with DCD. These factors include genetic disposition, social pressures, environmental constraints, and family structure and values. These factors interact to influence each child in a different way. If the influences are negative, the negative cycle from low motor competence, to hypoactivity and low physical fitness is reinforced (Figure 11.1). The results of poor motor coordination and the accompanying feeling of inadequacy are constantly reinforced in school-ground interactions. The long-term consequences include reduced motivation to participate in physical activity, fewer interactions with the environment, and, consequently, fewer opportunities to develop proficient motor skill or fitness. Parents, teachers, and peers often make negative judgments about the child's overall motor performance, reinforcing the child's desire to withdraw from activity. By contrast, if there are positive influences from family, friends, and community, this negative cycle can be broken.

HYPOACTIVITY AND DCD

A few studies provide support for lower levels of physical activity among children with DCD. An early study by Rarick and McKee (1949) contrasted a group of children with very low motor proficiency to a group with very high motor proficiency. The children with low motor proficiency were more interested in fine manipulative activities and tended to select passive activities for their after-school activity. This data is in keeping with the activity deficit hypothesis, put forward by Bouffard and colleagues (1996), that children with low motor competence are generally less active than children with high motor competence. More recent research lends

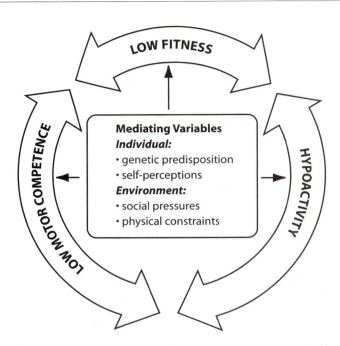

Figure 11.1 This model represents the continuous negative interaction between low motor competence, hypoactivity, and physical fitness. This negative cycle can be mediated by other factors that can increase or decrease involvement in physical activity.

further support to this concept, also known as "hypoactivity" (Bouffard, Watkinson, Thompson, Causgrove Dunn, & Romanow, 1996; Li & Dunham, 1993; Stratton & Armstrong, 1991; Thompson, Bouffard, Watkinson, & Causgrove Dunn, 1994). Children with poor coordination skills engaged in vigorous physical activity during school recess time for significantly less time (15.1%) than well-coordinated children (23.5%) and played on large playground equipment less often (Bouffard et al., 1996). During leisure time, they were not as active or vigorous as matched controls (Kuiper, Reynders, & Rispens, 1997). Even in structured physical education lessons, children with movement difficulties were engaged in moderately vigorous activity for less time (17.9%) than children with moderate competence (20.3%) or high competence (22.3%; Li & Dunham, 1993). Further, they were more likely to be off task and were usually less successful on assigned tasks (Thompson et al., 1994). Stratton and Armstrong (1991) measured heart rate in different ability groups during a physical education lesson. Children of low ability spent less time with their heart rate above 159 bpm (18.8%) than children of average (23.3%) or high ability (31.4%). These studies demonstrate the link among movement competence, habitual physical activity, and fitness in children. Children with low motor competence and low activity levels, generally, have low fitness levels.

The benefits of fitness and physical activity in minimizing the risk of disease and maximizing wellness have been clearly documented in children. Research has linked physical activity and high fitness levels in children and adolescents to reduced risk of cardiovascular disease (Gutin & Owen, 1999; Vaccaro & Mahon, 1989), reduced blood pressure (Dwyer & Gibbons, 1994), lower triglyceride and higher high-density lipoprotein cholesterol (HDL-C) levels (Armstrong & Simons-Morton, 1994; Raitakari, Porkka, & Taimela, 1994), reduced risk of obesity (Moore, Nguyen, Rothman, Cupples, & Ellison, 1995; Raudsepp & Jurimae, 1998), skeletal health (Bailey & Martin, 1994; McKay, Petit, Schutz, Prior, Barr, & Khan, 2000), and psychological health (Calfas & Taylor, 1994).

The decreased health status of children with low activity levels has been demonstrated in children with impairments that restrict their movement levels. Many studies have successfully tracked cardiovascular disease risk factors such as high blood pressure (Woynarowska, Mukherjee, Roche, & Siervogel, 1985), serum cholesterol and lipoproteins (Orchard, Donahue, Kuller, Hodge, & Drash, 1983), obesity (Charney, Goodman, McBride, Lyon, & Pratt, 1976), and low physical activity (Pate, Baranowski, Dowda, & Trost, 1996) in children. In other words, children who were high on risk factors maintained their standing relative to their peers over time. Patterns for life are well established at an early age. Low physical activity levels are linked to an increased risk of heart disease, a higher potential for obesity, and a higher risk of developing hypertension, osteoporosis, and insulin-independent diabetes mellitus (Ward, 1994).

Hypoactivity among children with DCD can put their long-term health and well-being at greater risk. More physically active children also have more opportunity to develop their muscular strength and endurance as well as their overall neuromuscular coordination. Increased physical activity should enhance their movement competence; by contrast, hypoactivity decreases the opportunity for children with DCD to reach their movement potential.

FATIGUE AND DCD

Inefficient movement patterns and mechanical inefficiency can involve high-energy demands. As a consequence, children or adults with DCD can fatigue much earlier than better coordinated people. In a study where muscle fatigue was estimated during anaerobic fitness testing, children with poor coordination had much higher levels of fatigue compared to the coordinated control group (O'Beirne, Larkin, & Cable, 1994). Levels of fatigue increased with age in the children with DCD but decreased in the control group. Fatigue reduces the ability to contribute joyfully and to participate enthusiastically in many daily activities. We have frequently heard children with DCD complain of tiredness after completing an activity. The early fatigue, accompanying the low levels of physical fitness, contribute to the discomfort and relatively low tolerance for physical activity exhibited by some children with DCD.

Teachers and coaches often perceive children with DCD as less active, even when their physiological load, as measured by heart rate, is actually higher. Because the movement patterns of these children are inefficient, higher fitness levels may be required to perform simple tasks that others take for granted (Ward, 1994). The mechanical inefficiency leads to earlier fatigue. Although fatigue has not been explored in children with DCD, it may have an influence on their participation in a variety of activities at home and at school as well as in the playground.

MEASURING FITNESS

The optimum measure of fitness is controversial, as is the means by which the data are reported. Many experts in the field recommend criterion-referenced standards to evaluate performance rather than relative to one's peers (Cureton & Warren, 1990). The logic is that standards are determined by what is considered a baseline for health. Unfortunately, the level of fitness necessary to maintain health over a lifetime is unknown, and some experts claim that insufficient evidence is available to link fitness in childhood to adult health. Consequently, the emphasis that should be placed on fitness testing in young children and adolescents is widely debated. Simons-Morton, O'Hara, Simons-Morton, and Parcel (1987) and Sallis and McKenzie (1991) argue that physical activity rather than physical fitness should be a focus in school-based physical education programs. It is generally agreed that physical activity and fitness are interrelated in children; however, the correlation is only moderate (Pate, Dowda, & Ross, 1990). Further, the information on levels of habitual activity in young children is sparse given the lack of acceptable and practical measures (Freedson, 1991). On the other hand, a number of fitness measures have high levels of reliability and validity with children (for an overview, see Safrit & Wood, 1995). Therefore, particularly for children at risk, such as those with DCD, the assessment and monitoring of fitness is important. Although norm-referenced standards for fitness evaluation are not widely used, the information provided is valuable with this group to detect individual differences and facilitate comparisons to the wider population. The information is also valuable to diagnose the child's current status and program appropriate intervention strategies.

Not only are children with DCD likely to be less fit, a true measure of their fitness is difficult given that many tests of fitness require a high degree of coordination. Similarly, a true measure of motor proficiency is hard to achieve, as many common test items such as standing broad jump require a high degree of motor fitness. Children with DCD perform motor tasks less efficiently, often with extraneous movements that increase the energy demands. The reduced movement efficiency contributes to a poor test outcome even though the child may be working as hard as a well-coordinated child. This is evident when heart rates are compared between well-coordinated and poorly coordinated children performing the same task (O'Beirne et al., 1994).

HEALTH-RELATED PHYSICAL FITNESS

Cardiorespiratory Endurance

Cardiorespiratory endurance, the capacity to participate in moderate to vigorous physical activity for a relatively long period of time, is generally low in children with DCD. This ability depends on the capacity of the body to remove waste products as well as supply vital oxygen and other nutrients to the muscles. Cardiovascular endurance depends on participation in regular physical activity, and our movement program records show that children with motor impairments can improve with training. Cardiovascular training is appropriate for most children and can be developed through fast walking, jogging, bike riding or swimming. It is a useful predictor of the body's long-term resistance to heart disease.

To date, we have not seen any reports of children with DCD performing the most popular laboratory test of cardiorespiratory endurance, a maximum oxygen consumption test (VO_{2max}) on a treadmill. Children with DCD who have coordination and timing problems would have difficulty performing this test because it is necessary to maintain a consistent rhythm and speed to run on a treadmill. The children would need to practice treadmill running prior to testing to develop both competence and confidence.

Common field tests of cardiorespiratory endurance include distance runs of 600–1600 m, a timed run (for example, 12 min), or a maximal effort, multistage run (ACHPER, 1996). Children with poor coordination generally perform poorly on these tests. Using an 800-m run from the Manitoba fitness test (Manitoba Department of Education, 1980), 15 of 17 children with DCD scored below the 50th percentile (Hammond, 1995). The median percentile for the group was 34. Using the same distance, Deschenes (1994) reported a significant difference in time between a well-coordinated and a DCD group. Of 28 children from our movement program timed on the 1.6-km run from the Australian Schools Fitness Test (Pyke, 1986), the majority were ranked below the 25th percentile (Larkin & Hoare, 1991).

An alternative test for those children who lack motivation or are unable to pace themselves over distance is a multistage, shuttle-run test that involves running in time with a cadence tape. Low fitness levels were reported for a group of nineteen 7–12-year-old children with ADHD on this test (Harvey & Reid, 1997). Like many children with ADHD, these children were below average in most fitness and fundamental movement skills. Our pilot data with children with DCD also indicate low fitness levels on a multistage shuttle run (Hands & Larkin, unpublished). As can be seen in Table 11.1 where recorded heart rates are similar for children with DCD and coordinated children performing the multistage shuttle run, the overall performance outcomes are very different. The coordinated children reached maximum heart rates after a longer time and were able to sustain the task longer. Again, there are some aspects of the multistage test that can confound the measurement of fitness in children with DCD. Anxiety about physical activity may complicate interpretation of heart rate responses and the need to pace the run may compromise the final level achieved. Our ongoing research with this test will increase our understanding of these limitations.

Cardiorespiratory endurance is claimed to be easiest of all physical fitness components to improve (Rintala, Lyytinen, & Dunn, 1990). A recent meta-analysis of the effects of exercise on health-related physical fitness in individuals with an intellectual disability showed large effect sizes for cardiovascular and muscular endurance (Chianas, Reid, & Hoover, 1998). This population generally demonstrates low motivation as well as some of the movement difficulties found in children and adults with DCD; yet aspects of their health-related fitness responded to exercise. Although we have not identified any formal studies looking at changes in

Table 11.1 Multistage Shuttle Run Levels, Peak Recorded Heart Rates (HR), and Time to Reach Peak HR for 8-Year-Old Boys with (*n* = 7) and without (*n* = 2) DCD

Group	Participant	Level*	Peak HR (bpm)	Time to reach peak HR (sec)
DCD	1	2.6	188	45
	2	2.6	200	110
	3	2.2	193	80
	4	1.6	177	70
	5	3.4	215	170
	6	3.2	207	30
	7	1.5	182	45
Control				
	8	4.5	212	170
	9	5.2	203	295

*The levels indicate an increase in running speed by 0.5 km/hr each minute.

cardiovascular endurance of children with DCD, measures taken at the beginning and end of the semester during a movement enrichment program indicated positive changes (Larkin & Hands, unpublished data). Prior to commencing the program, many children with DCD were unable to run the 800-m distance, preferring to walk or stop after a shorter distance. The inefficient movement patterns observed in these children require a high-energy expenditure. After a semester in the movement program children with DCD are usually able to complete an 800-m walk/run with greater ease in an improved time.

Body Composition

An individual's degree of body fatness helps predict vulnerability to a number of degenerative diseases such as high blood pressure, heart disease, and diabetes (Bar-Or et al., 1998; Gutin & Owens, 1999). Children and adolescents who have body fat levels above 25–30% have a greater chance of developing heart disease (Williams et al., 1992). Common field tests include body mass index (BMI), calculated by weight/height, or skin-fold thickness, measured with calipers. BMI, while being easier to derive, does not take into account differences between muscle mass and fat mass.

Hypoactivity among children with DCD could contribute to higher levels of body fat. Studies from a number of countries have reported higher levels of obesity in children with DCD or poor coordination. A recent longitudinal study of adolescents in Holland (Visser, 1998; Visser, Geuze, & Kalverboer, 1998) found that the group with DCD (*n* = 15) were significantly heavier than the control group (*n* = 16) when measurements were obtained monthly from 11:6 to 14 years of age. These adolescents had a higher Quetelet index (weight/height) indicating that weight rather than height was the contributing factor. In an Australian study, Hammond (1995) reported that 11 of 17 primary school children with DCD had higher than acceptable percentage body fat. All of the eight girls in the sample carried excessive body fat. Five of the sample (two boys and three girls) were classified as obese with a percentage body fat of 24 or more. Another Australian study showed that a group of 24 boys with DCD, in the 7–9-year age group, were heavier ($M = 30.9$ kg) than their coordinated age-matched peers ($M = 26.9$ kg; O'Beirne et al., 1994). Wasmund-Bodenstedt (1988) reported similar findings with a group of low motor achieving primary school children from Germany. The low achieving group had a mean percentage body fat of 21%, which contrasted to the 14% body fat of a high motor achievement group. In Harvey and Reid's (1997) study of children with ADHD and below average motor skill, BMI was average, but the sum of five skin-folds was above average indicating that these children were overweight.

In two studies from our research program, 36 children identified with coordination difficulties were clearly differentiated from their age-matched well-coordinated peers by heavier weight (Larkin, Hoare, & Kerr, 1989) and a higher endomorphic component in their somatotype (Larkin et al., 1989; Raynor, 1989). In these two studies, there were no differences between the coordination levels for the mesomorphy and ectomorphy measures. There are two issues that arise with increased body fat: the effect on health and the effect of the additional bulk on skill performance. In our earlier study (Larkin et al., 1989), there was a significant negative correlation between both endomorphy ($r = -0.49$) and mesomorphy ($r = -0.60$) scores and the distance jumped for the group of 20 children with poor coordination. The relationship suggests that the increased bulk, whether fat or muscle interfered with performance. For the well-coordinated group ($n = 20$), the relationship between endomorphy ($r = -0.05$) or mesomorphy ($r = 0.13$), and distance jumped was very low. Those children with DCD who are also obese find movement extra hard. They have a larger bulk to move with less power and coordination, and there will be a higher oxygen cost of locomotion.

Muscular Strength and Endurance

Children with DCD often have low muscular strength. Muscular strength is the capacity of a muscle group or muscle to exert a maximum force (Casperson, Powell, & Christenson, 1985). Poor muscle strength, in particular abdominal, may indicate a potential to develop musculoskeletal problems such as lower back pain. Good posture and correct pelvic alignment is also dependent on adequate muscle strength. Muscle strength also indicates a person's ability to perform many daily activities without risk of fatigue or injury. Muscular endurance is the ability of a muscle or muscle group to contract repeatedly over a period of time (Casperson, Powell, & Christenson, 1985). Improving muscular endurance requires continued or repetitive use of the muscle or muscle group. Consequently, the child who withdraws from movement is likely to have low muscular endurance.

Test items commonly used to assess muscular strength and endurance include push-ups, pull-ups, basketball throw, and grip strength. In our study of 85 children with coordination difficulties (O'Beirne & Larkin, 1991), the children scored from 0 to the 65th percentile rank for push-ups. The mean percentile rank for the group was 7, indicating that the strength and coordinative components of the test were very difficult for the group. Similar results (Hammond, 1995) were found using the flexed arm hang, a measure of upper limb strength, from the Manitoba fitness test (Manitoba Department of Education, 1980). The performances of the 17 children with DCD ranged from the 5th to the 62nd percentile rank using these Canadian norms. The group median percentile for the flexed arm hang was 32. Additionally, children with DCD or poor coordination have shown lower levels of grip strength when compared to well-coordinated peers (Larkin et al., 1989).

There are some studies that show strength differences for groups considered at risk for comorbid DCD. Beyer (1993) reported that boys with ADHD and no learning disorders (n = 56) had significantly lower measures of muscular strength than a group of boys (n = 60) with learning disabilities and no ADHD. The assessment was based on the Bruininks-Oseretsky (1978) strength subtest, which included the standing broad jump, sit-ups, and push-ups. However, grip strength in a group of children with ADHD was found to be above average (Harvey & Reid, 1997).

Data from a number of studies show that children with DCD, as well as children with other motor impairments, demonstrate low levels of abdominal endurance. In our studies that have looked at the abdominal endurance of children with DCD, we used the 60-sec sit-up test reported in the Manitoba fitness test. In a descriptive study of the abdominal endurance of 85 children with poor coordination, the percentile ranks of the children ranged from 0 to 40 with the group mean at the 15th percentile (O'Beirne & Larkin, 1989). In another study (Raynor, 1989) of 16 7-year-olds (eight girls, eight boys) with poor coordination, abdominal endurance measured using sit-ups was markedly lower (M = 12.6) than the age- and gender-matched well-coordinated group (M = 31.1). Hammond (1995), using a similar sit-up test, found that 17 children with DCD were ranked from the 4th to the 75th percentile with the group median at the 32nd percentile. The abdominal strength, measured by sit-ups, and arm strength, measured by push-ups, of children with ADHD, were poor and below average, respectively (Harvey & Reid, 1997). From the data available, it is clear that many children with DCD have low levels of abdominal endurance, although training can result in significant improvements.

Prior to testing for muscular endurance, children with DCD often need to relearn sit-ups to change from asymmetric and rocking patterns. They may also need additional muscular training to undo the effects of reduced activity. Many children with DCD initially find this task impossible to perform without some major modification. They are unable to isolate the abdominal muscles, finding the demands of both strength and coordination arduous. For these children, some light support on the back of the shoulders during the sit-up helps them to get "the idea of the movement." While a cadence tape is sometimes used to encourage rhythmical, consistent performance, children with DCD can find it difficult to keep up with the rhythm and the quality of performance is likely to further deteriorate.

Flexibility

Flexibility, the range of motion through which joints are able to move, varies quite markedly in children with DCD and may vary from joint to joint or between sides. Lack of flexibility can contribute to injury and long-term musculoskeletal problems, whereas excessive flexibility can result in joint instability and the potential to strain muscles or dislocate joints. Within the DCD population, extreme ranges of flexibility and inflexibility can be observed.

Sit and reach scores for 85 children with DCD ranged from 0 to the 95th percentile, with 44% scoring at or below the 10th percentile, and 73% scoring above the 75th or below the 25th percentile (O'Beirne & Larkin, 1991). Flexibility scores from another Australian study provided a range of percentile ranks on the sit and reach test from 25 to 97, with 10 of the 17 children with movement difficulties scoring at or above the 80th percentile (Hammond, 1995). Children with hyperflexible joints find it difficult to perform controlled movements in a consistent manner. On the other hand, some children are so inflexible they are unable to move their limbs in a way that enables them to perform a skill efficiently. For example, an efficient run requires a high knee lift and therefore some flexibility around the hip. Limited flexibility contributes to a low knee lift and a smaller stride length. In a sample of 19 7–12-year-old children with ADHD, where DCD may be comorbid, below-average measures on the sit-and-reach test were found (Harvey & Reid, 1997).

Flexibility is joint specific and therefore needs to be assessed at a number of joints. In our work with children with DCD, we have found some children to have adequate flexibility at the shoulder but not at the hip, and vice versa. Some children with DCD have decreased flexibility at the ankle and the knee (Larkin et al., 1989), and these findings could account for some of the difficulties these children encounter when running, jumping, and hopping. Flexibility can be improved by stretching. Exercises to improve flexibility are always included after preliminary warm-ups in our sessions with children with DCD. For those children with limited flexibility, further gentle and regular stretching is included in their program to reduce the limitations that they experience. For the children with excessive flexibility, activities are designed to enhance joint stability.

SKILL-RELATED FITNESS

Agility

Agility is the ability to change direction or body position quickly. Studies that have looked at agility in children with poor coordination indicate that these children have low levels of motor fitness in this area. This is logical given Butcher and Eaton's (1989) research that shows that a high activity level is associated with running speed and agility. In a descriptive study of 85 children with coordination difficulties, aged 7–11 years, scores between 0 and the 50th percentile were recorded on the agility run with a mean percentile rank of 8 (O'Beirne & Larkin, 1991). In another study, 59 children with movement difficulties scored between the 0 and 70th percentile on an agility run, with 71% falling at or below the 10th percentile (Larkin & Hoare, 1991).

Speed

Speed is the ability to perform a movement as quickly as possible and is a function of strength, coordination and agility (Rowland, 1990). Again, children with DCD perform poorly when speed is based on the 50-m sprint. Data from our research program showed that the 50-m run times for 85 children with poor coordination (aged 7–11 years) were ranked between 0 and the 40th percentile based on the ASFT norms (Pyke, 1986; O'Beirne & Larkin, 1991). In the Hammond study (1995), the 50-m run times of the 17 children with DCD were ranked from the 4th to the 75th percentile (based on the norms of CAHPER, 1980), with a median percentile rank for the group of 19.

Power

Measuring power, a combination of strength and speed, in children with DCD is difficult. While field tests such as the 50-m run, distance hop, or standing broad jump are practical and relatively easy to administer, they have great coordination and postural demands on the performer, and the measure of power is confounded by the coordination difficulties of children with DCD. For example, 30- and 50-m sprints are used to estimate anaerobic performance, but efficient running requires precise timing and positioning of the limbs, head and trunk control, and leg strength to propel the body forward. Despite these measurement difficulties, children with DCD perform poorly on tasks such as hopping, running, and jumping, which are considered as estimates of anaerobic performance. O'Beirne et al. (1994) found 50-m run times in a sample of 7–9-year-old boys ranged from below the 5th to the 65th percentile, with an average percentile rank of 10.6. Seventy percent of the boys scored at or below the 10th percentile.

Children with DCD also perform poorly on more controlled laboratory measures of anaerobic performance such as the Wingate Anaerobic Cycling Test (WAnT; Bar-Or, 1983, 1987). The advantage of the WAnT is that the positioning of the child on the bicycle ergometer reduces extraneous movements of the limbs, provides stability for the arms and trunk, and limits weight bearing. O'Beirne et al. (1994) found that 7–9-year-old boys with poor coordination achieved significantly lower levels of absolute and relative mean power when measured over the 30-sec period of the WAnT. These researchers also correlated performances on two tests of anaerobic performance—the WAnT and a 50-m run—for the poorly coordinated group and coordinated group. The control group showed a significant relationship ($r = -0.44$) between 50-m run time and peak power. The relationship ($r = -0.26$) between the two measures of anaerobic power was lower in the group with poor coordination indicating that we need to be cautious about estimating anaerobic power from field measures such as the 50-m run when we are working with children with DCD.

In summary, studies of children and adolescents with DCD have consistently reported lower health-related and skill-related fitness levels than the average child. For most fitness components, performance levels were significantly lower in the DCD population. The low levels of health-related fitness can contribute to early fatigue, while the low levels of skill-related fitness can limit motor skill development. The extreme ranges of flexibility identified through our research and clinical experience provide further evidence for subtypes of DCD and the need for different intervention strategies.

DEVELOPING FITNESS IN CHILDREN WITH DCD

Fitness can be improved. Children need to participate in regular, preferably daily, physical activity; however, for those with DCD, who find movement difficult and unenjoyable, more structure and direction is necessary. Our clinical experience with fitness assessment and programming for children with DCD has identified difficulties that can be avoided as well as some helpful hints.

Test Difficulties

• Bench stepping or sit-up tests that use a cadence tape can be difficult to interpret because many children with DCD also have poor rhythmic ability and find these tasks particularly difficult.

• Cardiovascular endurance runs of more than 800 m should only be used after a period of coaching and training. Most children with DCD have a higher energy expenditure than well-coordinated children and find long distance events extremely tiring. Further, such continuous running can reinforce inefficient movement patterns.

• Tests with many verbal instructions can overload or confuse the child. The translation of verbal instructions into action is difficult for many children with DCD particularly those who have problems with motor planning, therefore tests or activities with complex instructions should be avoided.

• A number of children with DCD suffer from other comorbid conditions and consequently have been assessed multiple times by numerous specialists. Some have developed an intense dislike of tests and laboratory conditions. Fitness testing in laboratories might enhance their stress level and therefore confound results. Providing a game style atmosphere can be helpful.

Teach the Test

Children will not produce their best result if they are unable to perform a test or are unaware of efficient strategies. Often the test needs to be taught prior to testing. Initially, time is spent with the child getting the idea of the movement. This is followed with further instruction and feedback to ensure that the task is performed efficiently. Until an acceptable level of performance is reached, measurement of fitness is confounded by the coordination problem. Interpretation of the test is difficult because the test cannot be considered a valid measure of fitness.

Plan for a Healthy, Active Lifestyle

• As practitioners, our overall goal should be to educate children about the value and enjoyment of regular physical activity so that they choose to lead an active lifestyle. Children with DCD can develop an intense dislike of physical activity, therefore practitioners need to work to ensure such children learn or rediscover the joy of movement.

• Teach children to understand and to monitor their bodies' responses to exercise. For example, when they run, their heart rate will increase and help provide their muscles with more fuel.

• Help children to find some developmentally appropriate activities in which they will enjoy some success, such as, walking, jogging, swimming, cycling, martial arts, or tee-ball.

• Encourage children to maintain a physically active lifestyle by encouraging participation in lifetime activities such as swimming, cycling, golf, ten-pin bowling, sailing, yoga, or weight training.

FUTURE RESEARCH

Future studies that clearly identify how physical fitness differs between children with DCD, those with DCD and comorbid conditions such as ADHD and Asperger's syndrome, and typical children are important. Findings may facilitate early diagnosis and better targeted remediation programs. Further, the link between movement competence and fitness (Marshall & Bouffard, 1997) needs to be made explicit. At present, it is simply implied through studies such as those presented in this chapter. Clarification of this relationship will increase the precision of our measurements of physical fitness and motor performance in children with DCD. Research investigating the difference in levels of perceived and actual exertion between children with and without DCD would be helpful in gaining a greater understanding of what children with DCD have to contend with. Too often, children with poor motor competence are perceived to be lazy or as not trying very hard.

While it is apparent that fitness in children with DCD is compromised by their condition, few studies have dealt with the long term consequences of DCD by tracking these children into adulthood. For example, what effect does movement fatigue have on activities of daily living? How does DCD affect a person's capacity to study? What is the health status of an adult with DCD? What percentage of adults with DCD suffer from hypokinetic diseases?

SUMMARY AND CONCLUSIONS

Intervention programs for children with DCD often ignore fitness development; however, sufficient evidence is available to indicate that most children with poor coordination have low fitness levels, which may compromise skill development as well as future health and well-being. The three-way interaction among motor competence, habitual activity level, and fitness necessitates comprehensive assessment and remediation strategies.

CHAPTER

12

Considering Motivation Theory in the Study of Developmental Coordination Disorder

Janice Causgrove Dunn and E. Jane Watkinson

The field of adapted physical activity has long had concerns about children who have significant difficulties learning and performing gross motor skills, but show no signs of overt neurological, general sensory, or intellectual impairments (Hulme & Lord, 1986; Wall, 1982). Over the years, a number of labels have been used to describe the motor difficulties experienced by these children, including clumsiness, physical awkwardness, movement difficulties, and, most recently, developmental coordination disorder (DCD).[1] Numerous studies have examined the social, emotional, and behavioral problems associated with motor incompetence, leading to a growing body of evidence suggesting that lack of movement skill may have damaging consequences for social and psychological development. The research also suggests that children who lack motor competence are at risk of

---

[1] In much of the research that we reviewed, participants were identified as having motor coordination problems, but the criterion of "interference in activities of daily living or academic performance" for the diagnosis of DCD (American Psychological Association, 1994) was not specifically assessed. Rather than assuming this criterion was met, we refer to participants in these studies as lacking in movement or motor competence, or as children with movement difficulties.

withdrawal from participation in physical activity, resulting in further impairment of motor skills and a negative impact on physical fitness and health.

The impact of motor incompetence depends largely upon the value that the child and his or her social milieu place on movement competence (Roberts & Treasure, 1992; Schoemaker & Kalverboer, 1994). For example, motor or athletic competence is highly valued in North America and is particularly important for boys (Chase & Dummer, 1992; Duda, 1987; Evans & Roberts, 1987; Weiss & Duncan, 1992). In fact, Chase and Dummer (1992) found that boys rated "being a good athlete" as the most important criterion for male social status. Given the research indicating that movement competence is positively related to social acceptance (Rose, Larkin, & Berger, 1997; Wright, Giammarino, & Parad, 1986), it is not surprising to find that children who lack movement competence frequently occupy marginal positions in their peer groups and have few playmates (Clifford, 1985; Cratty, 1979; Kalverboer, de Vries, & van Dellen, 1990; Shoemaker & Kalverboer, 1994). These children do not often participate in group games or team sports (Cantell, Smyth, & Ahonen, 1994; Evans & Roberts, 1987; Wall, Reid, & Paton, 1990). However, when participation in group activities does occur, children who lack movement competence are frequently the target of criticism and ridicule, and are often relegated to minor roles that provide few opportunities to interact with other children (Evans & Roberts, 1987; Portman, 1995; Shoemaker & Kalverboer, 1994). As play becomes more complex and demanding with age, the combination of increasingly poor motor performance, minimal enjoyment of physical activity, and socioemotional difficulties creates a disinterest in physical activity and a disinclination to choose to be involved (Cratty, 1994; Portman, 1995; Wall et al., 1990). In other words, children with movement difficulties are at risk of withdrawal from physical activity.

Clearly, withdrawal from participation in physical activities is not a constructive approach to coping with movement difficulties. Withdrawal contributes to a practice deficit (Bouffard, Watkinson, Thompson, Causgrove Dunn, & Romanow, 1996), which is likely to increase existing performance differences, and may exacerbate the problems that children with movement difficulties experience surrounding their participation in physical activity settings. Moreover, continued avoidance of active participation in physical activity is a major concern for professionals because of the negative impact of inactivity on physical fitness and health, feelings of unhappiness, exclusion, and isolation.

Evidence of withdrawal is seen in research indicating low levels of physical fitness in children with movement difficulties (O'Beirne, Larkin, & Cable, 1994; Smyth, 1992; Wall et al., 1990), although more direct evidence is revealed in research findings that children who lack movement competence are, on average, less actively involved in physical activity than their movement competent peers. Observations of play patterns of elementary school–aged children during recess reveal that children with low movement competence engage in significantly less vigorous play, and spend significantly more time away from the playground area than their peers (Bouffard et al., 1996). Children with low movement competence also engage in social play less often than their peers, and spend more time on their own. Similarly, observations of participation patterns during physical education classes reveal that children who lack movement competence are less likely to be engaged in assigned motor activities with success, more likely to experience difficulty with assigned tasks, and more likely to be engaged in off-task behaviors than their movement-competent peers (Causgrove Dunn, 1997; Thompson, Bouffard, Watkinson, & Causgrove Dunn, 1994).

Typically, in addressing this concern about movement difficulties leading to withdrawal from physical activity participation, the field of adapted physical activity has directed intervention strategies toward increasing the movement competence of the child. However, there are many psychosocial factors that may mediate the relationship between movement competence and physical activity participation. Well-designed psychological or social/environmental interventions may constitute another approach to the problem of withdrawal.

This chapter will explore the psychosocial factors that may influence the motivation and participation of children with DCD in physical activity settings along the continuum of structured and unstructured activity. Structured settings are those where participation decisions are made by someone other than the child and the child is expected to comply with the requests of the leader (e.g., school physical education). In contrast, unstructured settings are those where the child has the primary decision-making power and can make multiple decisions regarding participation and behavior (e.g., recess time at school). A number of motivational theories will be discussed, with particular attention to how they might apply to children with DCD. Throughout this chapter, we use theory to guide our thinking as we speculate how different tasks, environments, and patterns of perceptions might impact children's participation decisions. Many unanswered questions are posed about the relationship between the lack of movement competence characteristic of DCD and participation in physical activity.

USING MOTIVATION THEORY TO UNDERSTAND AND ASK QUESTIONS ABOUT PHYSICAL ACTIVITY PARTICIPATION PATTERNS OF CHILDREN WITH DCD

Motivation theory can facilitate our understanding of the factors that children consider when (1) deciding whether or not to take part in an activity and (2) making choices about their behaviors within an activity (e.g., how much effort to invest and whether to persist in the face of failure). Central to motivation theory is the notion of the self-system, and its relationship to actual competence and success in meeting task demands (Coopersmith, 1967). Common to the theories explored in this chapter is the construct of perceived competence. Perceived competence is an individual's perception of his or her success in domain-specific skills (Markus, Cross, & Wurf, 1990) and, thus, is a powerful mediator of motivated behavior (Eccles, Wigfield, Harold, & Blumenfeld, 1993; Harter, 1978; Nicholls, 1989). Perceived competence is an important factor that influences children's decisions to participate, to exert effort, and to persist in physical activities (Causgrove Dunn, 1997; Roberts, Kleiber, & Duda, 1981; Yun & Ulrich, 1997).

Harter's Competence Motivation Theory

Harter's "competence motivation theory" (Harter, 1978, 1981) attempts to describe and explain why people are motivated to participate in certain achievement domains. This model of competence motivation predicts that individuals who perceive themselves to be highly competent in a certain skill domain will persevere longer and sustain interest in mastering skills within that domain. Conversely, those who perceive themselves to have low competence will tend not to persist or maintain interest in the task. Perceived competence is conceptualized as multidimensional, comprised of specific perceptions in a number of domains (e.g., physical, social, academic). Harter suggests that cognitive appraisals of successful and unsuccessful mastery attempts form the basis of competence judgments in a domain. Sources of competence information can be internal ("I met my goal, I tried hard, I enjoyed it") or external ("My friends said I was good, no one made fun of my performance").

Children tend to rely on external sources of competence information (e.g., parents, coaches, teachers) until early adolescence when a developmental shift towards a preference for internal goals and performance standards occurs (Harter, 1978). It has been suggested that this decreased dependence on external information sources may enable older children to maintain positive self-perceptions and motivated behaviors (Frey & Ruble, 1990; Weiss, Ebbeck, & Horn, 1997). Research has shown that different levels of perceived competence are associated with different sources of competence information (Horn & Hasbrook, 1987; Weiss et al., 1997). Those children who are at risk (due to low self-esteem or low perceptions of competence) appear to find self-referenced information (e.g., self-improvement, effort) least salient to their own competence beliefs.

Given that perceptions of movement competence are, in Harter's view, largely based on the perceived success of mastery attempts in the movement domain, we would expect the physical competence perception of children with DCD to be low and to become increasingly so with age due to an extended history of failure experiences. The same reasoning would lead to the prediction that perceptions of movement competence vary with severity of the movement difficulties with more severe DCD being associated with more accumulated failure experiences during mastery attempts in the physical domain.

Several studies have found that children with movement difficulties have, on average, lower perceptions of physical or athletic competence than their movement-competent peers (Cantell et al., 1994; Causgrove Dunn & Watkinson, 1994; Rose et al., 1997; Schoemaker & Kalverboer, 1994; Ulrich, 1987; van Rossum & Vermeer, 1990). These findings suggest that children with movement difficulties have an accurate picture of their lack of actual competence in the motor domain. However, a closer look at the research reveals that this may not always be the case, and that the hypotheses regarding the relationships between age, severity of DCD, and perceived competence have not been strictly supported. For instance, while van Rossum and Vermeer (1990) reported that a group of grade 4 children who attended motoric remedial classes had significantly lower perceived athletic competence than their movement-competent peers, the relationship between perceived athletic competence and motor performance within the group who attended motoric remedial classes was nonsignificant. Similarly, Causgrove Dunn and Watkinson (1994) reported a nonsignificant relationship between perceived athletic competence and severity of movement difficulties for children in grade 4; however, this was not a consistent finding across all age groups included in the latter study. Among children in grade 3, perceived athletic competence decreased as severity of movement difficulties increased, as predicted by Harter (1978). In contrast, among fifth and sixth graders, the relationship was reversed with perceptions of competence increasing with the severity of movement difficulties. In an attempt to explain these unexpected findings, Causgrove Dunn and Watkinson postulated that older children with movement difficulties might have been using internal sources of evaluative information. It should be noted, however, that contrasting results have been reported by Ulrich (1987) and Rose et al. (1997), who reported that older children with movement difficulties have lower perceptions of competence than younger children.

Harter's (1978, 1981) theory also predicts a positive relationship between perceived competence and subsequent mastery attempts. In other words, children will generally select achievement tasks that demonstrate their competence and avoid tasks that demonstrate their incompetence. In support of this prediction, recent research examining the relationship between perceived competence and participation during recess has revealed that children in grades 1–4 tend to select playground activities (e.g., sliding, swinging, hanging, running, kicking) in which they feel more competent (Hilton, 2000; Watkinson et al., 1997; Watkinson, Causgrove Dunn, & Cavaliere, 2000). Interestingly, this tendency to approach tasks that demonstrate competence holds even in structured physical activity settings where children have limited choices regarding their participation. A study of participation behaviors of children with movement difficulties in grades 4–6 during physical education revealed that perceived competence was positively related to on-task behaviors, participation in assigned tasks with success, and persistence in the face of failure (Causgrove Dunn, 1997). Conversely, children with movement difficulties who had lower perceptions of competence spent more class time engaged in maladaptive (i.e., off-task) behavior than those with higher perceptions of competence.

Given that perceptions of competence are theoretically important predictors of motivated behavior in physical activity (i.e., engagement, effort, persistence), it is important to determine how children with DCD can develop and maintain positive self-perceptions. Based on Harter's (1978, 1981) theory, we might hypothesize that positive support from others for mastery attempts and encouragement to use internal information sources may contribute to positive performance expectancies, even in children who lack actual movement competence. However, the efficacy of these hypothesized recommendations as interventions intended to improve negative self-perceptions of children with DCD in physical activity settings has yet to be tested.

Eccles' Expectancy Value Theory

Eccles and her colleagues (Eccles et al., 1983; Eccles, Barber, & Jozefowicz, 1999; Eccles, Wigfield, & Schiefele, 1998; Wigfield, 1994; Wigfield & Eccles, 1992) have developed a model of achievement-related choices and behaviors that directly links the choices children make to their expectancies for success, and to the subjective values that they attach to the options perceived to be available. Thus, the model predicts that children with DCD are most likely to engage in activities that they believe they will be successful at, and that they highly value. Like Harter's competence motivation theory, this model assumes that beliefs about the self are highly salient in the choices children make about what to do and how to do it.

Expectancies

Eccles suggests that expectancies of success answer the question, "Can I do this task?" According to her model, expectancies are directly shaped by children's confidence in their abilities (perceived competence) and their perceptions of task difficulty, both of which are influenced by interpretations of past performances, perceptions of the beliefs and behaviors of socializers, and gender-role stereotypes.

Theoretically, children with DCD should have lower perceptions of ability and limited expectations for success across many tasks, due in part to their appraisals of the lack of success they experience in meeting task demands. In addition, negative evaluative information arising from others' appraisals will also contribute to negative expectancies of success in physical activity. This evaluative information is often received verbally, for example, in the form of teasing or as negative verbal performance feedback. However, negative evaluative information may also be behavioral, in the form of unsolicited assistance or in exclusionary behaviors like those described by a 6-year-old boy with movement difficulties in relation to the selection of teams on the playground: "the good players usually get picked first, which sometimes makes other kids left out because they get picked last if they're not good" (Evans & Roberts, 1987, p. 26).

Perceptions of task difficulty appear to have less relevance to choices than perceptions of competence, especially at younger ages (Wigfield, 1994). However, perceived task difficulty and perceived competence are not easily distinguishable in studies with children (Wigfield & Eccles, 1992). While our own research indicates that children as young as those in grade 2 can differentiate different playground activities in terms of both rankings and ratings of task difficulty, for some children these assessments may be largely driven by their own perceptions of competence (Watkinson & Causgrove Dunn, 2000).

Values

Values help children to answer the question, "Do I want to do this task?" Eccles and her colleagues have demonstrated that values may contain four motivational components: attainment value (the importance of doing well, the degree to which the task will contribute to the child's feelings about the self, and the extent it supports a child's desired self-schemata), intrinsic value or interest (the enjoyment one gets from the task), utility value (how the task relates to future goals), and cost (the negative aspects of doing the task). Each of these value components can positively or negatively influence achievement behavior and choice. Similar to expectancies, values are influenced by children's past affective experiences and their interpretations of the outcomes of past performances. Moreover, values are based on goals, which in turn are influenced by the cultural milieu in which the child lives.

Eccles suggested that values have a central role to play in young children's choice of activities, and that the intrinsic value of an activity may largely determine its importance to the child (Wigfield & Eccles, 1992). For example, Dwyer (1999) found that when children with varying playground participation patterns were asked why other children might choose to do certain tasks on the playground, most immediately responded "because it is fun." However, with further probing by the investigator, other values were voiced by the children, including attainment ("she wants to be as good as her friends"), utility ("she wants to be with her friends"), and cost ("they do it by themselves because they don't want other people to see them"). In other words, Eccles' four value components are evident in children's accounts of their participation in playground activities and in their explanations of other children's recess behavior, but enjoyment or interest appears to have primacy. Our own research confirms that children choose to engage in the "most interesting" or "most important" activities more frequently than the "least interesting" or "least important" activities when they go out to play at recess (Watkinson et al., 1997; Watkinson, Causgrove Dunn et al., 2000).

Values are not necessarily shared by all individuals in a cultural milieu. Rather, as part of the self-system, personal values differ from individual to individual. While most children may find certain activities enjoyable and interesting, a lack of movement competence may cause children with DCD to find these same activities less exhilarating and less interesting. Attainment value may also be lower for unskilled performers, so that, for many children with DCD, typical playground skills may be of little value to their self-schema. Furthermore, because the cost of a choice will be considered in decisions to participate in physical activity, children with DCD may choose not to take part in activities they would typically value for the enjoyment they provide, because they are unwilling to place themselves in situations where their performance can be ridiculed or negatively evaluated. As one boy put it when asked why "Johnny" wouldn't play tag if he were the worst person in the class, "[because] they'd try and make fun of him, like little jokes . . . like 'Johnny's It, Co-co fit. He's a naked idiot,' something like that" (Watkinson, Dwyer, & Nielsen, 2000).

Eccles' model suggests that both expectancy and value will have a direct effect on choice, on persistence, and on actual performance (through the mechanism of effort) in the physical activity domain. Task values especially influence intentions and decisions, rather than effort or persistence. Values may be particularly important to the decisions children make about joining physical activities in unstructured settings, because it is in these settings that children do not feel the need to comply with adult directions. Our research suggests that children's playground activity choices in free time are related to both their perception of competence and their perception of the value of the activity (Watkinson, Causgrove Dunn et al., 2000).

At the present time, however, the relationship between expectancy and value is not yet clear. According to Eccles' model, the relationship between expectancies and values should be weak in the early years, and then as children progress toward adolescence, the correlation between perceptions of competence in an activity and the value placed on it should increase. Our recent work with children in playground settings partially supports this theoretical prediction. Specifically, the relationship between children's expectancies (measured as perceived competence) and their perceived interest in specific playground activities increased with age, although the relationship between expectancy and perceived importance remained unchanged (Watkinson, Causgrove Dunn et al., 2000). Research also supports the positive relationship between expectancies and values (i.e., perceived importance of athletic competence) in children who lack movement competence; the higher the rating of importance, the higher the perception of competence in participants in grades 1–4 (Causgrove Dunn & Watkinson, 1994). Unfortunately, there was no analysis by grade in this latter study and therefore it is not known whether the strength of this relationship increased as children matured. Harter (1985) has suggested that a lack of synchrony in values and perceived competence will have a negative affect on both motivation and self-esteem. It is important for us to determine if this is typically the case for children with DCD or if they systematically devalue activities for which they lack competence.

In summary, both expectancies and values have a role to play in choices, according to expectancy value theory. When a child with a history of DCD asks "Can I do this task?" the answer is likely to be "No. I haven't been able to do it well in the past. The other kids teased me when I tried to do it. They think I can't do it, even though all of the other kids my age can do it." However, when the child with DCD asks "Do I want to do this task?" the answer is not as easy to predict. On the one hand, the child might value the activity for enjoyment and affiliation. On the other hand, the cost of taking part in the activity (discomfort, ridicule, scrutiny, negative appraisals) may substantially outweigh the enjoyment and utility (being with others). Indeed, Watkinson, Dwyer et al. (2000) reported one boy with movement difficulties as saying that, while his classmates valued sliding games on the equipment, he didn't because "people have to push people down. I hate those . . . because I'm always the one who gets pushed down. I'm the one who gets picked on."

Achievement Goal Approaches

Achievement goal approaches have been used to predict and explain cognitive, affective, and behavioral aspects of participation in a wide range of achievement situations. An underlying assumption of these achievement goal theories is that individuals strive to demonstrate competence or ability in achievement situations. However, the criteria used to evaluate competence in a particular situation, and therefore an individual's motivation and behavior in that context, are dependent on his or her goals for that activity (Ames, 1992; Dweck, 1986; Maehr & Nicholls, 1980; Nicholls, 1984, 1989; Roberts, 1992). In other words, variations in motivated behavior may not be a reflection of different levels of competence or motivation, but instead may be the result of different goals for participation.

Two different types of situational goals, or goal perspectives, have been identified. One of these perspectives is self-referenced, with a focus on performing tasks to completion, trying hard, acquiring new skills, and improving existing skills. This perspective is referred to as "task involvement" by Nicholls (1984, 1989), "learning goal" by Dweck (1986), and "mastery goal" by Ames (1984) and Roberts (1992). In contrast, the second goal perspective is norm-referenced and focuses on demonstrating superior ability relative to others or, failing that, on avoiding demonstrating low ability relative to others. This second perspective is referred to as "ego involvement" (Nicholls, 1984, 1989), "performance goal" (Dweck, 1986), "ability-focused goal" (Ames, 1984), and "competitive goal" (Roberts, 1992). For the sake of clarity, Nicholls' terminology will be adopted for the remainder of this chapter.

According to Nicholls (1984, 1989), task involvement is likely to promote positive perceptions of competence and motivated behaviors, even in individuals who recognize that they are below average in ability when compared to others. This is because children who are task-involved use subjective, self-referenced criteria (e.g., improvements in personal performance, learning, and mastery) to assess their level of competence. For a child with DCD in a physical activity setting, task involvement will likely lead to decisions to actively participate, assuming at least some improvements in skill and/or knowledge do occur. If the same child adopts an ego-involved goal perspective, however, competence assessments based on social comparisons with peers will likely result in perceptions of failure and incompetence, leading to withdrawal from participation (if possible). If complete withdrawal is not possible, more subtle avoidance strategies may be employed. In a physical education class, for example, the child may pretend he or she is not feeling well or has forgotten the appropriate gym clothing or equipment at home, take extended breaks to get a drink, or may simply try to maintain a physical position on the field or court that is as far away as possible from the center of the activity (thereby reducing the likelihood that anyone will involve the child in the play).

According to Nicholls' (1989) achievement goal theory, an individual's goal involvement is determined by his or her (1) goal orientation, (2) perception of the motivational climate, and (3) level of cognitive development.

Goal Orientation

Goal orientation refers to an individual's dispositional preference for task- and/or ego-involved goals. More specifically, task orientation refers to a tendency or proneness to approach tasks with a focus on improving skills, trying hard, and learning new skills. Ego orientation refers to a dispositional tendency to approach activities with the goal of demonstrating superior performance relative to others. However, because task orientation and ego orientation are independent, individuals have varying levels of predisposition toward both types of goals.

Research indicates that task and ego orientation reflect different theories of achievement, different beliefs about the causes of success, and different views about the purposes of participation in an activity. For example, task orientation is positively related to beliefs that success in physical activity is due to intrinsic interest, motivation, effort, and cooperation (Hom, Duda, & Miller 1993; Newton & Duda, 1993; Roberts, Treasure, & Kavussanu, 1996; Treasure & Roberts, 1994; Walling & Duda, 1995). In contrast, ego orientation is positively related to beliefs that success is due to ability, deception and taking an illegal advantage (i.e., cheating), as well as external factors (Hom et al., 1993; Newton & Duda, 1993; Roberts et al., 1996; Treasure & Roberts, 1994; Walling & Duda, 1995; White & Zellner, 1996). Individuals who are highly ego-oriented are also more likely to endorse the legitimacy of aggressive and injurious acts in sports than people with low ego orientation (Duda, Olson, & Templin, 1991; Dunn & Causgrove Dunn, 1999). With reference to beliefs about the purpose of participation in physical activity, task orientation is positively related to the purposes of personal development, fitness, the promotion of lifetime health, and preparation of good citizens, while ego orientation is positively related to the purposes of improving social status and enhancing self-esteem (Papaioannou & Macdonald, 1993; Treasure & Roberts, 1994).

Goal orientations are presumed to develop over time and to be influenced by socializing adults. Over time, parents, teachers, and coaches play significant roles in the development of goal orientations by making approval or reinforcement dependent upon outperforming others, or alternatively upon effort and personal improvement. Research into the criteria parents use to assess their children's performances (Roberts, Treasure, & Hall, 1994), as well as studies examining the relationship between parents' and children's goal orientations (Duda & Hom, 1993; Ebbeck & Becker, 1994) suggest a tendency for parents to evaluate their children's ability according to their own goal orientations, and then to influence the development of their children's goal orientations by providing feedback consistent with their evaluation.

Cognitive Development

A child's understanding of the concept of ability also influences goal involvement. Nicholls (1978, 1989) described the developmental changes that occur in children's understanding of the concept of ability as a process of differentiating the concepts of luck, difficulty, and effort from ability. Until about 8 years of age, children do not understand the concept of normative difficulty. Prior to this, task difficulty and ability are confounded, in that hard tasks are those that are "hard for me," and easy tasks are those that are judged "easy for me." The concepts of ability and luck continue to be confounded until approximately age 9, when children finally recognize that effort and ability do not influence the outcomes of "luck tasks." Finally, effort and ability are not completely differentiated in all children until about 12 years of age, at which time children develop the mature or adult understanding of ability as current capacity. Prior to this, effort is ability; people who try harder are seen as having more ability. It should be emphasized that almost all children have acquired the adult (or mature) conception of ability by 12 years of age (as opposed to *at* 12 years of age), but many children gain this understanding at an earlier age.

Nicholls (1989) suggests that an undifferentiated conception of ability causes younger children to approach achievement situations throughout the elementary-school years with the goal of increasing mastery, and to assess their competence through self-referenced judgments (e.g., "am I getting better at this?"). For young children with DCD, an undifferentiated conception of ability may enable more positive perceptions of competence, based on self-referenced performance improvements (assuming this occurs), and the understanding that better performance in the future simply requires more effort. Once the mature conception of ability is developed, an older child with DCD realizes that ability can only be accurately assessed in relation to the ability of others (i.e., through normative evaluation). The nature of one's understanding of the concept of ability does not, however, wholly determine which goal perspective will be utilized in a particular situation (Nicholls, 1990, 1992). Virtually all children have developed a mature conception of ability as current capacity by about 12 years of age, but there continues to be considerable variation in the extent to which individuals view superior ability as necessary for success. In other words, individuals who are capable of judging their performance and/or ability from a more differentiated perspective do not always choose to do so (Nicholls, 1989).

Perceived Motivational Climate

The third factor influencing an individual's goal involvement in a particular situation is that perceived motivational climate of the activity (Ames, 1992; Nicholls, 1989; Roberts, 1992). Motivational climates are also influenced by the actions of socializing adults, though it has been suggested that the children themselves contribute to the climate also. Ames (1992) and Nicholls (1989) suggest that in classroom and sporting environments, for example, parents, teachers, and coaches structure motivational climates by providing instructions, feedback, rewards, and explicit expectations for children. Children assess the situational goal structure established for the activity and adopt a consistent goal of action. Situations that emphasize the learning process, maximal effort, and personal mastery are referred to as having a "mastery climate" and are likely to promote task involvement. Conversely, situations that are constructed to emphasize normative evaluation (e.g., focus on interpersonal competition, social comparison, normative feedback), tests of valued skills, and increased public self-awareness, have a "performance climate." A performance climate tends to promote ego involvement (Nicholls, 1984, 1989).

It does not appear, however, that situations contain a general motivational climate that is salient to all individuals. Research in physical education reveals that students perceive differential expectations and treatment by teachers toward high and low achievers, illustrating that it cannot be assumed that cues and demands are perceived the same by all people in a particular situation (Martinek & Karper, 1984, 1986; Papaioannou, 1995). Even when instructions and feedback are consistent for everyone in a particular situation, there are differences in the particular cues selected by individuals and individual differences in how those cues are interpreted (Ames & Archer, 1988). Nicholls (1989) has suggested that the cues selected, and the manner in which they are interpreted, are influenced by the individual's goal orientation. In support of this view, several studies in physical activity contexts have shown positive associations between individuals' goal orientations and their perceptions of the motivational climate (Ebbeck & Becker, 1994; Kavussanu & Roberts, 1996; Seifriz, Duda, & Chi, 1992). In addition, there is evidence that goal orientations influence preferences for different types of performance-related information; individuals high in ego orientation requested more normative information than individuals high in task orientation (Butler, 1993). In situations where participants' goal orientations are in conflict with the motivational climate, Treasure and Roberts (1995) suggest that the goals selected by each individual depend upon the relative strength of his or her goal orientation compared to the motivational climate. In other words, the stronger an individual's predisposition toward task or ego involvement, the less likely that situational cues will override it. Conversely, the weaker an individual's goal orientation, the more easily it can be overridden by situational cues. As a result, situational characteristics may be more influential in determining the goal involvement of children and young adolescents than older adolescents and adults, because children have not yet developed their personal theories of achievement and, therefore, may have relatively weak goal orientations (Treasure & Roberts, 1995, p. 479).

In an effort to test the predictions of achievement goal theory outlined in the preceding pages with children who lack movement competence in a structured physical activity situation, Causgrove Dunn (1997, 2000) examined the relationships among goal orientations, perceptions of the motivational climate, and perceived competence in participants from grades 4 to 6 in physical education. As predicted by Nicholls (1989), highly task-oriented children with movement difficulties perceived the situational goal structures of their physical education classes to be more mastery oriented than those with low levels of task orientation. In turn, the perception of a mastery motivational climate was positively associated with perceived competence (Causgrove Dunn, 2000). In contrast, highly ego-oriented children perceived the situational goal structures of their physical education classes to be more performance-oriented than those with low levels of ego orientation. Perceptions of a performance climate were negatively associated with perceived competence. Perceived competence was positively associated with adaptive participation behaviors (e.g., staying on task, persisting with assigned tasks despite difficulties) and negatively associated with off-task behaviors (Causgrove Dunn, 1997). Also in accordance with achievement goal theories, the perception of a performance climate differentially affected participation behaviors, depending on the individual's perceived competence. For children with movement difficulties who had low perceptions of competence in physical education, increasing levels of perceived performance climate were associated with increasingly maladaptive behavior patterns. These findings are in agreement with the recommendations of achievement goal theorists, and suggest that a physical activity program designed to maintain or enhance positive self-perceptions and active participation by children with DCD should be structured to emphasize subjective self-evaluations based on effort, improvement, and mastery. However, as is the case with other motivation theories discussed in this chapter, these recommendations have yet to be systematically tested in the form of an intervention study. It is not yet known whether physical activity programs designed to emphasize a mastery climate will improve negative self-perceptions and reduce maladaptive behaviors of children with DCD.

Goal Structure Theory

Goal structure theory (Ames, 1984; Ames & Ames, 1984a, 1984b) describes the relationships among children in achieving the goals of a particular activity, and the motivational outcomes that different relationships (or goal structures) elicit. As such, it is another approach that considers the context in which learning and performance take place. The goal structures conceptualized by Ames and her colleagues were based on their study of the classroom climates that differ essentially in the degree to which students are rewarded for, and dependent on each other for, capable contributions.

Competitive Climate

A competitive climate is a situation in which students "work against each other such that the probability of one student achieving a goal . . . is reduced by the presence of capable others" (Ames & Ames, 1984b, p. 536). Competitive activities are ubiquitous in structured physical activity classes. On the playground they are largely, though not entirely, represented by typical sports and games such as soccer and baseball. The nature of competitive settings leads to normative assessments of ability or self-other comparisons that require both competence and effort to avoid failure (Nicholls, 1989). For children who lack competence and thus have low success expectancies, a competitive activity may be intimidating. Moreover, if the activity is not highly valued or is not perceived to support achievements that will lead to attainment of the social goals, it is unlikely that a decision to take part would be made.

Cooperative Climate

Cooperative structures are those in which "the probability of one student receiving a reward is enhanced by the presence of capable others" (Ames & Ames, 1984b, p. 536). These situations are characterized by shared goals, helping behavior, interdependence, and self-group comparisons. A common goal can only be achieved in this setting if it is attained by all of the participants. Because each performer plays a role in the outcome of the group, individuals feel a moral responsibility to pull their own weight. The climate of this kind of goal structure is one in which individuals support and encourage each other, but each individual is expected to contribute an effortful performance (Johnson & Johnson, 1985). A meta-analysis of studies concerning cooperation indicates that cooperation promoted higher achievement and greater group productivity, and promoted more positive social relationships within the group than competition (Stanne, Johnson, & Johnson, 1999). Such analyses are based on group statistics, however, and may mask a person by treatment interaction that would be especially interesting to those who are concerned about children outside the average (Bouffard, 1993).

Cooperative activities are very frequently used in structured activity classes, and take many forms on the playground, including tag games and stunts such as swinging and hanging in which pairs or groups act together to accomplish a goal. Pedagogical experts often recommend the use of cooperative structures to increase opportunities for skill practice and to foster social inclusion (Kirchner & Fishburne, 1998; Nyisztor & Rudicle, 1995), especially for "differently abled" students (Sherrill, 1993). However, Ames and Ames (1984b) suggest that cooperative structures may encourage children to evaluate their own contributions to the group. For a child who lacks movement competence, this evaluation may lead to negative affective outcomes (particularly when the group fails). In other words, for children who have difficulty making capable contributions toward the group goal, a cooperative goal structure may not be as facilitative of involvement as many practitioners think.

Individualistic Climate

Individualistic climates are those in which success is "neither diminished nor enhanced by the presence of capable others" (Ames & Ames, 1984b, p. 536). It is a situation in which the goals of participants are unconstrained by the goals of others, where independence, individual effort, and self-self comparisons are typical. Individualistic structures are typically adopted in activity settings to foster skill practice and problem solving. Sherrill (1993) recommends that competition against the self, and other forms of individualistic structure, should be used to facilitate the development of more positive self-concepts in children who lack movement competence.

Research has shown that children can perceive the three goal structures described by Ames and Ames (1984a, 1984b) in structured physical activity settings (Cavaliere, 1999). Moreover, it appears likely that children take the goal structure of the playground activity into account when they decide to join or not join an activity. Interviews with children who do not take part in many of the activities of their peers at recess indicate that the psychological cost of taking part in competitive or cooperative activities, especially if they are open to the scrutiny of peers, may be too high for some children (Watkinson, Dwyer et al., 2000). For example, one child attributed his avoidance of tag games to the cost of ruining the game for the whole group because of his inability to run fast enough to avoid being "it" all the time. Obviously, contexts can have a powerful influence on children's participation decisions.

Consideration of the Person-Task-Environment Interface in the Study of DCD

Research has begun to explore the relationship of a child's psychological makeup and his or her perception of the performance climate. However, it is still unclear how these relationships are affected by the actual activity choice or the specific context in which the child is participating. Will perceived ability influence motivation and behavior in individual activities such as free play in the same way that it does in sports and games, or dance? Are there aspects of specific activities that make them more or less likely to produce positive motivational orientations for all children, regardless of their actual movement competence? Do children who lack actual movement competence learn more, or feel more positive about themselves in certain activities or certain active settings? Is it possible that children with DCD are awkward in some psychological or social contexts and not others? According to ecological psychologists, the movement performance of children exists within a context that has physical, social, and affective constraints and affordances (Davis & Burton, 1991; Davis & van Emmerik, 1995a, 1995b). In Gibson's (1979) terms, the environment provides "affordances" to living creatures who perceive and act on those affordances according to their perceptions of themselves. The person is conceptualized as a living system driven by information and constrained by physical and social structures and systems. Physical structures include the space, equipment, relative size of objects, weather and other environmental influences. Social constraints include the nature of the social group in which the behavior is taking place, the behaviors of significant others in the social group (teachers, parents, peers), and the relationships of the participants in the group to each other. Social constraints or affordances detected by the affective system contribute to decisions about participation. In other words, the social setting in which the behavior will take place is assessed relative to the affective or psychological properties (constraints or affordances) of the participant to determine whether these properties afford the attainment of personal goals. In spite of the current popularity of the ecological approach, few attempts have been made to capture the essential features (beyond teacher behavior) of the setting that are perceived by the participant. Virtually no studies have examined participation outcomes in physical activities as the product of psychological or affective constraints and affordances, social or environmental constraints and affordances, and physical constraints and affordances.

SUMMARY AND CONCLUSIONS

The motivation theories discussed in this chapter suggest that decisions by children with DCD to participate or withdraw are at least partially driven by self-perceptions and perceptions of the activity context. Specific decisions and behaviors are mediated by expectancies and values in a particular activity, by conceptions of ability and competence, and by motivational orientations that may be moderated by perceptions of the climate and the goal structure of the activity. These psychosocial factors are complex and difficult to assess, but may be responsive to interventions designed to change or maintain positive and adaptive perceptions. Put differently, it may be possible to influence the participation decisions and behaviors of children with DCD by addressing their perceptions of themselves or by tackling environmental factors that may lead to positive and adaptive decision-making, in addition to changing their movement competence. An ecological task analysis approach, which considers all aspects of the child, including psychological and motoric capacities, along with the task itself and the social and physical environment in which it is performed, may be a fruitful approach to the study of children with DCD.

CHAPTER

13

Families As Partners

Sharon A. Cermak and Dawne Larkin

When a child is struggling at home or at school, there is often an impact on family functioning. Difficulties with motor coordination affect not only those with the condition but also their families (Chesson, McKay, & Stephenson, 1990; Chia, 1997; Sprinkle & Hammond, 1997). To enhance our understanding of the impact of developmental coordination disorder (DCD), clinicians and educators need to understand the implications from the child and family perspective (Cohn & Cermak, 1998). Brown and Barrera (1999) emphasize the importance of understanding the child within the family and the family within the community when assessing the child's and the family's needs. Miller and Hanft (1998) emphasize that partnerships with families that accommodate cultural and ethnic aspects are essential for developmental assessment. Using a systems approach facilitates the identification of family resources and concerns (Seligman & Darling, 1997). It is important to develop a "parent-professional partnership" model in which the parent's and child's perspective is highly valued. Including the family can help educators and therapists to design interventions that are congruent with parents' values and needs (Cohn & Cermak, 1998; Cohn, Miller, & Tickle-Degnen, 2000). However, Lawlor and Mattingly (1998) point out that there are many unresolved dilemmas with family-centered care, so it is necessary to ensure that the families want to be involved with their child's intervention

In this chapter, we focus on understanding parents' perceptions of the problems experienced by the child with DCD. We deal with the parents' contributions to the diagnostic process, and their perceptions and concerns about the motor skills and social participation of their child. We address the important issue of physical activity and the implications for the family and child. Finally, we focus on the resilience and coping strategies of families and their expectations for their child with DCD.

THE DIAGNOSTIC PROCESS

Identification of a child's motor problem is often difficult. Chesson and colleagues (1990) reported that many mothers of children with motor learning difficulties knew that there their child had a problem, but they could not specify it. Because parents did not know whom to consult, there were a number of unsuccessful contacts with health professionals (Stephenson, McKay, & Chesson, 1991). Many parents indicated that the child's problem was a source of stress in the family (Chesson et al., 1990), as was the diagnostic process (Chia, 1997; Stephenson, McKay, & Chesson, 1990). However, identification of the motor problem produced varied effects ranging from relief to reluctant acceptance and even denial.

Chia (1997) reported similar findings using a questionnaire with eight parents of boys aged 7–10 who had dyspraxia and were referred for occupational therapy. Parents identified concerns about understanding their child's diagnosis. For some parents, having a diagnosis was a relief. One parent said, "At last somebody believed me. I have been concerned for months" (Chia, 1997, p. 106). For others, the process of uncovering a diagnosis was stressful and anxiety provoking. Short and Crawford (1984) also emphasized the positive outcomes from the identification of children's movement problems. Parents of elementary school children indicated that the knowledge of their child's coordination difficulties increased their understanding of the child, and "they realized their children were not lazy, slow or inattentive and were then able to be more realistic in their expectations" (p. 36).

The Dyspraxia Foundation (1998), a support group for parents of children with dyspraxia, was interested in diagnosis of dyspraxia and sent a questionnaire that was completed by 454 members of the group. Although 65% of parents realized their child had difficulties by the time the child was age 3, less than 10% of the children were diagnosed by age 3; 56% were diagnosed between ages 4 and 11 years, with 75% of the children not diagnosed at the time they started school. Results of another questionnaire completed by 114 parents whose children had DCD or other mild movement impairments indicated that it took an average of 19–24 months and three professionals to obtain a diagnosis (Ahern, 1995). One-third of parents surveyed had concerns about their preschool child's progress and had sought help, however, appropriate tests were not carried out until difficulties were experienced at school several years later.

In a qualitative interview of 11 parents of children with movement difficulties, Ahern (1995) examined factors that induced parents to seek professional help for their child's difficulties with motor coordination. One of the most common motor problems described by parents was their child's inability to ride a tricycle. Ten out of 11 parents particularly noticed this. Poor balance was described in connection with climbing and playing on playground equipment such as slides and monkey bars. Many parents indicated that their child had difficulty coordinating walking and running, and said their child "looked funny" or fell over often.

Research to date indicates that identification of movement difficulties is often a long and stressful process. For example, the data from the Dyspraxia Foundation (1998) indicated that 3 years was the average age for parents to report that they were aware their child was having difficulties, while the average age for diagnosis of dyspraxia was $6\frac{1}{2}$ years. Factors that can contribute to these delays in diagnosis include family dynamics and differences in parents' observations (Chesson et al., 1990); parents' concerns about the motor behaviors and the effect they have on the family (Stephenson et al., 1990); the position of the child in the family; the gender of the child (Stephenson et al., 1991; Revie & Larkin, 1993); and parents' or professional's limited knowledge about the condition and its long-term consequences (Fox & Lent, 1996).

Once a child's difficulty is identified and diagnosed, families seek information about their child's condition. Stephenson and colleagues (1991) emphasize the importance of giving this type of support to parents. This provides the family with control and a way for them to focus on helping their child. In a survey of parents of young children with disabilities (Humphry & Case-Smith, 2000), parents reported that they desired information and that the information should address the following concerns, in order of priority:

1. The child's disability
2. The services available for the child
3. The future
4. The services for the parents
5. General child development
6. Services for the siblings

Parents want information for themselves and also so that they can explain the child's needs to other family members and professionals (Stephenson & McKay, 1989).

PARENT PERCEPTIONS AND CONCERNS

Parents' reports of the movement competence of their children with DCD are generally quite accurate (Hoare, 1991). Interviews and questionnaire data from parents provide insights into their perception of their child's motor behavior. Hoare reported that 58% of parents with children in the group with DCD ($n = 74$) thought their child had below average handwriting; only 8% reported above average handwriting. In comparison, 13% of the parents of the control group ($n = 71$) rated their child's handwriting below average and 43% rated it above average. Fifty percent of the parents of the children in the group with poor coordination rated their child's manual dexterity below average, and 45% of parents rated drawing/painting below average. It was clear from the ratings that many parents recognized the difficulties their children were experiencing with movement as 74% indicated that their child had below average coordination.

While most parents are aware of their child's abilities, there are cases in which parents perceive their child's motor development to be appropriate when their child is performing below his or her peers (Abbie, Douglas, & Ross, 1978; Gubbay, 1975). For example, in Gubbay's survey of 63 children with motor difficulties, 39 parents indicated that their child was average or above average at sport while 24 parents ranked their child's sporting ability as below or well below average. If a child has a significant delay in one area such as language, a mild delay in the motor area may not be noticed, and motor skills may even be considered a strength. For some children with DCD, the gap between the child's abilities and the expected performance may not become apparent or problematic until the child enters school and the expectations change (Humphry & Case-Smith, 2000).

Within multicultural societies, there are differences in motor expectations, and these can contribute to different expectations about motor competence (Cintas, 1995; Hopkins & Westra, 1989). At times, this creates discrepancies between parent reports and societal or peer evaluations. Families from different cultures often have different perspectives on child rearing, health care, and disabilities. For example, in some cultures, parents may expect a child to begin feeding himself with a spoon at 18 months of age and dress independently by age 4. In other cultures, parents may feed the child until he or she is old enough to use a spoon without spilling food, or they might continue to dress the child for an extended time (Henderson, 1995). Similarly, culturally based beliefs affect the manner in which families adapt to a child with a disability, and these beliefs also influence the family's level of trust and use of professionals (Seligman & Darling, 1997). Professionals working with children and their families need to be aware of differences in lifestyle or in parent-child interaction that may affect perceptions of the child's problems and acceptance of professional recommendations (Seligman & Darling, 1997).

SOCIAL PARTICIPATION: A VALUE AND A CONCERN

How do the parents see the social participation of children with DCD? Parents often indicate that their child with movement problems has difficulties in the social domain, and are concerned that their child has few social contacts with other children (Schoemaker & Kalverboer, 1994). They express sadness that their child is not invited to birthday parties (Chia, 1997) and indicate that their child has no friends (Taylor, 1990). In a survey of 74 parents of children with poor coordination, 31% of parents indicated that their child had below average popularity; 28% reported below average social interactions; and 24% indicated below average attitude to others. Sixteen percent of parents indicated that their child had below average levels of cooperation and 15% reported below average conduct (Hoare, 1991). These numbers contrasted markedly with the control group in which the percentages ranged from 1% to 4%. For overall social behavior, 22% of parents of the children with poor coordination replied that their child was below average, while 1 out of 71 parents from the control group replied that their child was socially below average. A higher percentage of the control group was reported by their parents to have above average social behavior (55%, popularity, to 69%, attitude to others) compared to parent reports for the group with DCD (21%, popularity, to 42%, conduct).

Some parents are concerned with their children's aggression and indicate that their child's movement problems interfere with social participation. Gibson (1996) identified that children who were physically incompetent often became frustrated. In Gibson's study, one mother reported that her child "gets angry and frustrated at school. If he hasn't managed to do his work, he'll come home and take his anger out on us. He flies into a temper" (p. 103). Chia (1997) found that most parents reported feeling isolated and felt that the community did not seem to have an understanding of the stresses experienced by families who have children with dyspraxia. Parents expressed feelings of mental and emotional exhaustion, guilt, frustration, and resentment. Parents reported that their child's condition affected both their leisure activities and that of their children. Parents commented that "they were too tired to entertain or visit friends because of the high level of attention that they needed to give to their child" (Chia, 1997, p. 107). It is not surprising that parents of adolescents who had motor difficulties indicated that they experienced higher levels of family and health related stress than parents of a control group (Larkin & Parker, 1999).

Parents express concerns for the psychosocial well-being of their child with DCD. Ahern (1995) found that a high percentage of parents (65%) believed they needed to protect their child with movement difficulties from having his or her feelings hurt by others. The words from a young boy exemplify the effect of poor motor skills on social standing and self-esteem:

> They always pick me last. This morning they were all fighting over which team had to have me. One guy was shouting about it. He said it isn't fair because his team had me twice last week. Another kid said they would only take me if his team could be spotted four runs. Later, on the bus, they were all making fun of me, calling me a "fag" and "spaz." There are a few good kids, I mean kids who aren't mean, but they don't want to play with me. I guess it could hurt their reputation. (Levine, Brooks, & Shonkoff, 1980, p. 83)

Cohn (2001) described a qualitative research study of 16 parents whose children, ages 4–10 years, were receiving occupational therapy. When asked, "At what point did you decide to seek therapy for your child?" there was a common concern related to their child's ability to participate in the social contexts in which they live, learn, and play. All the parents interviewed worried that their children were not "fitting in" or "keeping up" with their peers. One parent expressed concern because her daughter was not engaged in playing with other children. Although most parents think about their child's academic performance, parents of children with DCD often are more concerned with their child's social world.

Information from the family assists in developing a general profile of the social problems that the child is experiencing. For example, Reuben and Bakwin (1968) reported a case of a bright 10-year-old boy whose "clumsiness was a source of distress at home at the dinner table and in dressing" (p. 605). Identifying difficulties with using a spoon, fork, and knife at a developmentally appropriate age, and difficulties with dressing suggests a motor problem. Further probing can add weight to meeting DSM-IV criteria that the motor problem interferes with the child's activities of daily living. Moreover, the motor problems may have social implications that can be identified during parent interviews: How do the parents respond to the problems with eating? How do the grandparents respond? Do the siblings react? Does this problem change the social behavior of the family? For example, does the family stop going out to nice restaurants with their children? Is the child teased by peers at school for messy eating?

THE FAMILY AND PHYSICAL ACTIVITY

An important part of parenting is managing a child's movement opportunities (Sprinkle & Hammond, 1997). Parents make choices about toys, friends, and experiences that can help or hinder their child's ability to acquire new movement skills. In addition, shared recreational and leisure activities form the basis for many family traditions and result in a sense of family unity and identity (Humphry & Case-Smith, 2000). Oftentimes, the skills and interests of a child limit family activities (Chesson et al., 1990). For example, children with DCD may avoid or not want to participate in physical activities such as hiking, camping, or biking. Parent's efforts to protect their child with DCD from physical harm can also influence participation in physical activity. Sprinkle and Hammond report an incident where parents protected their child by providing a confined space for long periods of time. They did not understand the motor problem or realize that limiting movement could further constrain motor development.

Generally there is an assumption that family involvement in physical activity influences the activity of the children (Anderssen & Wold, 1992; Brustad, 1993). If this is the case, then parents with DCD who have withdrawn from a physically active lifestyle may not provide the experiences and modeling for their children. In turn, this could lead to a deprived movement environment for the child and compromise motor skill development. Very little research has looked at the relationship of parental coordination and physical activity with skill and activity in children who have DCD. In an early study, Rarick and McKee (1949) described factors that were different between 10 third-grade children with very high levels of motor proficiency and 10 third-grade children with very low levels of motor proficiency. These groups were selected using tasks such as running, jumping, throwing, striking, catching, side-stepping, and balancing (primarily gross motor activities) that typically identify children with DCD. Only 3 of the 10 children in the group with very low motor proficiency had one or both parents actively participating in athletic activities, while 9 of the 10 children in the group with very high performance had one or both parents active. None of the children from the group with low motor proficiency had frequent active play with their parents in contrast to 8 children in the group with high motor proficiency. In addition, the play facilities in the home more frequently were adequate for children in the high motor proficiency group than the low proficiency group. And, although twice as many members of the low-proficiency group lived near playgrounds, fewer of the low-proficiency group were regular attenders.

There have been remarkable changes in the influences on children's lives since this early study. Television and computers have become a part of daily life and our society has become more sedentary. In a recent study by Hoare (1991), there was no significant difference between the time spent on sport and recreation by the families of children with DCD and families of a control group. Of note was that 22% of families from the DCD group and 21% of families from the control group reported that they seldom spent time in family recreation; only 4% of the parents of the group with DCD and 11% of the control group families reported daily recreation. Another study also found no differences between the reported physical activity of parents of adolescents who had a history of movement difficulties and parents of the control group. However, there was a significant relationship between parents and adolescents with movement difficulties, whereby parents who perceived more barriers to participation in physical activity were more likely to have children who perceived more barriers (Larkin & Parker, 1999).

It is possible that decreased parental participation in motor activities with their children is due to the children's poor motor skill and reluctance to engage in this type of activity. Alternatively, poor coordination of the parent might contribute to decreased activity by the parent. For some families, there is a familial tendency for coordination difficulties or DCD. In a number of families with a child with DCD, a parent will indicate that they have similar problems (Hoare, 1991). In some families, there are siblings as well as a parent with motor difficulties. Involving the family in a movement intervention program can improve the outcome for the child with DCD and the family as well (Larkin & Parker, 1996). However, Thursfield (1980) cautions that some parents have unrealistic expectations or demonstrate overt rejection of their child. In these circumstances, parental participation in the intervention process could have negative consequences.

The value of physical abilities varies within and across cultures, influencing the parent's perceptions of whether there is a "disability." Many parents do not understand the contribution of regular physical activity to the growth and development of the child, particularly the musculo-skeletal and the cardiovascular systems. It is important for the clinician and educator to help parents and children make these links so that both the child and the family can recognize the benefits of engaging in regular physical activity. We have instances where families have increased their activity level and expressed pleasure in their continued physical activity as a function of their initial involvement in their child's intervention program (Larkin & Parker, 1996).

RESILIENCE AND COPING

It has long been recognized that a child's development is strongly influenced by the child's caregiving environment and family system. A number of factors appear to affect the response of family members to the child's motor difficulties resulting in positive and negative influences on the family and the child. Some families create wonderfully supportive systems where there is a good balance between the child's strengths and limitations and his or her interaction with the family. These parents counterbalance some of the negative environmental influences that the child can experience through interactions with the peer group at school. Although these families may still experience initial and ongoing problems, they enjoy their child's accomplishments and appreciate their child's growth.

Alternatively some families do not understand the motor difficulties of the child and consequently react negatively to the clumsy behavior (Sprinkle & Hammond, 1997). In some families, parents may provide support while siblings tease the child. The response of siblings to the child with DCD has varied, with a range of relationships and emotions (Chesson et al., 1990; Gibson, 1996). Relatives also can have positive or negative influences. All these relationships affect how the family copes.

Compare the grandfather who takes his grandson with DCD fishing with the grandparents who make the parents and child feel unwelcome because of spills at the meal table. Stephenson and colleagues (1991) emphasize that "an important part of therapeutic intervention may be increasing children's self-confidence and reducing intra and extra family tensions" (p. 91).

The perceived coordination level of family members and their successes or failures in the motor domain can have important influences on family coping strategies. Problems have emerged from families where the father has been an excellent sports person and his son has DCD and is unable to meet the father's expectations. A phrase repeatedly overheard is "when I was your age I could. . . ." Some parents who had poor motor skills when they were young but who were able to achieve with extra effort feel that their child could also do better if he or she just tried harder. Other parents recognize the challenges that their child is facing and are extremely supportive, providing gentle guidance and encouragement as the child struggles to master everyday motor skills.

Chesson and colleagues (1990) identified differences in parental relationships toward the child who had motor/learning difficulties, when compared to their relationships with siblings. These included parents treating the child differently, showing more anger or frustration, greater protectiveness, less patience, or making more allowances for them than for their siblings. Similar findings are reported in other studies (Ahern, 1995; Gibson, 1996; Sprinkle & Hammond, 1997).

Sometimes marital relationships have been affected by problems associated with having a child with DCD or mild motor impairment. Chesson et al. (1990) found that "the two most frequently reported sources of marital strain were: (i) factors associated with the identification and acknowledgement of the child's problems; and (ii) approaches to child handling and management" (p. 129). From interviewing parents of 31 children with motor difficulties, parents of 10 children indicated that their marriage had been negatively affected by stress related to the child's difficulties. Family dynamics differ so markedly that responses can range from meeting what is oftentimes an ongoing challenge to finding a source of strength in the intervention process.

PARENTAL EXPECTATIONS FOR INTERVENTION: HOPES AND REALITIES

Cohn and colleagues (2000) stated that it is important to develop goals and objectives that are congruent for parent's hopes for therapy outcomes. When examining parent's hopes for change with occupational therapy in children with sensory modulation disorder, parents expressed both child-centered outcomes and parent-centered outcomes. Three interrelated child-centered themes emerged: social participation, self-regulation, and perceived competence. Parents hoped that their child would fit into the school, community, and family context, and develop acceptable ways of regulating behavior.

While parents valued increases in their child's self-worth more than they valued increased skill, they recognized that their child's improvements in skills and engagement in activities was enabled by therapy and contributed to their child's reconstruction of self-worth (Cohn et al., 2000). In another study, parents perceived that occupational therapy helped their children to take more risks. They reported that it improved self-confidence, which contributed to "a willingness to try new things; acceptance of help; increased perseverance and achievement" (Stephenson et al., 1991, p. 106). Parent's also report that movement programs help their child with motor difficulties improve in a range of motor, social, and cognitive skills (Abbie et al., 1978; Cantell, Larkin, & Hands, 1999). In response to intervention programs parents indicated positive changes in their children's physical coordination, behavior, self-confidence, concentration, willingness to try, and ability to mix.

In several studies (Cohn et al., 2000; Stephenson et al., 1991), two themes related to parent-centered outcomes emerged: the desire to learn strategies to support their children, and personal validation of the parenting experience. These were clearly linked to their children's construction of self-worth. Parents valued the support, information, and strategies learned to enhance their parenting. Parents found that by understanding their child and understanding why things were difficult, they were able to develop more realistic expectations for their children and themselves. They found that they were better able to advocate and communicate with school personnel. Parents reported being more sensitive to their children's needs and were able to provide better support for the child's present and future development.

SUMMARY AND CONCLUSIONS

In summary, it is clear that families have remarkably different dynamics that can influence the social and physical world of the child with DCD. It is important to explore the parents' values and beliefs as well as their knowledge of their child's motor and social difficulties. A family-centered understanding of contextual issues and problems experienced with activities of daily living provides valuable information about the parent's perceptions and concerns and aids the diagnostic process. By identifying the goals, values, and desires of the parents as well as those of the child, we can engage the parents and child as partners in the intervention process in a way that matches the family resources.

PART

VI

Interventions for Developmental Coordination Disorder

CHAPTER

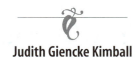

14

Developmental Coordination Disorder from a Sensory Integration Perspective

Judith Giencke Kimball

While the term developmental coordination disorder (DCD) has become the internationally accepted name for the symptoms displayed by the child with difficulty in coordination, most of the work by occupational therapists using a sensory integrative (SI) approach utilizes the term "developmental dyspraxia." Whether this term is synonymous with DCD is debatable, but it is clear that the symptoms described in SI literature represent at least one subgroup of DCD.

DEFINITION

Ayres defined developmental dyspraxia as "a motor planning problem" (1979, p. 91) and as a "disorder of sensory integration interfering with ability to plan and execute skilled or non-habitual motor tasks" (1972a, p. 165). She stated that "praxis is a uniquely human skill that enables us to interact effectively with the physical world" and "is one of the most critical links between brain and behavior. Praxis is to the physical world what speech is to the social world. Both enable interactions and transactions." (1985, p. 1). It is "really, a kind of 'intelligence' or human competence, but our usual interpretation of the word 'intelligence' does not necessarily include praxis" (1985, p. 7). Ayres stated that "praxis and motor function are not synonymous," that "in treating dyspraxia, the emphasis is on ideation (generating an idea), concept formation, and planning; whereas in treating a neuromotor problem, the emphasis is on motor execution" (1985, p. 2).

Individuals who are dyspraxic have difficulty initially planning a nonhabitual motor act and also have difficulty internalizing the plan of the movement they want to accomplish. As a result, they cannot effectively call on that plan in a situation where the common components of previous learning could be extracted and used as a basis for new learning, thereby increasing the efficiency of new motor learning (Kimball, 1993, 1999). "Praxis is not a question of whether the child can accomplish the movement, but whether he can accomplish it with integration and quality" (Kimball, 1993, p. 109).

THEORY

A short synopsis of the evolution of the thinking and research in sensory integration (SI) provides the rationale for treatment of children with dyspraxia using an SI frame of reference. In-depth discussion of SI theory may be found in Ayres (1985), Fisher, Murray, and Bundy (1991), Kimball (1993, 1999), and Parham and Mailloux (2001). The seminal work in the development of the theory explaining the etiology and the treatment of dyspraxia from a sensory integration framework was done by A. Jean Ayres beginning in the 1960s (Ayres, 1965) and continuing through the 1980s (Ayres, 1972a, 1979, 1985, 1989). Ayres (1965, 1972a) recognized that, as our understanding of neurobehavior is refined, SI theory and implications for practice will also change. The work initially begun by Ayres has been continued by numerous occupational therapy researchers and clinicians (Fisher, Murray, & Bundy, 1991; Cermak, 1991; Kimball, 1993, 1999; Clark, Mailloux, & Parham, 1989; Parham & Mailloux, 1996; Wilbarger & Wilbarger, 1991).

One of Ayres' major contributions to the understanding of coordination problems in children is the concept that dyspraxia is more than a motor coordination difficulty. She hypothesized that dyspraxia reflects inefficiencies in the central nervous system (CNS) that result in less than optimal integration of sensory input and a decreased ability to utilize that input to produce the desired actions on the environment. These praxis-related coordination problems have far-reaching consequences. They influence the child's ability to organize, and to start, stop, and sequence motor activities, and also may influence the child's ability to do the same with cognitive activities (Kimball, 1993, 1999).

In developing sensory integration theory, Ayres (1965, 1966a, 1966b, 1969, 1972b, 1972c, 1977, 1978, 1989) conducted a series of factor analytic and cluster studies in which she identified different types of sensory integration dysfunction. Although each study made its individual contribution and there was variability among studies, common factors emerged. A praxis factor was consistently identified in almost all studies. Praxis (motor planning), assessed by having the child imitate nonmeaningful positions assumed by the examiner, was repeatedly linked with difficulty processing information through the tactile and kinesthetic senses (e.g., poor tactile and kinesthetic discrimination) and, to a lesser extent, the vestibular-proprioceptive senses. Ayres termed this "developmental dyspraxia." Ayres (1972a) suggested that praxis or motor-planning ability depends in part on a well-developed body scheme. The most recent standardization of the Sensory Integration and Praxis Tests (SIPT; Ayres, 1989) resulted in new and revised methods to test dyspraxia, enabling differentiation of types of practic abilities (Fisher & Murray, 1991, p. 10).

Ayres (1972a) discussed the differential contributions to praxis of the alert/arousal component and the discriminative component of each sensory system, with particular attention paid to the tactile/kinesthetic, proprioceptive, and vestibular systems. Ayres (1972a) suggested that, when the alert/arousal component is not contributing in an optimal way, issues such as sensory defensiveness (sensory system modulation problems) may develop. When the discrimination component is not functioning optimally, there is inadequate support for development of normal practic abilities. These theoretical explanations have been expanded by others. In Table 14.1, the functions addressed in SI are divided into three areas. Praxis has always been viewed as an end product ability that relies in part on the adequate processing of underlying sensory/motor processes. These underlying processes are delineated as "functional support capabilities," a term coined by Kimball (1993) (for a listing, see Table 14.1).

Evaluation of children using the Sensory Integration and Praxis Tests (Ayres, 1989) and other assessments (e.g., Dunn, 1999; Miller, 1988; Parham, 1987) reveal many combinations of difficulties. Some children show difficulty with sensory modulation as their primary problem. This difficulty regulating sensory information to produce an appropriate adaptive response may result in sensory defensiveness (Dunbar, 1999). Other children show primary problems in motor planning (dyspraxia) and still others manifest a combination of problems. When difficulty in sensory modulation is seen as part of the child's condition, it must be treated first or concurrently in order to optimize treatment, because difficulty with sensory modulation may mask the emergence of practic and other abilities (Dunn, 1999; Kimball, 1993, 1999; Miller et al., 1999; Stallings-Sahler, 1998; Wilbarger & Wilbarger, 1991).

SENSORY DEFENSIVENESS

Wilbarger and Wilbarger (1991, p. 1) define sensory defensiveness as "the overactivation of our protective senses." Kimball (1993, 1999) explains that sensory defensiveness results from a modulation problem in sensory processing. Information from sensory systems registers in an additive fashion in the nervous system to contribute to the total picture. If the sensory systems input results in a high level of arousal, this activates the primary survival response of the organism, a fight, flight, or freeze response. If it is not possible to fight or flee, the high level of arousal does not dissipate easily, leaving the individual with increased anxiety, difficulty completing adaptive responses in the environment, and a central nervous system that is on a heightened level of alert. In this state, the individual is more likely to respond in a survival mode to a sensory input that normally would not be interpreted as a threat and might even seem trivial to the observer. Thus, the term "sensory defensiveness" (SD) is often used. A more complete description of SD (also

Table 14.1   Sensory Integrative Functions

Sensory Modulation ⟶ Functional Support Capabilities ⟶ End Product Abilities*

Sensory System Modulation
- Manner in which sensory system processes input
- Influences ability to use the information processing component optimally
- Influences and influenced by arousal level
- The way in which the sensory system processes input affects the quality of a child's ability to respond adaptively

Under or overreactivity to sensory information in tactile, auditory, visual, vestibular, olfactory, or proprioceptive systems can result in problems in:

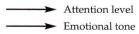 Attention level

⟶ Emotional tone

Functional Support Capabilities
- Information processing component of sensory systems—discrimination of sensory information
- Underlies and provides support for the end-product abiliites
- Helps integrate and modulate input from the arousal/reactivity components of the sensory system
- Integrates the information/discriminative components of sensory systems

Includes:
- *Suck-swallow-breathe synchrony:* support for biting, chewing, phonation, vocal abilities, and postural control
- *Sensory discrimination:* ability to perceive through touch and other sensory systems, and to define the spatial and temporal qualities of the environment
- *Cocontraction:* stabilizes joints for use; contributes to balance and movement patterns important for praxis
- *Muscle tone:* provides basis for equilibrium, movement, and praxis
- *Proprioception:* relates to understanding of body's position in space
- *Balance and equilibrium:* responsible for ability to maintain posture and to move through the environment
- *Lateralization:* development of hand dominance
- *Bilateral integration:* ability to use both sides of the body together in action; includes midline crossing

End Product Abilities
- Reflect integration of sensory system modulation levels and functional support capabilities

Includes:
- *Praxis:* planning the course of action, including sequencing
- *Form and space perception skills:* basis for some aspects of academic skills
- *Behavior:* cognitive, social, and environmental; also need to consider sensory modulation and functional support antecedents
- *Academics:* should be viewed in relation to other end-product abilities
- *Language and articulation*
- *Emotional tone:* includes stress level and self-esteem; closely related to sensory modulation
- *Attention and activity level:* includes self-control and ability to stay focused cognitively and motorically
- *Environment mastery:* ability to produce an appropriate adaptive response with appropriate praxis, emotional tone, activity, behavior, and academic level

*In order to produce the desired adaptive response, an individual must be able to modulate sensory information and have reasonable functional support capabilities. This model is presented as a linear model for simplification, although it is recognized that the process is not linear and there is an interplay among systems.

called "sensory modulation dsyfunction") and its treatment can be found in a number of publications (Kimball, 1999; Miller et al., 1999; Wilbarger & Wilbarger, 1991).

FUNCTIONAL SUPPORT CAPABILITIES

Once treatment for difficulty in sensory modulation (if present) has been addressed, the treatment for dyspraxia is begun. Treatment for dyspraxia using a SI frame of reference initially focuses on facilitating improvement in the functional support capabilities (FSCs). Deficits in functional support capabilities are viewed as key components contributing to poor praxis (Ayres, 1972a, 1985). The ten functional support capabilities are listed in Table 14.1. They are mainly physical capabilities that underlie and support praxis and other abilities. They help integrate the two distinct types of sensory systems input, alert/arousal, and discrimination, through providing avenues for modulation of alert/arousal input and avenues for interpretation of discriminative input. A sensory integration frame of reference utilizes therapeutic activity specifically to increase the child's functional support capabilities that are hypothesized to improve those functions thought to contribute to good praxis. For example, an activity that includes challenges to proprioception and balance would help improve functioning in those areas as well as increase muscle tone and cocontraction, all in preparation for an activity demanding more difficult motor planning. Functional support capabilities are also incorporated into therapeutic activities aimed specifically at improving praxis. Take the example of a child working on the timing and sequence of catching a ball. Practice and analyzing the skill into its component parts are commonly used in other frames of reference, such as motor learning, to improve the skill of catching. In SI and in the ecological framework, different sizes of balls would be used to improve practic abilities through variety in visual/spatial attributes. To improve the child's praxis, proprioceptive input is varied using different weights of balls, and vestibular/balance input could be added by having the child swing straddling a bolster swing. All this adds multiple sensory systems and the opportunity to increase integration of those senses (SI), with adaptive responses resulting in increased support for accomplishing praxis. The types, intensity, frequency, and duration of sensory input are carefully evaluated and modified so "disintegration" does not occur. Success is an important ingredient for praxis and self-esteem.

TREATMENT OF DYSPRAXIA

Dyspraxia is seen as one of the "end products" that may be influenced using a sensory integration frame of reference. Many therapists feel that influencing the development of practic abilities has far-reaching effects on the other end products, although much of this needs to be empirically examined (Ayres, 1972a, 1985; Kimball, 1993, 2000). It has been previously stated that having good practic ability influences more than just movement; it contributes to the ability to start, stop, sequence, and organize in cognitive action realms. Being able to start, stop, sequence, and organize has a great influence on the quality of the child's participation in his or her daily activities that utilize these abilities.

THE ENVIRONMENT: PHYSICAL AND EMOTIONAL

In treatment using sensory integration, the environment is used as a catalyst in the facilitation of sensory integration. Therapists make use of the environment to create challenges, enhance organization, and develop an inner drive and patterns of successful interaction in order to enhance the competence of the child (Burke, 1998).

Occupational therapy using a SI approach has been done traditionally in a clinic environment because it is easier to accomplish therapeutic goals. The processes to achieve the goals include the following:

1. Increased intensity of selected sensory input
2. Many affordances for the child to select activities that will provide enhanced sensory input
3. Opportunity for adaptive motor responses

The child's natural environment also provides many opportunities to improve practic abilities as they are embedded in the child's normal occupations, especially play and school. Common to SI activities is some form of intense movement or vestibular/balance input. This necessary intensity can be accomplished through therapy or play equipment suspended from the ceiling (or a tree or outdoor play structure). Traditionally, the types of equipment suspended have included the following: a net swing or hammock suspended from one or two points, a tire swing, a platform swing, a trapeze bar, a bolster swing, and a flexion swing. Also used is anything upon which the child can sit and bounce (therapy ball), stand and bounce (trampoline) or pull with arms and get a rebound such as a shock cord. The environment also is filled with movement-based toys such as scooter boards to ride around the room and down the ramp, ball type games, riding toys that can be driven by using arms alone, and a bubble ball container to jump into or lie in.

The therapist desires that the environment enable the provision of a variety of sensory inputs. Besides equipment, this can include different heights as can be found in lofts, climbing structures, hiding structures, and ramps (inclines) and different surfaces as can be constructed with varying thickness, heights, and weights of mats or foam. Other differences can be found in varying light, sound, and fragrance. Sensory integration is different from a sensory stimulation approach because in sensory integration, the sensory input is coupled with an adaptive motor response initiated and carried out by the child. It is believed that this linking of sensory processing and adaptive motor responses is needed for optimal sensory integration to occur (Ayres, 1972a; Kimball, 1999, 2000).

While providing the physical environment for SI challenges is essential, providing the emotional environment is equally essential for successful treatment. Participation of a knowledgeable therapist is necessary to assure physical as well as emotional safety. Good relationships between the child, therapist, and parents are needed and must be carefully fostered. Environments must be set up to provide the "just right challenge" physically and emotionally to improve sensory integration and praxis as well as the self-esteem that comes from the child's participating fully, successfully, and joyfully in his occupation of play.

TREATMENT PROCESS

As stated previously, sensory modulation problems are addressed first in the treatment process, as a modulated central nervous system has the best chance of successfully completing occupational demands. This is followed by work on the functional support capabilities, which should be paired initially with less complex motor planning. For example, the child with low muscle tone and poor cocontraction could use heavy joint and muscle work (proprioception) combined with movement (vestibular) to increase feedback to his or her joints and muscles, thereby increasing the tone and cocontraction. An example would be the child pushing himself across the floor prone on a scooter board and pushing large blocks over, or using shock cord (elastic) to pull himself while lying on a platform swing. These activities have only simple practic requirements, but provide the preparation of the underlying neural process thought to facilitate the development of praxis (Ayres, 1972a, 1979, 1985; Kimball, 1993, 1999). After or concurrent with the increased input to underlying sensory processes (FSCs), activities with more complex practic components are facilitated.

The following are basic tenets of sensory integration to facilitate the development of praxis:

1. Treatment is child-oriented and, when possible, child directed. The child is enticed to engage in activity, usually not formally directed. There are two reasons for this: (a) the child's volitional engagement in occupation will increase his motivation and emotional involvement which will lead to greater success, and (b) the child must initiate his own body movements in order to activate the neural mechanisms of feed forward and efferent monitoring if practic abilities are to be improved.

2. Treatment is aimed at underlying deficits rather than specific behavior or skill development. The purpose of using a sensory integration approach is to build a repertoire of motor responses based on good or improved functioning of the functional support capabilities, which support the child's improvement in the process of motor planning (versus a particular motor skill). Unlike some motor learning approaches (see Chapter 16), treatment in SI traditionally has not been based on repeated practice of the same task. Sensory integration relies on the building of motor patterns by using multiple contexts, and changes in the surface characteristics of the task (e.g., throw a bean bag in a box, throw a ball in a box). The therapist initially elicits an outcome, then slightly changes the task characteristics to meet the outcome requirements. In this way, the child must change some part of the adaptive response, thus building a motor repertoire. For example, the child rides down the ramp on a scooter board and crashes into a padded wall. He shows good ability to extend his back (prone extension) while moving down the ramp and can get his hands out (protective extension) to stop himself before hitting the wall (both FSCs). In addition to crashing into a pad, other activities the child could perform during

the riding down the ramp include hitting a suspended ball with two hands, pushing aside plastic bowling pins or picking up bean bags and throwing them into a target. Two activities and then three activities in a row performed before hitting the wall would greatly add to the practic challenge and help build praxis.

3. Use of the body senses is emphasized in SI. All sensory systems are believed to influence each other, therefore treatment is multisensory. Several sensory systems may be needed to get the desired response, thus the term "sensory integration." For example, Shelly is a 7-year-old first grader who is having problems with fine motor and gross motor skills. Her teacher is particularly concerned with her handwriting. Shelly has an immature grasp, holds the pencil very tightly, and presses down so hard that the pencil lead breaks. She has low muscle tone, poor cocontraction, and poor postural stability. Shelly reported that "writing makes my hand hurt." Rather than practice handwriting, the occupational therapist using a SI frame of reference provided FSC activities in numerous sensory areas prior to handwriting. These included hand games with squishy Play-Doh and resistant theraputty (proprioception and tactile); doing chair or wall push-ups (proprioception); writing on paper taped to the blackboard or an easel (proprioception and visual); using markers with thicker points than a pencil and vivid color (visual); and even scents in the ink (olfactory). Breathing activities and songs were also added. A pencil grip was available when she desired it. When possible, the occupational therapist added movement activities (vestibular) in the morning, but most writing activities were preceded with only one or two of the above suggestions because of time constraints and fitting into the environment of the class. With this variety of sensory input, Shelly made improvements in printing and showed greater endurance; her teacher began incorporating some of the activities into the regular classroom routine.

4. Adaptive responses must be within the child's developmental level while stretching him or her a bit for growth (the achievable challenge). If a child is pushed too hard, rather than sensory integration, you will achieve sensory "disintegration" as the child becomes frustrated and fails. It is important to elicit adaptive responses to the environment in the natural occupations of children, play, self-care, and work (school).

5. While adaptive motor responses are desired, adaptive emotional and ideational responses are just as important. The child needs to know what he or she wants to do to act on his environment. Verbalizing it before he or she does it may help develop praxis. As starting, stopping, and sequencing are problematic for children with dyspraxia, at first, the child may need help to initiate sequences or cues as to where and how to stop.

While the above are the basic tenets of the SI frame of reference, the following case study describes its use.

Case Example

Mike was a 9-year-old third grader referred for occupational therapy at his school. Mike had difficulty in school with math, spelling, handwriting, following directions, finishing tasks, paying attention, and organizing work to start and sequence. He could not skip, do jumping jacks, jump rope, blow bubbles with gum, or put together puzzles. His favorite pastime was watching television. His mother reported that Mike did not like to participate in any activities requiring gross motor coordination. When the family went for walks or sledding, Mike would complain of fatigue and refuse to continue participating. When sitting at his desk at school or at the kitchen table, he often would hold his head up with his hands. He did like to be in the water, but had a very difficult time learning to swim, as he could not put the strokes together. Mike's mother and teacher both reported that he showed a disorganized approach to tasks. WISC-III intelligence testing revealed a Verbal IQ of 110, Performance IQ of 72, and Full Scale IQ of 90.

Results of the occupational therapy evaluation showed that Mike did not have difficulty in sensory modulation. However, Mike had lower than normal muscle tone and poor cocontraction. His typical posture was stooped shouldered with his head forward. He was overweight and large for his age. He showed poor ability to catch his balance in prone, sitting, and standing, and often was not able to get his hands out to catch himself when he fell. He showed poor stability of proximal muscles resulting in lessened ability to hold a stable upright posture around mid-line, resulting in constant wriggling. These factors also contributed to Mike's easy fatigue. Mike's practic abilities were poor. He had great difficulty with alternating forearm rotation, serial finger thumb opposition, and jumping jacks. When the jumping jack activity was broken down into parts, hands only and feet only, he still could not accomplish it. He could not hold his body up against gravity while in the "superman" position on his stomach or while totally flexed on his back. He was not able to flex his body enough to get his feet off the floor in order to swing hanging from a trapeze, and he had difficulty holding his body weight while trying to just hang onto the trapeze bar in spite of normal muscle strength. His ability to start, stop, sequence, and organize an activity was compromised.

Mike's occupational therapist at school focused on helping Mike meet his educational needs. The occupational therapy program at school incorporated principles of sensory integration including having Mike do "readiness" activities before a fine motor related task such as handwriting, and before transitioning to a new activity. These activities included using theraputty, wall or chair pushups, isometric activities with hands and arms, and helping the teacher or janitor with any heavy work activities such as taking the chairs off the desks in the morning. The school occupational therapist also worked on gross motor coordination mainly using a scooter board as the school did not have suspended equipment.

While principles of sensory integration can be incorporated into school-based practice, most school systems do not have the physical environment to support sensory integration procedures. Mike's school-based occupational therapist referred him to a private occupational therapist in order to address more specifically his SI problems. Private occupational therapy initially focused on increasing functional support capabilities especially muscle tone and cocontraction so Mike could move his body against gravity. Activities included those with vestibular and proprioceptive sensory input, starting with simple practic challenges such as sitting or lying on various moving pieces of equipment (e.g., a platform swing and a bolster swing) and keeping his balance. Later, a more difficult practic challenge was added such as batting balls or picking up objects from the floor while swinging. After holding his body weight with his arms and flexing his feet on the floor to swing on a trapeze, Mike progressed to swinging over objects while keeping his feet up, and then to swinging over objects and letting go at the proper time to crash land in mats.

Mike's mother reported that after several months of individual treatment, Mike was able to join the family in sledding. He could pull his sled up the hill for the first time, and lasted over one hour without complaining of fatigue. His ability to actually start his homework and organize himself also improved. Mike's teacher reported that Mike showed gains in math skills. One of Mike's goals for himself was to improve his swimming, as he really liked spending his summer days at the pool. After preparatory work on functional support capabilities to provide facilitatory input, the therapist provided consultation to Mike's swimming instructor on the practic abilities inherent in swimming. Mike's father stated that Mike improved much faster in swimming during the summer that he received therapy than in previous summers, and he was able to coordinate his strokes well enough to pass an intermediate level swim test.

EFFECTIVENESS RESEARCH

Occupational therapy using sensory integration has gained popularity as an approach to remediation of disorders of sensory modulation and developmental dyspraxia (Vargas & Camilli, 1999). However, there exists controversy regarding the documented effectiveness of this approach. There have been a number of published literature reviews of research examining the efficacy of sensory integration. Some have examined effectiveness with a particular population of children such as those with mental retardation (Arendt, MacLean, & Baumeister, 1988) or with learning disabilities (Hoehn & Baumeister, 1994; Polatajko, Kaplan, & Wilson 1992; Schaeffer, 1984). Others have reviewed sensory integration efficacy with multiple populations (Cermak & Henderson, 1989; Miller & Kinnealey, 1993; Ottenbacher, 1982, 1991; Spitzer, Roley, Clark, & Parham, 1996; Vargas & Camilli, 1999). Overall, the results of research across studies have not yielded consistent findings. When considering the effectiveness of sensory integration approaches for children with DCD (or dyspraxia), it is critical to examine the effectiveness of intervention with that population. However, most research on the effectiveness of sensory integration has included a broader variety of participants, such as children in the general category of learning disabilities or the general category of sensory integration dysfunction. Because not all children with learning disabilities have sensory integration problems and not all children with sensory integration problems have dyspraxia (Cermak, in press; Missiuna & Polatajko, 1995), it is not possible to draw conclusions about the effectiveness of sensory integration procedures for children with dyspraxia (or DCD) from these studies.

Research is now beginning to look at specific types of sensory integration dysfunction in specific clinical populations such as sensory modulation disorders in children with Fragile X (McIntosh, Miller, Shyu, & Hagerman, 1999; Miller et al.,

1999; McIntosh, Miller, Shyu, & Dunn, 1999). Similar research is needed with the DCD population. We need to examine whether the population of children with DCD and the population that occupational therapists refer to as developmental dyspraxia are the same or different populations. Evidence suggests that DCD is a heterogeneous group, with different subtypes (see Chapter 3). We need to ascertain whether children with motor planning problems and difficulty integrating information through their somatosensory senses are a valid subgroup of children with DCD. We need to examine whether and in what ways children with DCD and/or developmental dyspraxia benefit from sensory integration procedures. We need to compare the effectiveness of SI to other intervention strategies, such as task specific interventions (see Chapters 16 and 17) or motor learning (see Chapter 15). We need to identify which approaches work for which children and for which outcomes. We also need to scrutinize SI treatment studies to be sure that what is being called SI really meets that criteria (Kimball, 1988). It is highly likely that many do not.

SUMMARY AND CONCLUSIONS

Developmental dyspraxia, as defined within the context of the sensory integration framework, can be considered as a subtype of DCD. Using a sensory integration approach for the treatment of praxis is a complex process aimed at improving underlying problems such as sensory modulation where necessary, and functional support capacities which influence praxis. Sensory integration procedures focus on improving praxis to enable the child to more fully participate in his or her daily occupations of play, self-care, and school/work. Successful treatment of practic problems may have a profound effect on a child's life, improving not only his or her coordination, but influencing other areas such as self-esteem and organizational abilities, thus enriching the quality of life for the child and his or her family.

CHAPTER

15

Integrating Motor Learning Theories into Practice

Cheryl Missiuna and Angela Mandich

Many different types of intervention approaches for children with developmental coordination disorder (DCD) have been developed and researched over the years. Recently, with the increased emphasis on evidence-based practice, we have seen a trend toward examination and comparison of the efficacy of particular approaches. In a review of many of the approaches that have been used with children with DCD, Sigmundsson, Pedersen, Whiting, and Ingvaldsen (1998) concluded that it may be the teacher or the underlying teaching principles, not the specific intervention method, that accounted for any positive treatment effects. In this chapter, current motor learning theories are examined in order to identify and describe the principles that can be used to guide intervention with children with DCD.

MOTOR LEARNING THEORIES: PAST AND PRESENT

The motor learning theories that guide practice today have emerged gradually as either a compilation of, or a reaction to, older theories of motor learning and motor control. Most of the motor learning theories that we consider to be "classic" in terms of their contribution to the field originated about 30 years ago in an era when it was believed that sensory input simply elicited stereotypical movements known as reflexes. At that time, changes in motor behavior were thought to reflect the maturation of a central nervous system that was hierarchically organized. As the cortex gradually assumed control of motor functions, primitive reflexes were believed to be inhibited or integrated in order to form the basis of more functional movement patterns (Kamm, Thelen, & Jensen, 1990). The Closed-Loop Theory of Adams (1971) is recognized as the first more comprehensive explanation of motor learning. While he agreed that the central nervous system controlled the execution of movement based upon sensory feedback, he proposed that errors in motor performance were compared with existing memory traces. When you practiced a given movement, the memory trace would become stronger and the accuracy of the movement would increase. This emphasis upon learning from intrinsic and extrinsic feedback was an important step forward; however, Adams theory was criticized as it could not explain movements that were made in the absence of any sensory input or feedback (Shumway-Cook & Woollacott, 1995).

Hierarchical models continued to dominate our understanding of motor learning and skill development throughout the 1970s and 1980s. In his schema theory, Schmidt (1975) proposed that new movements were created using a generalized motor program that was derived from similar types of movements that had been made in the past. The child stored in memory the initial conditions of any particular movement, the specific parameters that were used to make it, the outcome, and the sensory consequences of the movement. When a novel movement was required, the initial conditions and desired outcome would be recognized and a schema from a similar type of movement would be selected and put into place. A motor program would be generated and the response specifications evaluated through feedback from the body and the environment. This type of mechanism was described as "open loop," since preprogrammed instructions were formed and sent outward to effect movement. The schema would, however, be modified by the movement experience, and the detailed aspects of movement such as the specification of parameters of force and distance would become more refined with continued practice of the movement. Schmidt's schema theory contributed to many of the motor learning principles used today regarding optimal practice schedules and feedback about the outcome of the movement (knowledge of results). Over the next decade, Schmidt's theory was developed and modified (Schmidt, 1988, 1991). Although other theories have also been advanced, the underlying premise has remained fairly similar.

As we moved into the 1990s, we began to see the strong emergence of dynamical systems theories in the motor learning field. Rejecting the concept of a centralized, hierarchically organized set of motor programs, dynamical systems theorists argued that movement development is an emergent property of the interaction of multiple, cooperative systems (Thelen, Kelso, & Fogel, 1987). With each new stage of a child's development, movement problems arise and the central nervous system must evolve dynamically to address them (Eliasmith, 1998). There is considered to be a need for heterarchical cooperation among the subsystems of the learner, the action goal, and the context in which the task is to be performed. Factors within the child that influence this interaction include the child's biomechanical, neural, and physiological capabilities but also his or her cognitive problem-solving abilities and experience with the task (Ulrich, 1997). In order to facilitate motor learning, it is necessary to identify the factors that may be changed in order to move the system forward to the next level of performance (Burton & Miller, 1998). Thelen (1995) has suggested that variables such as physical growth and biomechanics may be more important for motor learning in infancy and that factors such as experience, practice, and motivation may be more influential when the child is older. Ultimately, according to dynamical systems theorists, children will learn functional motor behaviors as they discover the fit between their capabilities and the goals that they wish to achieve.

It is interesting to note that it is only the most recent of motor learning theories, the dynamical systems theories, that have finally been able to address a problem posed back in 1967 by Bernstein as the "degrees of freedom" problem. Bernstein (1967) pointed out that, within a hierarchical, centrally programmed system, there were far too many independent coordinates (e.g., joints, individual muscles) to be controlled during every single movement. Effective movement involves the coordination and control of sets of muscles in order to allow stabilization of some joints and movement of others. Dynamical systems theorists agree with Bernstein's proposition that groups of muscles spanning across several joints are constrained to act as functional units, referred to as "coordinative structures" or "movement synergies," which represent the child's preferred strategy to solve a task in the most energy-efficient way (Thelen, 1995; Ulrich, 1997). Acceptance of the idea of synergies and of the interaction between the child, the action goal, and the features of the environment are critical to understanding principles of motor learning today.

The most recent advance in motor learning theories is reflected in Gentile's (1998) proposition that both implicit and explicit learning processes take place in parallel during the acquisition of a functional motor skill. The explicit process is a conscious mapping of a set of correspondences between the child and the environmental conditions in order to achieve the action goal. The idea is that the child puts into place a movement structure that is "in the ballpark" and is good enough to meet the task demands. More specific processes such as muscle contraction patterns, stabilization and positioning of joints, and response to gravity and other forces are only crudely organized at first, but, with continued practice, become more controlled and finely tuned. These changes in the organization of force components increase performance efficiency but are not conscious and are therefore considered to result from implicit learning (Gentile, 1998). Gentile's (1998) contribution brings us to the point of considering the key principles that guide intervention from a motor learning perspective.

PRINCIPLES OF MOTOR LEARNING

The basic premise of motor learning theories is that movement skill can be improved through the provision of appropriate practice and timely feedback. Research within this field has indicated that decisions about the scheduling and variability of practice experiences and about the kind of feedback that will be most useful depend upon the stage of the learner and the type of task to be learned. Specific intervention techniques may also differ depending upon which type of motor learning, implicit or explicit, requires facilitation. Four key variables—stage of the learner, type of task, scheduling of practice, and type of feedback—will now be described and discussed with regard to what is known about children with DCD.

Stage of the Learner

Fitts (1964) and then Fitts and Posner (1967) described three stages of acquisition of skilled movements. In the first stage, the cognitive stage, the child gets the general idea of the movement, bringing to that situation any factual information or background knowledge that is applicable to that task. It is a stage characterized by large variability: the child may use awkward body postures, error rates are likely to be high, and the child may not be aware of what needs to be improved or changed. Colley (1989) indicates that this is the stage during which the child has the greatest need to attend to and integrate information from the environment. The second stage, the associative stage, is the phase during which the child learns to perform the skilled movement with some degree of accuracy. This stage is characterized by fewer errors and the child is able to use error information to correct movement patterns. In the final autonomous stage, the skill is able to be performed fluently and automatically. Slow improvement is still possible at this stage, and the child can usually detect his or her errors and make the appropriate corrections.

Children with DCD have been described as having difficulty learning novel motor tasks, executing new motor skills, and generalizing learned motor skills to new situations (Ayres, 1985; Denckla, 1984; Goodgold-Edwards & Cermak, 1990). It is probable that these children have difficulty establishing the timing and sequencing of the synergies of movement (Blanche, 1998) and that the early cognitive stage of learning will often need to be the focus of intervention.

Type of Task

From a motor learning perspective, it is important to classify motor skills across a number of dimensions since each of these is relevant to the way in which the intervention session will need to be structured.

1. *Gross motor—fine motor.* The first type of classification of motor tasks describes the type of muscle groups that are required to perform the skill (Magill, 1998). Most gross motor actions such as walking and running use large musculature and are considered to be fundamental skills. Fine motor skills usually require greater control of small muscles including those of the hands and fingers. Van Wieringen (1988) drew a similar distinction when he suggested that skills such as crawling and walking are phylogenetic skills that rely on existing coordinative structures that are shared by all humans. Other skills such as handwriting and playing piano are ontogenetic: they have to be taught and tend to be culturally bound.

2. *Simple-complex.* Simple motor tasks such as reaching for an object require a decision followed by a sequenced response. More complex tasks such as handwriting require the integration of information from a variety of sources and the application of underlying rules that guide performance (Colley & Beech, 1989). This way of thinking about tasks parallels the open-closed loop distinction described by

Adams (1971). In an open loop task, a motor program is put into place before the action begins and it is not modified during performance of that task. An example of this would be throwing a ball. In a closed loop task, such as cutting out a shape with scissors, the child has to continue to monitor and respond to feedback received intrinsically from the body and extrinsically from the environment.

3. ***Discrete-serial-continuous.*** Some tasks require a single discrete movement with a clear beginning and end point. An example of this would be depressing the space bar on a keyboard. Other tasks are considered to be serial because a series of distinct movements need to be combined to achieve the action goal; for example, typing a sentence contains a series of discrete movements. At the other end of the continuum are continuous motor skills, such as swimming, that contain movements that are repetitive but do not have a distinct beginning and ending (Magill, 1998). Tasks that are discrete or serial can be practiced in parts, but tasks that are continuous usually need to be practiced in their entirety.

4. ***Environment changing—stationary.*** The difficulty of learning a task is influenced tremendously by the extent to which the task is predictable. When the environment is changing or variable, the child has to learn the movement and also learn to monitor the environment in order to adapt to change. Running on rough terrain or playing soccer are examples of tasks in which the environment is constantly changing. This concept is not to be confused with the open and closed loop features of a task as described above. Brushing one's teeth or playing the piano are tasks in which the child must monitor sensory feedback during the task (closed loop), but the environment remains stationary (Sugden & Sugden, 1990).

Children with DCD typically have less difficulty with phylogenetic skills but seem to have more trouble with learned tasks that require greater precision and hand-eye coordination. Continuous, closed loop tasks and situations in which the environment is changing require the child to expend resources monitoring intrinsic and extrinsic feedback during performance of the task and present a great challenge for these children. The impact of the child and/or the environment being stable or moving is so critical for children with DCD that it served as the theoretical underpinning for the section of the Movement Assessment Battery for Children (Henderson & Sugden, 1992) that asks about children's areas of task difficulty.

Practice

One very important consideration in motor learning is the practice schedule. Two aspects of the scheduling that have received much attention in the literature are decisions about whether the order of tasks that are practiced should be random or blocked and whether tasks should be practiced as components or in their entirety.

Random vs. Blocked

There is little question that blocked practice, repeating the same task over and over again, leads to improved performance on an immediate basis. If the emphasis is on learning, however, then random practice is much superior both with regard to retention and also transfer to novel, more complex, tasks (Lee, Swanson, & Hall, 1991). Random practice seems to encourage learners to compare and contrast the strategies that they are using to perform different tasks. If a movement problem can be solved by simply recalling the most recent solution to it, then the cognitive effort involved in problem solving and in developing a plan of action is bypassed (Lee, Swinnen, & Serrien, 1994).

Part or Whole Task

Adams (1987) indicated that the most bewildering body of literature in the motor learning field had to be "the field of part-to-whole transfer, which asks whether the most efficient way to learn a task is to practice repetition of the whole task or to practice subtasks" (p. 45). Theories which suggest that automatization occurs through the chunking of smaller parts into larger parts support an approach that incorporates practice of subcomponents of the task. A contrasting view has been proposed by Marteniuk (1986), who believes that action plans develop based upon the child's perceived goal of the task and previously acquired movement capabilities. Learning is modified through a comparison of the results of the movement to what was desired. This idea has been supported by Singer and colleagues (Singer, 1988; Singer & Caraugh, 1984), who suggest that, during the learning phase of a complex motor task, various cognitive processes need to be activated and controlled at the appropriate moment in time. This latter argument supports a whole task approach. Research on this issue suggests that it may be the type of task that is of greatest relevance to the part-whole decision (Shumway-Cook & Woollacott, 1995). If the task is one in which coordination, sequencing, and timing is involved, then whole task practice will be more effective. If a task is discrete or contains distinct parts, then individual movements can be practiced as part-tasks but should then be combined into whole-task practice. A child learning to play hockey could be taught to shoot on goal as a discrete task, for example, but the movement of hitting the puck would then need to be combined with skating toward the goal.

The reasoning behind the guidelines outlined above is important to understand when considering intervention with children with DCD. While there is no doubt that repetition of a task results in motor improvement, it seems that it is actually the child's cognitive processes that are affected by the repetition (Lee et al., 1991). Practice involves the child's repeated attempts to solve a goal-related movement problem based upon previous experience with that problem. It is the problem-solving activity that is engaged in by the learner that contributes to how well the skill is eventually learned (Lee et al., 1991). Bernstein's (1967) early view of the role of practice was quite profound in that he emphasized that practice should not consist of repeating the means of solution but of repeating the process of solving the movement problem. It would seem that most complex tasks should be practiced as whole tasks with the child's attention directed to the relevant part in order to guide the solution. If generalizability is the goal, practice sessions should progress from more constant to changeable environmental conditions so that the child acquires the ability to solve increasingly varied movement problems.

Types of Feedback

Different types of feedback contribute to the process of learning a motor skill. Feedback can be either intrinsic or extrinsic to the child with the latter type of feedback focusing either on the child's performance (knowledge of performance) or on the results of their motor behavior (knowledge of results).

Intrinsic Feedback

Intrinsic feedback is inherent within a task and is received from any of the child's sensory systems through the normal production of movement (Schmidt, 1991; Shumway-Cook & Woollacott, 1995). For example, when a child is handwriting, they receive information from their body as they perform the task. "I feel my feet flat on the floor, my back against the chair, my hand holding the paper. I can see the pencil move. I am holding the pencil very tightly." In children, intrinsic feedback is generally not perceived consciously unless external direction is provided that asks the child to attend to it. Gentile (1998) cautions that, when handling techniques or manual guidance are used, the therapist becomes part of the regulatory conditions of the task, and this alters the intrinsic feedback available to the child. Movements that are physically guided by the therapist may interfere with the implicit learning that is needed for children to generate their own movement structures. Again, it is the cognitive effort associated with learning to interpret one's own intrinsic sources of feedback that appears to influence learning of a skill (Lee et al., 1994).

Extrinsic Feedback

Extrinsic feedback is provided by the therapist or by observing the results of one's actions and generally supplements the intrinsic feedback that is available. Extrinsic feedback serves to increase the rate of skill acquisition and can be provided either in the form of knowledge of performance or knowledge of results (Magill, 1998; Schmidt, 1991). As a general rule, feedback should be precise and provided frequently in order to increase a child's motivation to continue to work on a task; however, extrinsic feedback should usually be delayed a few seconds in order to permit the child to process intrinsic feedback first (Poole, 1991).

Knowledge of performance (KP) refers to the type of feedback provided regarding the process or pattern of movement that is used to achieve the goal (Schmidt, 1991; Shumway-Cook & Woollacott, 1995). Knowledge of results (KR) refers to the type of extrinsic feedback that focuses on the outcome or success of the action. Both are important types of feedback because they motivate the learner and are used to guide change. The scheduling and frequency of extrinsic feedback is of concern if learning, rather than improved performance, is the aim. Feedback should typically be provided quite soon after a movement, but not immediately, as one does not want the learner to become reliant on the information (Miles Breslin, 1996). For a similar reason, feedback should not be provided on every movement attempt in order to give the child an opportunity to learn to monitor the outcome of the movement pattern him- or herself.

With children who are learning motor skills in a typical fashion, intrinsic feedback often provides sufficient error information and extrinsic feedback, in the form of knowledge of results, is not required or may be of only minimal assistance. Children with DCD often have difficulty establishing movement synergies, however, and extrinsic feedback may be a key to identifying and correcting error patterns. It has been proposed that these children do not solve movement problems in a typical way and that extrinsic feedback that focuses the child's attention on important sensory cues, specific aspects of the task, and features of the environment may be important (Lefebvre & Reid, 1998).

THE IMPORTANCE OF MOTOR LEARNING PRINCIPLES FOR CHILDREN WITH DCD

Hypotheses concerning possible causal mechanisms in children with DCD have been outlined in earlier chapters and interventions to address some of these impairments have been described. While the ability of each approach to "fix" the underlying impairments may be open to debate, few would argue that there is a need to intervene in order to prevent some of the secondary effects of the disorder. Children with DCD spend less time engaged in physical activity (Schoemaker, Hijlkema, & Kalverboer, 1994) and lack fitness and strength (O'Beirne, Larkin, & Cable, 1994). They tend to avoid motor activities and, therefore, have fewer opportunities to practice motor skills: lack of competence and lack of motivation thus combine and result in lack of participation (Bouffard, Watkinson, Thompson, Causgrove Dunn, & Romanow, 1996; Wall, Reid, & Paton, 1990). Movement education approaches used with this population must provide "optimally challenging, success-oriented and joyful experiences for children with DCD" (Rose, Larkin, & Berger, 1998, p. 325) in order to break this vicious cycle. It would seem to be imperative to begin with action goals and tasks that the child wishes to learn and to find a way of helping the child solve those movement problems. Children with DCD do not appear to have the basic skills required to analyze task demands, interpret appropriate cues from the environment, use knowledge of performance to prepare for upcoming actions, or adapt to situational demands (Goodgold-Edwards & Cermak, 1990; Lefebvre & Reid, 1998). Therefore, the principles of provision of feedback at the right stage of learning and providing problem-solving movement opportunities make sense.

MOTOR LEARNING PRINCIPLES: APPLICATION

From a motor learning perspective, the therapist or movement educator's role is to evaluate, and then facilitate the development of the postural control and movement synergies that are necessary for the child to achieve a functional action goal (Blanche, 1998). Although specific treatment protocols have not been described in the motor learning literature, a number of authors have discussed the series of steps involved in implementing motor learning principles (Davis & Burton, 1991; Larin, 1998; Yang & Porretta, 1999). These authors describe the importance of beginning with a clear identification of the action goal. The most obvious way to do this is to simply ask the child what he or she wishes to or needs to be able to do. The movement educator then specifically delineates the required movement and its function.

The second step involves the educator performing an analysis of the goal or task that the child has selected, by simply watching the child perform the task. Burton and Miller (1998) have described a systematic process within which the analysis can be conducted, called "ecological task analysis." In contrast with traditional task analysis, in which the task or goal is analyzed in isolation, ecological task analysis focuses on the dynamic aspects of movement behavior by examining the limitations and enablements of the child, the environment and the task as they interact. There is no assumption of a single best solution for task performance. Multiple solutions are possible and are determined by the unique reciprocal relationship between the constraints of the environment, the child's capabilities and attributes, and the goal or intent of the action (Burton & Davis, 1996). The child is asked to perform the task a few times, using whatever movement skill or form he or she prefers. The outcome of each movement choice is recorded and analyzed. Following this observation, the therapist will also be able to describe the action goal with regard to the task classification described in an earlier section. In addition, the therapist will need to establish the function of the task, which elements of the task and/or environment are invariant and which are modifiable, and identify the link between each of these features and the capabilities of the child. For example, if the function of the task is to catch the ball, the educator might determine that the distance and force with which the ball is thrown, the size, and texture of the ball are variables that can be modified during the early stages of learning. The child with balance and coordination problems might begin to learn to catch while in a seated position with a large nerf ball tossed gently toward him or her.

When the ecological task analysis is complete, the therapist or movement educator will develop a plan for intervention. Taking into consideration the stage of the learner, the therapist will develop a plan that will consider the frequency and type of practice and feedback that will be required to learn the task. The context will also be determined: in most instances, a "multicontext" approach is optimal so the child will be more likely to learn and generalize the motor skill (Toglia, 1991). This means that the task may need to be presented in a variety of ways and in a number of settings.

Within a motor learning model of practice, the therapist may use a variety of techniques including verbal instructions, positioning, and demonstrating movement strategies. Verbal instructions will focus on the correspondence between the child and objects in the environment and will emphasize key movement features that are directly related to achievement of the functional goal (Gentile, 1998). Generally, verbal instructions about the entire movement should be provided first, followed by breaking the task down with an emphasis on only one or two essential elements at a time (Larin, 1998). Based upon the results of research on feedback, some trial and error should be permitted without feedback in order for the child to attempt to solve the problem himself.

Physical handling is another technique that can be used to guide a child's body position or to promote movement; however, the extent to which manipulation should be used is a subject of some debate (Nicholson, 1996). It has been suggested that providing manual guidance may be helping during the early stages of learning because it can guide selective attention and help the child organize and plan the movement. As discussed earlier with regard to intrinsic feedback, others feel that guidance or facilitation of movement should be used as little as possible because the therapist rapidly becomes part of the environment and this alters the intrinsic sources of feedback that are available to the child (Gentile, 1998).

Demonstration or modeling is another therapeutic technique that is congruent with a motor learning perspective. Observing another person performing the motor skill can be useful to help children attend to environmental cues and essential features of the task. With children who have a low level of skill, watching a peer or another individual who is in the early learning stages has been found to be more effective than observing a skilled performer (Lee, Swanson, & Hall, 1991). Observational learning may be enhanced by verbal instruction to focus the child's attention.

Modern perspectives of motor learning recognize that learning only takes place when there is evidence of a relatively permanent change in the child's ability to respond to a movement problem or achieve a movement goal. Therefore, motor learning must be evaluated through tests of retention and transfer, not just immediate changes in motor performance (Ma, Trombly, & Robinson-Podolski, 1999). Therapists who use motor learning principles during intervention will not be satisfied with the child demonstrating acquisition of the original action goal during the therapy session. In order to test whether motor learning has actually taken place, the therapist must create an opportunity for the child to demonstrate that learning during a subsequent session (retention), on a closely related task (transfer), or in a different setting (generalization). As described in an earlier section, application of the principles of motor learning is quite different if immediately improved performance is the goal of intervention. In nearly all cases with children with DCD, however, learning that is permanent and generalizable will be the goal of both child and therapist.

Case Scenario

Jordan is an 8-year-old boy who was referred to occupational therapy for assessment and intervention due to coordination problems. Jordan was described by his family physician as having "poor fine and gross motor skills" and was given a diagnosis of developmental coordination disorder. Although Jordan reached all developmental milestones within normal limits, he had difficulty acquiring many seemingly simple tasks of daily living. Riding a bike, learning to tie his shoes, buttoning his shirt, playing catch and cutting his food were all challenging activities. Presently, he is having difficulty writing his letters, and complains that his hand tires easily. In gym class, he cannot keep up with his peers and on the playground he fails to participate in activities like dodgeball and baseball. He reports, "I am always the last one chosen for the baseball team." Results of standardized testing on the Movement Assessment Battery for Children place Jordan in the 1st percentile for his age. Based on assessment results and the functional problems described, a motor learning approach was selected for intervention.

In order to motivate Jordan to participate in therapy, he was asked to identify two action goals that he wanted to work on. Jordan identified (1) playing baseball with the kids at recess and (2) getting better at cursive writing.

Considerations from a Motor Learning Perspective

Jordan is in the cognitive stage of skill acquisition. He has the general idea of what is required to play ball and to write but variability is great. His posture is awkward, he has difficulty coordinating movements and his error rate is high. He does not know why he cannot throw the ball or keep his letters oriented to baseline. He is having difficulty integrating cues from the environment and needs the therapist to direct his actions.

The therapist completes an ecological task analysis and determines the specific movement patterns that are not working well for Jordan. First, they will work on throwing and catching the ball. Jordan is going to learn to throw a softball a distance of 6 feet in a stationary environment. As Jordan improves his skills the therapist will increase the complexity of the activity—in this case, distance thrown—and move to an environment where the path of the ball for Jordan to catch becomes more variable. At this early stage of learning, it is important to find the "just right challenge" for the child.

An analysis of handwriting indicates that Jordan has difficulty stabilizing and cocontracting the joints of his fingers in a dynamic fashion. During therapy they will focus on increasing Jordan's attention to feedback while learning the letters g, c, a, d, that share common strokes. As Jordan masters these letters, others will be added. Once Jordan is able to form all the letters, maintaining accurate size and shape, intervention will focus on joining the letters, spacing, and finally increasing the speed of his writing.

Feedback will be provided by the therapist and will focus initially on intrinsic feedback, emphasizing the position and feeling of his hand and arm when he throws the ball. When he is writing, attention will be directed to the sensory information available regarding his body position, pencil grip, and position of the paper ("you are holding the pencil too tight," "your wrist will need to move so you can write all the letters in this word"). The therapist may provide additional proprioceptive and sensory input by physically guiding the child through the movements so the child gets the feel of them. The therapist may also demonstrate the movement and provide verbal instructions or cues. Verbal instruction will be straightforward and direct, defining the key points of the movement ("keep your elbows bent," "keep your eyes on the ball").

The therapist, in the form of knowledge of results, will also provide extrinsic feedback ("your letters are falling below the line, the words are too close together, the spacing of the words needs to be a finger distance apart"). It is best to provide feedback intermittently so the child does not become dependent on the therapist. Knowledge of performance focuses the child on developing the proper movement patterns ("follow the movement through the arc when you throw the ball"). Through feedback and grading the task, the child develops the proper movement patterns required for execution. Once the basic movement patterns have been established, the therapist uses practice to ensure learning takes place. The activity will be varied slightly each time in order to get Jordan to keep solving a slightly different movement problem. Transfer and generalization, measures of motor learning, will be ensured by changing environments and tasks: from the stable environment to the baseball field, from the therapy room to the classroom, and from cursive writing exercises to classroom assignments.

MOTOR LEARNING: FUTURE DIRECTIONS WITH CHILDREN WITH DCD

The principles of motor learning reviewed in this chapter can be used as guidelines for therapists and educators when working with children but have not yet been elucidated sufficiently to form a specific protocol for intervention. While the application of motor learning theories makes intuitive sense with children with DCD, research will be required to examine their efficacy. Intervention protocols have been developed and researched with children with DCD which use motor learning principles in combination with other theories that emphasize the role of cognitive processes in movement skill (Mandich, Polatajko, Missiuna, & Miller, in press; Missiuna, Mandich, Polatajko, & Malloy-Miller, in press). One example is the Cognitive Orientation to Occupational Performance (CO-OP) protocol that has been developed and investigated by the DCD Research Group in Canada (Miller, Polatajko, Missiuna, Malloy-Miller, & Mandich, 1999; Polatajko, Mandich, Miller, & Macnab, in press.

In CO-OP, using the principles of motor learning, the therapist focuses on the functional movement goal and helps the child to discover the relevant aspects of the task, to examine how they are currently performing the task, to identify where they are getting "stuck," and to creatively think about alternative solutions. In this cognitive approach, though, a global strategy based upon the problem-solving structure first outlined by Luria (1961) and developed by Meichenbaum (1977) is used to provide a consistent framework within which task-specific strategies are revealed. The environment is structured so that children can discover strategies that help them to become more aware of their performance. For example, performance requirements (e.g., you need to reach out with both hands to catch a big ball), intrinsic feedback (e.g., you need to hold the pen more firmly), or of the variable aspects of the task (e.g., little balls are harder to catch than big ones). Specific cognitive strategies that seem to be particularly successful with children with DCD have now been identified and described (Mandich, 1997; Polatajko et al., in press).

Another major difference in the cognitive approach is the style of interaction that is used by the therapist. In motor learning, the therapist gives verbal instruction that guides and directs the child's movements. In the cognitive approach, the therapist never presents information but, instead, uses questions to help the child discover the problems, generate solutions and evaluate their application in a supportive environment. This style of interaction is called "mediation" and is described in detail elsewhere (Missiuna, Malloy-Miller, & Mandich, 1998). An additional focus in the cognitive approach is on having the child verbalize the strategies that appear to guide or change his or her motor behavior. For example, a child who is learning to roller blade might tell himself "ankles up" as his cue to co-contract his ankle muscles and keep his body upright. Once a strategy is found to be helpful, the therapist uses questions to help the child "bridge" or generalize that strategy, eliciting from the child other times and situations in which that strategy might apply, for example, skating or walking on a balance beam (Polatajko et al., in press).

SUMMARY AND CONCLUSIONS

Motor learning theorists today believe that movement skill development occurs when the child encounters, and figures out solutions to, movement problems. The solutions emerge when the multiple systems within the child interact cooperatively with the functional task within the context of the environment. It is the role of the therapist to analyze the movement problem, or action goal, from an ecological perspective considering the variable features of the task, child and the environment. When the movement synergies that the child is using have been identified, the therapist will structure the task and environment in order to facilitate the provision of extrinsic and intrinsic feedback within a practice schedule that is optimal for the type of task. While specific intervention protocols have not yet been developed for children with DCD, therapists and movement educators can use an understanding of the principles of motor learning to structure their session and guide the selection of techniques that will be used. Children with DCD will benefit from this approach if the emphasis is upon varying the practice circumstances so that each repetition of the action goal becomes a new problem-solving opportunity. Research is needed to examine the specific components of motor learning theory and their effectiveness with children with developmental coordination disorder. Future work in this area will also examine the role of cognition and use of cognitive strategies in facilitating motor learning.

CHAPTER
16

Task-Specific Intervention for Children with Developmental Coordination Disorder: A Systems View

Dawne Larkin and Helen E. Parker

Task-specific intervention is one of many approaches designed to improve the motor performances of children and young adults with motor learning difficulties. Among the earliest reported programs was Lippitt's (1926) series of exercises to improve the coordination and balance of children and college students with "poor muscular coordination." However, the idea of task-specific intervention is not new. In 1951, Lafuze used this approach with college women with low motor ability. Her fundamental motor skills program, which included running, jumping, throwing, and striking, resulted in improvements in motor performance as well as increased knowledge of skills. The multifaceted task-specific intervention that we present here focuses on helping children with developmental coordination disorder (DCD) achieve efficient, fluid motor performances of tasks that are both culturally appropriate and personally meaningful. Using this method, the child learns how to perform a focal task efficiently while also learning underlying movement principles (implicit knowledge), such as absorbing force or stance positioning, that might carry over to a cluster of related tasks. In this chapter, we discuss the theoretical and practical implications of task-specific learning, an approach that we have been using successfully for many years with children with DCD and other motor difficulties.

The multifaceted approach we take to task specific learning is convergent with a broad systems framework espoused by von Bertalanffy (1968) as well as the dynamical systems framework applied to motor development (Clark, 1995; Parker, 1992; Thelen & Ulrich, 1991) and to motor rehabilitation (Scholtz, 1990; Shepherd & Carr, 1991). It is also consistent with the ecological approach to motor behavior (Davis & Burton, 1991). The framework allows us to plan our intervention strategies in a coherent and principled way, one that is theoretically relevant but practically viable. We believe that the emergent change in motor behavior of each child with DCD is a function of multiple interactions. This is in line with the concept of equifinality, "the same goal may be reached from different initial conditions and in different pathways" (Bertalanffy, 1968, p. 132). There are multiple learning pathways that the practitioner and child can take to achieve an optimal solution to the motor problem/task and to developing a positive involvement and attitude to physical activity.

Although we emphasize task-specific learning, we acknowledge that this is but one approach to helping children with DCD improve both their motor skills and general participation in physical activity. There are a number of approaches (Henderson & Sugden, 1992; Miyahara, 1996; Sigmundsson, Pedersen, Whiting, & Ingvaldsen, 1998; Sveistrup, Burtner, & Woollacott, 1992; Wall, McClements, Bouffard, Findlay, & Taylor, 1985; also see Chapter 15) that might be implemented in parallel or in sequence to further enrich the child's motor development. Prior to further discussion of the practical aspects of the task-specific learning approach, we will explore some of the theoretical influences and assumptions that guide our approach and briefly discuss the movement efficiency and the diverse effects of DCD on the growing child's learning and performance of motor skills.

DIFFERENT SYSTEMS FRAMEWORKS— THE INTERACTION OF CONSTRAINTS

We base our intervention on a broad systems framework incorporating many influences. During the 1970s and 1980s, new approaches emerged based on Bernstein's (1967) seminal ideas of the complexity, nonlinearity, and interactivity of motor control processes and Gibson's (1966) ecological psychology principles of direct perception and organism-environment interaction. These ideas acknowledged the complexity of the physical action system and described how control of motor skill arises from nonlinear and nondeterministic interactions between such systems. Genetics, structure, function, and experience all interact to produce the final motor behavior. "Subsystems are equal contributors in principle, although the system stability may be more sensitive to some elements than others" (Thelen & Ulrich, 1991, p. 34), and this sensitivity may change throughout the motor learning process. This was a break away from the unidirectional, brain-to-behavior, top-down, specified control model of motor behavior that ignored the way that the details of action evolve in response to the influences of both internal neural input, and external gravitational and inertial forces (Bernstein, 1967). These contextual and probabilistic models of motor behavior development are better placed to explain what initially appear as inconsistencies, for example, why there is no consistently identified damage to the motor areas of the brain in children with DCD.

In the early 1970s, Gentile and Higgins worked on a task taxonomy that linked the performer and the environment. Using this framework, tasks were classified as closed or open, according to the stability of the performance environment (Gentile, 1972; Higgins, 1977). A more complex two-dimensional system evolved that included two aspects of the environmental context and two aspects of function of the action. Combining the different performance environments of closed or open and intertrial variability with the two-task functions of body transport (stationary or moving) and object manipulation revealed 16 task categories of varying complexity (Gentile, 1987; Higgins, 1977). This taxonomy provided a coherent instructional framework for task selection and task progression, and currently influences our task-specific approach to children with DCD where we generally focus on closed skills or simplify the environment in the early stages of skill acquisition. The framework continues to serve motor skills teachers well and is currently incorporated into the Behavior Checklist of the MABC (Henderson & Sugden, 1992). However, it does not include factors related to the learner's attributes that are equally important to task selection and instructional design—physique, fitness, cognition, and motivation.

Important learner attributes, such as these, were incorporated in Newell's (1986) interactive constraints model of motor coordination. His model highlighted three sources of influences whose interactions both enable and constrain the final motor performance. The sources of constraint include organismic constraints (the performer's neuromotor plant, physique, fitness, maturation, and motivation), task factors (discrete-continuous, fine or gross-motor, simple-complex), and environmental factors (open-closed, sociocultural context, on land or in water, instructional factors). The systems model provides a relatively simple, yet useful, framework for the practitioner seeking to accommodate key performance factors in planning individual task specific instruction (Figure 16.1).

At the sociocultural level of a systems perspective, there are a number of important questions that influence the choice of motor tasks to be taught to each child. What focal tasks to choose? Where to start and how to progress? What skills does the child need to fully participate within his or her current cultural context? What lifetime motor skills can he or she learn that will contribute to future health and well-being? What skills does the child want to learn? What is the current level of performance in those skills? Each are important questions that any motor skills teacher or therapist in school or clinical settings must answer to plan appropriate motor skill interventions based on tasks that are meaningful for the child.

In using this approach, the teacher consciously assesses both the performer's limitations and attributes. Is the child overweight? Does the child have low flexibility? Does the child have cognitive impairment? Is the child reluctant to try motor skills? Does the child listen well? Further, Bernstein's (1967) insight about the influence of context-conditioned variability on task performance means that there will be no single, definitive approach for instructing skills to all children. Coaches, teachers, and movement therapists need to appreciate how the individual's unique makeup shapes the learning process. Fundamental to our task-specific teaching

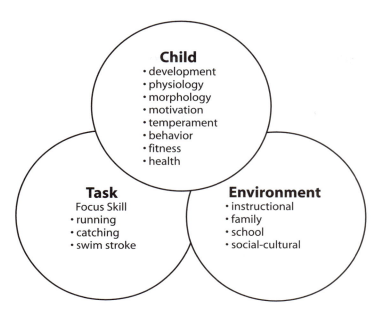

Figure 16.1   Systems model for task-specific instruction and learning.

approach is consideration of the interacting constraints, structural, physiological, cognitive, and motivational that the child with DCD brings to the learning setting.

Finally, at the task level, particular intervention strategies for the teacher or therapist become evident. For example, Bernstein's (1967) idea that a perturbation (change of action) in one part of the movement will have consequential effects on other parts of the movement. In order to teach motor tasks to children with motor learning difficulties, it is essential for the movement specialist to have an in-depth understanding of the important details of the action dynamics (for more, see Arend & Higgins, 1976) and the contribution they make to performance outcome. For example, Oslin, Stroop, and Siedentop (1997) reported carry-over benefits of practicing one element of the overarm throw (the step) on the improved efficiency of other throw components in preschool children.

The reflective teacher assesses the nature of the task to be learned and the performance environment that best enables the action to be performed safely within the child's limitations (e.g., in-water practice to support excess body weight, mats to cushion landing, trampolines/rebounders to assist with flight). Diagnostic analysis of the respective impact of these multiple sources of constraint on motor coordination add levels of insight for effective task-specific teaching and learning.

OPTIMIZING IN TASK-SPECIFIC INSTRUCTION/LEARNING

A key goal of task-specific instruction is to optimize the manner of performing a focal skill given the constraints of the child's motor ability, fitness, and motivation.

Note, we prefer to use the term "optimal" rather than "best" in describing the manner in which the task is performed. This is based on improving the energy efficiency of performance as influenced by the interactions of neuromechanical, physiological, and social factors.

While movement efficiency is a system goal in learning, children with DCD by no means achieve energy efficiency in motor performances. When left alone, they develop inefficient movement patterns. When these patterns become habitual, they will feel comfortable to the child, despite the poor action effect. As Ellfeldt and Metheny (1959) commented many years ago, "He may 'feel' the difference between two performances, but he cannot perceive good movement kinesthetically until he produces it. He cannot predict the outcome of performance from the 'feel' during production until he determines what cues from kinesthesis, touch, and pressure correlate with good performance. Otherwise, old errors feel good" (p. 244). Targeted, corrective teaching can eliminate such inefficiencies from the movement by highlighting the feel and outcome of more effective movement. The inefficient pattern should be corrected as early as possible before the ingrained bad habit feels "natural" and thus becomes resistant to correction.

A poorly executed task is seen as "clumsy," based on qualitative criteria such as poor flow, timing, and sequencing. Different types of incoordination are observed in children with DCD, from the overly constrained to the overly variable. In 1940, Bernstein (1967) pointed to the overly constrained inefficiency with which novices execute tasks. "When someone . . . first attempts to master the new co-ordination, he is rigidly, spastically fixed and holds the limb involved, or even his whole body, in such a way as to reduce the number of kinematic degrees of freedom which he is required to control" (p. 108). This is one of the general types of movement patterns that we see with DCD. At the other extreme, we often see children with DCD whose movement shows total lack of constraint. Such children display extreme variability in repeated attempts at a task, with successive performances lacking even "ball park" adjustments to task goal and purpose. Both types of incoordination require additional energy to control movement and thus lead to earlier fatigue than would normally be expected.

Touwen (1998) highlighted the developmental importance of adaptive variability, the process of choosing the appropriate movement strategies to specific situations and environmental goals and purposes. Children with DCD often have great difficulty using adaptive strategies. At another level, Touwen also described what he termed "primary variability" in infants with even mild developmental disorders. Children with DCD characteristically lack both adaptability and variability in motor behavior. Such limitations are addressed explicitly within the task-specific framework.

The teaching of swimming strokes probably provides one of the most instructive lessons in how task-specific teaching optimizes performance. Children and adults who are not taught to swim rarely achieve an efficient stroke. They tire easily and look awkward. Swimming instruction turns this around. Thus, our aim in task-specific instruction is to teach the child with DCD to perform culturally normative tasks in mechanically efficient ways, so that the child feels good performing rhythmically, enjoys performing the task, and looks coordinated rather than clumsy, and consequently is no longer subject to peer ridicule.

HOW DOES DCD EXPERIENCE ALTER THE SYSTEM?

From a broad systems perspective, there are many functional levels from the neuro-physiological to the psychosociological, where limited and unpleasant movement experiences can change the developmental pathway of the child with DCD. The mutually constraining effect of experience and development is most sharply drawn in such children. Some of the experiential variations that might compromise their motor skill learning are the following:

- Neuromotor and perceptual-motor subsystems may be "inexperienced," and the tuning of these systems will be limited (Sporns & Edelman, 1993).
- The musculo-skeletal systems of children with DCD develop differently due to a lack of appropriate levels of stimulation. Poor muscular power and limited flexibility result from a more sedentary lifestyle (O'Beirne, Larkin, & Cable, 1994).
- Morphological variations, particularly joint laxity or excessive body weight, can make performance and learning of locomotor skills more difficult.
- Low levels of cardiorespiratory endurance, motor fitness, and strength (see Chapter 11) may compromise skill development and contribute to early fatigue in the learning environment.
- Implicit knowledge of motor tasks, such as an understanding of the regulatory features of the environment (Magill, 1998), can be poorly developed and contribute to additional frustration during motor skill learning.
- Explicit knowledge about physical activities is compromised by limited motor experiences and withdrawal from the movement culture.
- Parents who have experienced motor learning difficulties report that a negative attitude to physical activity can arise as a function of experiences with others, and the difficulty and frustration associated with motor skill learning (personal communications).
- Increased anxiety about physical activity, reported by girls with low levels of coordination (Rose, Berger, & Larkin, 1999), can interfere with skill acquisition.
- Low motivation for physical activities contributes to movement withdrawal and a negative cycle of nonparticipation and even lower motivation.
- Reduced perceptions of movement competence and confidence, expressed by the "I can't do it" syndrome, slows learning.
- The quality of social support from family and friends can result in positive or negative contributions to skill development (Rose, Berger, & Larkin, 1994).

Identifying such experiential constraints can be done in the context of the task specific approach and the intervention can target the child's needs directly or indirectly. One of the strengths of the broad systems framework is that it is multidimensional, incorporating complex interactions in a systematic way. This allows the movement specialist to select relevant, specific tasks and to methodically plan appropriate instructional progressions. Our approach to task-specific teaching and learning is defined, as much as possible, by child-centered needs.

USING THE TASK-SPECIFIC APPROACH

Our work focuses on 5–12-year-old children, those in the first six years of schooling. The motor tasks we teach are those typical to most Australian children in this age bracket and, in that sense, are developmentally and culturally appropriate. They are tasks that most children want to learn. These tasks include a range of motor skills, such as running, hopping, skipping, jumping, rope skipping, ball skills, hitting skills, bicycling, and swimming.

Although whole skills are learned, what has been termed a whole-part-whole approach is sometimes used with complex tasks and a part-whole-part approach is used with swimming strokes. Where possible the child attempts the actual task (e.g., the overarm throw), while the teacher focuses on actions of the body components (that is, of the feet and legs, arm, trunk), task elements (for example, preparatory wind-up, action to ball release and follow through), and task dynamics (control of force, time, direction and amplitude; see also Laban notation). Where appropriate, sensorimotor elements are also explicitly addressed: Does that feel better? Watch the ball all the way! Feel the stretch! Collier and Reid (1987) reported the success of using extensive, complementary physical, visual and verbal prompts with autistic children in learning a motor skill. From our experience, using a similar approach with children who have DCD results in skill progress.

Verbal mediation is also used within the task-specific context. The child has the opportunity to teach the teacher or to repeat what the teacher has said. Of course, an ability to describe the task often does not parallel the ability to perform the task in a coordinated fashion—a divide in procedural and declarative knowledge levels (Leonard, 1998; Wall et al., 1985). For example, some children with DCD involved in a landing skills program (Larkin & Parker, 1998a, 1998b) were able to verbalize movement cues taught but were unable to implement them.

Although the task-specific approach is structured, we also encourage guided exploratory approaches to task performance. For example, exploring different ways of holding a bat, exploring different ways of hitting a ball, exploring different stride lengths, exploring different ways of using the arms to assist locomotor activities, exploring which is the better side to hold a bat, or which hand feels better when throwing a ball. There are some benefits from this guided exploration. It explicitly contrasts differences in positioning and action that are felt by the child and, with guidance from the teacher about the effectiveness of the performance (e.g., "that is a much better throw"), sensitizes them to what a better way will feel like (Ellfeldt & Metheny, 1959). Generally, a more cost-effective performance is achieved as the child starts to get a more comprehensive understanding of the dynamics of the body. They begin the process of exploring motor solutions within the focus task in an effort to establish a more efficient style. This is congruent with Bernstein's (1967) view linking motor learning with the process of task exploration. Practice "does not consist in repeating the means of solution of a motor problem time after time, but in the process of solving this problem again and again by techniques which we changed and perfected from repetition to repetition" (Bernstein, 1967, p. 134).

With our multifaceted task-specific approach, we also target important motor fitness elements that support effective task performance. For example, the child who has limited lower leg strength and power, compromising the development of a more efficient running stride, is given strength-building activities to practice (e.g., leaping and bounding games). The child is also encouraged to participate in other lower limb strength-enhancing activities (e.g., beach walking with the family). In essence, using a dynamic, flexible, yet structured, multidimensional perspective can redirect the emphasis of the learning situation while a specific task remains the focus of instruction.

HOW LONG DOES IT TAKE TO LEARN A TASK?

The motor learning literature is not definitive about the time it takes to master a motor skill (Kelly, 1989). There is very little research that has looked at the time it takes children, whose motor learning ability is considered typical, to learn different motor tasks to a level considered efficient and effortless. The time for task mastery is contingent on multiple factors; Newell's (1986) model identifies three key sources of constraint. For children with DCD, defining the standards that meet a criterion of mastery is problematic. When we say "learn," what do we mean? We are looking for a level of performance where the child moves efficiently, the movement is relatively effortless, and the performance is consistent if the environment is closed or the task is consistently successful if the environment is open.

The case studies from Marchiori, Wall, and Bedingfield (1987) suggest that it is difficult for children with DCD to achieve efficiency and consistency in a closed skill despite many trials of continuous practice. Data from our own studies (Larkin & Parker, 1998a, 1998b; Revie & Larkin, 1993) indicate that the time varies according to the task and the individual child. With task-specific teaching of two-foot landing to 7–9-year-old children with DCD, we saw limited improvements in performance after six 15-min sessions of intensive teaching and feedback. With specific teaching of tasks such as throw and distance hop or kick and bounce and catch to young children with DCD, Revie and Larkin (1993) found improvements to be specific to the task actually taught. That is, over eight 20-min sessions, the taught throw and hop skills improved but not the non-taught kick and bounce-and-catch skills. The opposite was true for the reverse intervention group. The degree of improvement in the taught skills was quite varied, however, with the individual improvement in throwing distance, for example, ranging from 0.8 to 10 meters. This highlights a wide range in speed of learning among children in the DCD group with some responding particularly well to specific teaching and others less so. Werner and Rink (1989) reported that their four experienced, second grade teachers effected a reduction in landing force from jumping from most children over six weeks of instruction. However, they also reflected that after completing the unit of instruction twice, teachers reported that they still needed more time to teach effective landing to a reliable standard. Teacher competence was also an issue.

Little is known about the constraint of age on skill development in children with DCD, but it needs to be considered. For example, Parker and Blanksby's (1997) longitudinal tracking of typically developing preschool swimmers at a community swim school illustrated the constraint of age in attaining water confidence tasks and basic locomotor skills. Water confidence was passed by 2- and 3-year-old learners in 22 weekly lessons, double the number needed for 4-, 5-, and 6-year-olds. Basic locomotion skills were passed in a further 44 lessons (2-year-olds) and 35 lessons (3-year-olds) compared to the 20–24-lesson range for 5–6-year-old learners; older learners attained mastery even more rapidly. Little research has looked at the effect of age constraints and motor skill learning in children, especially those with DCD.

In summary, developmental, experiential, and task difficulty factors all impact the pace of learning. Combined with the constraints arising from the child's motor learning difficulties, the instructional time required for a child with DCD to master a motor task becomes very difficult to determine. We emphasize to teachers that their aim is to advance the child's performance towards optimal, efficient execution, no matter how small the steps are.

USING A TASK DIAGNOSTIC MATRIX TO TEACH SPECIFIC TASKS

The teacher's goal is to break down inefficient movement habits and establish more efficient movement patterns. To do this, we observe current performance abilities within a task-diagnostic matrix, determine the causes of inefficient movement, and begin the process of instruction and practice so that the child can learn a more efficient movement pattern.

To complement the task diagnosis, teachers using the task-specific approach should also evaluate the general behaviors of the child during activity sessions. Such behaviors as hyperactivity, impulsiveness, temper outbursts, interruptions, attention span, attention to instructions, and conceptual understanding are monitored. There are some extremely bright children with motor learning difficulties whose declarative knowledge is remarkable. They understand aspects of the physics of motion and are very competent with the sequential ordering of the task components but nevertheless fail to establish flow. Thus, the behavioral information is an essential part of modifying instruction to meet the child's individual needs, cognitive attributes, frustrations, motivations, and personality.

The task-diagnostic matrix incorporates analysis of the focus task—components, phases of action, dynamic elements, related fitness requirements, and the performer's physical attributes and component actions and behavioral analysis. This matrix allows the teacher to determine a more optimal instructional sequence and approach for the individual child. Tables 16.1, 16.2, and 16.3 provide examples of the type of breakdown necessary for effective instruction.

Running

Through analytical observation of the child running, the teacher notes low knee lift, mid-foot landing with no toe-off, limited use of the ankle, limited flight phase

Table 16.1 Task Diagnostic Matrix for Running

Learning Goal	Components	Phase of Action	Dynamics	Motor Fitness
To run with speed and efficiency	Leg action Arm action Head and eyes Trunk posture Breathing rhythm	Support Recovery Flight Landing	Speed Stride length Step width Amplitude and direction of forward knee swing Amplitude and direction of arm swing	Leg strength Hip flexibility Anaerobic power Endurance

Table 16.2 Task Diagnostic Matrix for Two-Hand Catching

Learning Goal	Components	Phase of Action	Dynamics	Perceptual-Motor Fitness
To catch a large ball with the hands	Hand posture Arms action Head posture Fixation/focus Stance	Tracking Contact and grasp Reception	Positioning and timing with respect to ball Stance adjustment Amplitude of "give"	Visual motor match Hand eye coordination Anticipation Visual fixation and tracking skills

Table 16.3 Task Diagnostic Matrix for Freestyle Swim

Learning Goal	Components	Phase of Action	Dynamics	Motor Fitness
To stroke smoothly with unilateral breathing for 5 m	Body position Hand posture Arms action Head position Isolation of head action from trunk posture during breathing	Pull Arm recovery Kicking Head turning to breathe in Breathing out	Temporal asymmetry of hand action "Flow" Spatial positioning of hands with respect to body and legs Timing Amplitude	Strength of arms, wrists, and fingers Shoulder flexibility Trunk stability Hip mobility and knee stability Aerobic fitness Vital capacity

and shortened stride, excessive trunk rotation with arms flailing across body, and uncontrolled head rotation and instability.

Common problems include the following:

- Head instability—does not constrain degrees of freedom
- Trunk rotation—inertial qualities of the system override stability
- Arm swing—overconstrained or uncontrolled
- Knee lift—low strength, short stride with established habit
- Landing—heavy, heel strike; stiff ankle positioning
- Propulsion not using ankle extensors—fails to utilize degrees of freedom

Catching

Common problems include the following:

- Arm/hand preparation—stiff posture, degrees of freedom overconstrained
- Tracking—watches thrower not ball; shuts eyes as ball approaches; turns head away, fails to account for the regulatory aspects of environment
- Stance—feet remain stationary, does not adjust body position to path of ball
- Hands in reception—too far apart for small ball, do not adjust to temporal or spatial constraints
- Arms in reception—remain extended, do not give to absorb impact

Swimming

Common problems include the following:

- Leg kick—kick from knee only (knee flexion-extension), cycling action, scissoring as trunk twists
- Head—lifts head forward to breath; block twisting with trunk
- Body position—more vertical than horizontal in water, twisting along vertical axis
- Arm action—uneven pull in alternate arm action; elbow skims water in low recovery, short underwater pull
- Whole stroke—arrhythmic, head turn, trunk posture, arm action and leg kick deteriorate when whole action is attempted

DOES THE TASK-SPECIFIC APPROACH WORK?

Although there is limited research supporting the task-specific approach, there is some published support for it with children with DCD (Revie & Larkin, 1993) and young adults with low motor ability (Lafuze, 1951). The continuous monitoring of progress in case studies in our motor learning program provides further evidence, albeit at a weaker level. Case reports on children's progress at the completion of each 11-week block contain information on skill and fitness improvements made and each child's attempts are logged in weekly qualitative and quantitative evaluations.

Our task-specific approach involves constant feedback and positive support for the child's attempts. The feedback focuses on the task efficiency by giving knowledge of performance to the learner (e.g., "What great long strides!! Well done") to converge with the child's new proprioceptive feeling from using a better running technique (i.e., good knee lift forward).

The case studies of motor skill learning (Marchiori et al., 1987) in two boys with movement difficulties clearly indicate how difficult it is for children with DCD to attain a proficient level of skill, even in a closed environment and after 1,200 trials. These researchers used high-speed filming to monitor changes in the boys' hockey slap shot performances, which were still exceptionally variable from trial to trial and the velocity of the puck and stick head remained low by comparison to unpracticed age matched controls. Marchiori et al. (1987) point out that performance feedback was provided by parents who were given key cues; however, the quality and amount was not monitored.

Our experiences indicate that the quality of feedback that the child receives is dependent on both the teachers' explicit, deep knowledge of the skill they are teaching and their ability to observe the fine detail of the movement. In turn, quality and timely feedback contributes to the gradual sculpting of a more optimal skill performance for that individual. Constant teaching and re-teaching, reinforcing the small gains, translate over the longer term to better performance in the focus tasks and a child who is happier to engage in movement and physical play.

To date, there is limited evidence of transfer of training using task-specific approaches, although early studies indicated that measures of motor ability such as balance and agility improved (Lafuze, 1951). Women with low motor ability who were exposed to a basic skills program showed improved performance in motor ability, specific games activities, and attitude to physical education (Broer, 1955). Despite criticisms about the development of "splinter skills" with a task-specific approach, it appears that there is some carryover into the more general motor domain. Broer suggested two factors that may contribute to more general improvements: the application of some of the principles of movement (e.g., transfer implicit knowledge between tasks) and increased self-confidence. There is a clear need for more systematic study of the factors that contribute to and the degree to which more general benefits accrue from the task-specific approach.

EXPANDING THE TASK SPECIFIC APPROACH FOR OPEN ENVIRONMENTS

Initially, the task-specific approach focuses on efficient closed skill performance. However, this is only a beginning to developing skill for games and sport for children with DCD. We also explicitly develop skill adaptability to handle open environments. After the initial stage of teaching more efficient movement, we teach the child to work in an open and predictable environment and then move on to a less predictable environment. We then take the next step of incorporating the "closed" focus skills into more complex, "open" games. In the more traditional models of task-specific teaching, the skill environment can be overly restrictive for developing team game activities and "game sense" decision making. The lack of simulation of a game's spatial, temporal, and teamwork and social requirements limits the child's preparedness for playing team games.

We overcome this limitation through a skill extension program that uses modified games in small groups with a higher student to staff ratio than in the intensive, individualized focus skills program. The modified games context adds an additional layer of complexity to motor skill performance as preparation for modified sports such as tee-ball, mini-tennis, minkey (modified field hockey), soccer, volleyball, and badminton. The children are taught to deal with the dynamic spatial and temporal demands of the environment as well as other players who have slower and less predictable motor skill. The modified games extension program has an additional benefit of providing the context for the development of social skills that are an important part of game playing.

At all levels of programming, we emphasize the importance of the joyful interplay between the child and teacher. Fun is paramount for these children for whom movement performance is hard work and difficult. A key underpinning philosophy is for teachers to make learning both fun and meaningful to the child with DCD.

STRENGTHS OF THE TASK-SPECIFIC APPROACH

Task-specific instruction within a broad systems framework focuses on learning useful and functional skills, specifically those that are meaningful to the play culture of children. Learning motor skills to a standard that allows the children to participate in play in a real way, to be included, and to experience the joy of physical activity, establishes physical activity as a habit—a way of daily life.

At the personal level, the children experience a sense of achievement in the motor domain—"I can do it; I am not hopeless." These movement successes build on success, reinforcing further attempts and building movement confidence—"I want to play."

From a functional perspective, learning specific tasks cements foundation skills. Initially, the skills are closed in nature to accommodate the movement difficulties; however, practice variations stimulate adaptation to more open performance environments. Although "specific" at one level, these well-performed skills provide precursor experiences that enable other extension skills to be acquired, albeit slowly. The individualized planned progression is methodical, with achievable goals at every step of the way. The instructional sequence allows for advancement and revision, this being crucial for cementing both skill and implicit movement knowledge.

Finally, the approach facilitates socially appropriate behavior by initially working in a teacher/student dyad and progressing to learning in pairs and small groups. As progress is achieved in skills such as listening, timely responding, following instructions, answering and asking questions, turn taking, sharing space and equipment, cooperating and competing, and greater awareness of others around in the space, the child's readiness for the social interaction in games grows.

SUMMARY AND CONCLUSIONS

Although at a practical level task-specific instruction appears to be a relatively successful strategy to use with children with DCD, gathering empirical support within a systems framework for further advancement of instructional practice is important. We require studies to investigate the degree of transfer of skill learning possible in children with DCD, both among skills of similar type, and within increasingly complex performance environments for skill adaptation.

There is a need to systematically identify control parameters (critical factors that both "push" and "draw" the system) that contribute to the development of more efficient movement patterns in children with DCD. We must also consider what instructional sequence is optimal for the child?

Research is needed into the different movement constraints (e.g., fitness, morphology) that contribute to the difficulties with motor learning. This links to the issue of characterizing and defining subtypes in DCD that have been investigated using other frameworks (Wright & Sugden, 1996; Hoare, 1994). Whereas all children with DCD are inefficient movers, some are overstable, rigid, and stiff in performance, while others are unstable, fluctuating, and variable. Identifying the different coordination patterns and why they are so different will help to build more effective intervention strategies.

CHAPTER

17

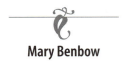

Hand Skills
and Handwriting

Mary Benbow

The fun and games of childhood may seem more like hard labor to a child diagnosed with developmental coordination disorder (DCD). In the early histories of children diagnosed with DCD, one often hears about delays in acquiring skills such as dressing, feeding, cutting, pouring, and bathroom hygiene. Skills mastered without attention or effort by their siblings and peers were often long-term struggles for them to acquire. While their age-mates enjoyed skilled activities such as ball games, running, and tricycles, they were not able to join in the fun. These children were reluctant to attempt new motor challenges that intrigued their peers. They tended to stick with a few well-practiced activities that they felt comfortable doing. The early paucity of activities further delayed developing the most basic gross, fine, and visual motor control. Help was seldom sought until the child experienced failures with higher level preschool activities such as cutting with scissors or coloring.

A child with normal intelligence and free of neurological disease who has marked impairment in the development of motor coordination interfering with academic achievement or activities of daily living satisfies the American Psychiatric Association (1994) diagnostic criteria for DCD. As more early education settings employ educator/occupational therapist/speech therapist teams, children with coordination disorders are being identified earlier. Though the criteria for the diagnosis remain the same, the manifestations of this disorder change with each stage of development. Skilled programming and intervention should begin as early as possible for a child at risk to avoid unrealistic expectations and repeated failures that can lower a child's motivation and spirit. Secondary difficulties of self-esteem, social acceptance, coping strategies, and willingness to try can often be more detrimental than the primary motor problem. In this chapter, discussion is limited to the development of hand skills and the teaching of handwriting.

PRESCHOOL YEARS

A preschool child with a coordination disorder is at a distinct disadvantage as soon as he or she enters preschool. The ideal preschool experience for the child would be one that provides motor training and supervision in kinesthetic, fine motor, and noncompetitive gross motor activities. Additionally, the preschool should program sufficient time for social skills awareness and sensitivity training, problem solving, and language skills, including telling and listening to stories. Each child's unique interests should be developed and areas of competence should be acknowledged and valued.

Kinesthetic Activities

Developing body and spatial awareness using simple kinesthetic games fascinates children and builds confidence in the child with a motor disorder. Doing activities with the eyes closed tends to reduce stress and increase enjoyment. Preschoolers enjoy the following kinesthetic activities:

a. **"Object placement sensitivity."** The child is seated at a table to play. Have the child place a small toy anywhere within easy reach. The child should withdraw his or her arm to his or her side, close his or her eyes, and reach to retrieve the toy. Increase the challenge by having the child place the toy with one hand, close his or her eyes, and retrieve it with the other hand.
b. **"Alternate stacking."** The child is seated at a table to play. Locate about a dozen poker chips or checkers of two different colors. Pile one color to the right and the other color to the left of the child's midline within the working area. With his or her eyes closed, the child should build a stack as tall as possible using alternate hands to create a striped tower. Typically the non-stacking hand will be substituted for vision in this task. Dismantle the tower, separating the colors, and try again for a higher tower.
c. **"Dropping/catching."** The child can stand or sit. Flex both elbows to 90 degrees. Both hands should be positioned at midline, one palm up and the other palm down and ready to drop and catch the falling object. After closing his or her eyes, the child should drop a weighted object (e.g., rock, golf ball) from the upper to the lower hand. Increase the skill demand by positioning the hands farther apart and/or dropping a lighter object such as a Ping-Pong ball.

Graphic Activities

Graphic activities should be directed to working on a vertical plane (chalkboard or easel) while standing. Standing allows more natural weight shifting for balance through the trunk, pelvis, and lower extremities, and frees the arms and hands for their best performance. The vertical writing surface will require positioning the wrists into extension to work. The extended wrist position will facilitate movement of the thumb into abduction with rotation for distal digital holding of short pieces of chalk or crayons. The shoulders, which are rotary joints, allow freedom of movement in all directions. The drawing surface should be large enough for the child to enjoy full bilateral vertical, horizontal, and diagonal excursions. The impermanence of chalkboard expression can lower performance anxiety by allowing the child to erase anything that he or she is not happy with and try again. Working with both hands simultaneously will help the child develop the feel for his or her preferred hand. Hand preference should emerge from large scale graphic exploration and other bilateral symmetrical skills before the child is expected to do paper and pencil work at a desk.

Gross Motor Activities

All children in the preschool should participate in gross motor activities, making use of playground equipment. If the child is physically or socially unsure of him- or herself, adult support and assistance is often required to encourage the child's participation. Playground activities provide the base for fine motor learning expected in the classroom. Laterality, balance, and control of the trunk, shoulders, and arms are the foundation for mastering fine motor skills. Gross motor skills used in riding bicycles or other riding toys are especially important. Additional coaching may be needed for the child with DCD so that he or she can enjoy these activities and be socially part of the gang.

PRIMARY SCHOOL

The developmental skill level of each child entering school typically is assessed during kindergarten screening. Each child's level in gross motor, language, social, and fine motor development should be known and respected by professionals who work with them.

Gross Motor Activities

A major goal of physical education should be physical fitness and motor confidence. Motor confidence is built on the functional control of the trunk, eyes and limbs. Wisely selected and adapted sports activities that benefit all children are crucial for the child with coordination problems. Of greatest value are the noncompetitive activities that demand bilaterality and variations of thrust and counterthrust such as skipping, throwing, and soccer. Getman (1992) suggests soccer as the ideal activity. Rules should be adapted so all children can benefit from the game and enjoy their participation. He promotes this game, as it provides the greatest opportunities for basic bilaterality and balance of the supporting structure, the total upright body. Visually guided control of the ball must come from the feet, legs, head, shoulders, and sometimes the hips. The players learn to anticipate the ball's trajectory and plan their movements while constantly maintaining the best possible integration of bilaterality and equilibrium. The game requires the added skills of stopping, starting, timing, and changing sequences of movements in the effort to avoid the goalie and put the ball into the net. The use of both body sides in a soccer game, adapted to be within the child's level of skill and enjoyment, should enhance complementary use of the upper limbs.

Kinesthetic Activities

Kindergarten and first grade youngsters enjoy time spent at a chalkboard. Younger children have more success if they draw symmetrical designs on a chalkboard using two short pieces of chalk, one held in each hand. Typically, a 5–6-year-old child will be able to copy a heart, apple, house, and diamond to his or her satisfaction using both hands but will be less successful when using one hand. Once he or she has drawn the design with his or her eyes open, the activities can be made more engaging by adding the challenge of repeating a design with the eyes closed, using kinesthesia.

Children enjoy "chalkboard sports." These are games such as baseball or hockey that have a spatial component. After drawing a baseball diamond shape and labeling home plate, first, second, and third base, have the "batter" use chalk and move around the shape for a single or double hit or a home run. Once he or she develops sensitivity for the distances, have the child close his or her eyes and move the chalk from home plate to the appropriate base for a single, double, triple, or home run.

Target skills can be improved while developing a child's kinesthetic sense. Gather 8 to 10 objects of the same weight and size to be pitched at or into a target. With eyes open have the child practice enough to gain the feel of the position and power required to hit the mark. Maintain the position of the child and the target to continue the game with eyes closed.

Graphic Motor Activities

When difficulties and deficits arise in educating young children, a typical response is to "do more of it, earlier." Instead, it should often be "do less of it, later." An obvious indicator for delaying paper and pencil tasks is lack of hand preference. Extra time should be given to the child who has movement problems, who is known to be late in establishing hand preference. Many alternatives to writing are educationally sound and should be substituted for printing in the primary grades. Anagrams placed along a ruler or magnetic letters aligned on a metal surface can be used to make letter sound combinations or spell words. A set of magnetized words, sold as "instant poetry kits," or "Magnetic Storytime," is an educational and enjoyable way for a child to use his or her verbal skills before he or she is ready to print or write. Flannel boards with Velcro-backed symbols are readily available and should be used functionally and creatively in primary classrooms. Chalkboards and Magna Doodles work well when a horizontal writing surface is unsuitable for the child's level of wrist and hand development. Simple math lessons can be done orally, by using counter pieces, or by sticking a star or peel-off sticker to indicate the correct answers. Printing on ruled paper is a skill that should be delayed for many entering kindergarten children. It is important for the child to master readiness skills before handwriting instruction is initiated (Alston & Taylor, 1987; Wright & Allen, 1975). These writers have found that, when handwriting instruction is premature, children become discouraged and develop poor writing habits, which later become difficult to correct. Readiness factors involve a number of sensorimotor systems. Writing letters and numbers requires integration of the visual, motor, sensory, and perceptual systems. Visual and fine motor coordination is needed to control writing implements. Lamme (1979) identified six underlying skills that should precede handwriting instruction. These are (1) fine motor development, (2) eye-hand coordination, (3) the ability to hold utensils or writing tools, (4) the capacity to smoothly form basic strokes such as circles and lines, (5) letter perception, including the ability to recognize forms, notice likenesses and differences, and infer the movement necessary for the production of the form, and (6) orientation to printed language, which requires the visual analysis of letters and words and right-left discrimination. Beery (1997) and Benbow, Hanft, and Marsh (1992) suggest postponing formal handwriting instruction until the child can complete the first nine designs in the Developmental Test of Visual-Motor Integration (VMI). The ninth design, an oblique cross, includes diagonal lines that are required for printing 12 capital letters of the alphabet. Weil and Amundson (1994), while examining 60 typically developing kindergarten children (aged 54–64 months), found that children who were successful in copying the first nine designs produced significantly more letters than those who had not reached this level of skill on the Developmental Test of Visual-Motor Integration (VMI). In this study, Weil and Amundson found that kindergarten children were able to copy 78% of the letters presented, despite having received no formal training. Based on their results, they suggest that most typically developing kindergarten children should be ready for printing instruction in the latter half of the kindergarten school year.

McHale and Cermak (1992) examined the amount of time spent on fine motor activities in classes from grades 2, 4, and 6. They found it to be 31–60% of the school day. Eighty-five percent of the fine motor activities consisted of paper and pencil tasks. For children with fine motor coordination problems, it appeared that more time and energy was spent on the motor challenge than on the cognitive challenge.

UPPER EXTREMITY SUPPORT FOR HAND SKILLS

Hand skills depend on the interaction of all joints of the upper extremity—scapulo-thoracic, glenohumeral, elbow, and wrist. Each upper extremity joint should allow fluid movement into its mature patterns (external rotation, extension and abduction) while the hands are being used. The ideal time to observe these skills is while the child is engaged in activities with his peers. If there seems to be a significant problem in skills, more formal testing is often required to establish specific developmental goals. I have found it helpful to note the use of each upper extremity joint as the child is engaged in familiar activities, providing a systematic observation and consultation scheme to explain why certain skills are too challenging and need to be modified or delayed. Adapted or bypass strategies for classroom tasks should be understood and appreciated by professionals to save the child from feeling "stupid" or appearing unwilling, rather then unable, to perform skilled tasks. The range of motion (ROM) and utilization of all joints should be noted in order to include activities that will meet the child's specific needs. In children who are experiencing fine motor problems and/or delays, it is common to find the shoulder joint slightly biased toward internal rotation, adduction and/or flexion; the elbow toward pronation and/or flexion; and the wrist toward flexion and ulnar deviation. In addition to full ROM, all proximal joints must provide a stable base of support for the joints distal to them to enable their functional control.

Shoulders

Strengthening and stabilizing the shoulder complex should be a primary, specified goal in physical education. Activities requiring weight bearing, climbing, and compression are ideal for developing these proximal joints. Playground supervisors should be made aware of the children who need encouragement and assistance in using gross motor equipment for climbing and strengthening.

Elbow

It is helpful for adults who supervise primary activities to observe if the child turns his or her hands from full palm down to full palm up position in order to do activities using deft movement patterns. Rotation at the elbows allows the child to inspect or manipulate a toy or tool at the most natural and comfortable angle. Lack of utilization of the elbow can be observed when the child positions the scissors wrong side up for cutting, is unable to turn a door knob far enough to open the door, or has difficulty in rotating the forearms to play "Itsy Bitsy Spider."

Activities that include full use of elbow rotation include (a) games where the hands, or a paddle or racket, are used to tap objects upward from a palm-up position, (b) guiding a metal object along a track, printed on stiff card stock, from beneath with a magnet held in a three jaw chuck grip (Figure 17.1), and (c) balancing a metal Slinky® on both palms and shifting it up and down without grasping the ends of the spirals. If the child is unable to do these activities because he or she cannot rotate into or maintain the palm up posture, he or she should be referred to a therapist to assess and, if indicated, increase range of motion at the elbow joints.

Wrist

Children with fine motor problems often compensate for lack of stabilization of the wrist in the extended position by flexing the joint to stabilize it bone on bone. This wrist posture limits the wrist/finger joint interplay needed for grip strength and skilled use of the fingers. Specific activities that require full wrist extension with stabilization include (a) lacing toys, (b) mural painting on newsprint taped to the floor, and (c) drawing, coloring, or writing on vertical surfaces (easel or chalkboard) above eye level.

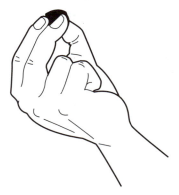

Figure 17.1 Tripod grasp with the dominant hand in a full palm up position below the card. Used with permission from Zaner-Bloser, Inc.

Wrist/Thumb

When the wrist is stabilized in extension, it facilitates abduction of the thumb metacarpal from the plane of the palm so that the thumb can rotate to oppose any of the four digits. Diametric (pulp-to-pulp) opposition allows for the distal manipulation of tiny objects held within the fingers and thumb. Lack of development of the wrist extension/thumb abduction with rotation is indicated when (a) the child fails to wrap the thumbs for added strength while trying to support his or her body weight on an overhead bar or Jungle Gym, (b) when the child is unable to round thumb and index finger to make a smooth circular "OK" sign, and (c) when he or she picks up small objects by pressing the thumb against the lateral surface of the index finger. Incomplete abduction of this mobile thumb joint results in a posture that cannot be adequately stabilized for distal manipulation (Kapandji, 1982). Inefficient use of the thumb may be due to incomplete ROM at the carpometacarpal joint (the saddle joint) at the base of the thumb. Joint mobilization techniques can be used by an occupational or physical therapist to increase ROM allowing full expansion of the thumb-index web space for diametric opposition. Activities to develop wrist extension/thumb abduction skills include (a) holding a drinking straw in the recessive hand, and gradually advancing a 15–20-inch piece of round plastic string through the length of the straw by feeding it along, using translation (extension) movements away from the palm with the index and thumb pulps (Figure 17.2); (b) working on an Etch-a-Sketch® or Magna Doodle® with the frame attached to the wall above eye level (a higher position will require greater wrist extension to reach the knobs, eraser bar, or marker magnet); and (c) outlining before coloring a design with the paper or page taped to a vertical surface, such as a glass sliding door or window.

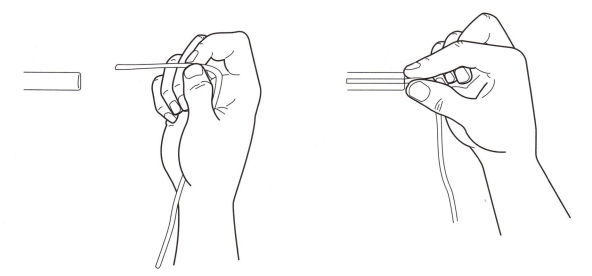

Figure 17.2   The thumb and index finger move from full flexion to full extension in a needle threading motion. Used with permission from Zaner-Bloser, Inc.

REFINEMENT OF HAND SKILLS

Arches of the Hand

Tubiana (1981) states that the arches of the hands direct the movement and grade the power of the fingers. The hand's great adaptability for cupping and flattening depends on its fixed and mobile units. Fixed elements include the distal row of carpal bones and the central attached metacarpals of digits II and III. The small degree of movement at the fixed junctures allows stability without rigidity. The mobile elements include the four fingers and the peripheral metacarpals of the thumb and little finger. When the hand is cupped, the palm structures should be mobile enough to form a deep hollow at the base of the long finger and a deep gutter between the two sides of the hand. The arches provide the unique ability of the human hand to manipulate objects of many sizes, shapes, textures, and weights.

Hand skills depend on the arches. Although there are three identifiable arch systems, they tend to blend together as the hands are being used. There are four longitudinal arches made up of the three bones of each finger plus its metacarpal bone. Longitudinal arching, an extrinsic muscle action, is used in scratching, raking or gathering multiple objects into the palm. There are two transverse arches. The arch at the metacarpal phalangeal (knuckle) level is very mobile and active in holding and manipulating small objects. The transverse arch at the distal wrist level is fairly stable but allows drawing the peripheral metacarpals on the two sides of the hands together for firmer grasping or cupping the hand. There are four diagonal arches, or arches of opposition. They are made up of the two bones of the thumb plus its metacarpal as it opposes each of the finger tips. The diagonal arches are active in holding, stabilizing and directing tools as an extension of the hand. A diagonal arch (the knife holding posture; Figure 17.3) has the index finger extend along the top of the blade to direct its movement while exerting downward pressure with the handle stabilized against the heel of the hand.

Lack of development of the arches can be seen in hands that appear flat at rest and have poorly defined thenar and hypothenar eminences over the metacarpal bones of the thumb and little finger. The child will appear awkward in such skills as picking up small objects without curving the fingers and thumb for tip to tip opposition, failing to create a hollow with the hands in which to shake dice, and making vertical jagged lines when intending to make small circular movements with a pencil or marker.

A number of activities will develop arches, including the following:

• Cup the hand in a palm up posture, so that a deep hollow is formed at the base of the long finger; grains of rice or sand should be slowly spooned into the hollow, stabilizing the arch and increasing it as more material is added.

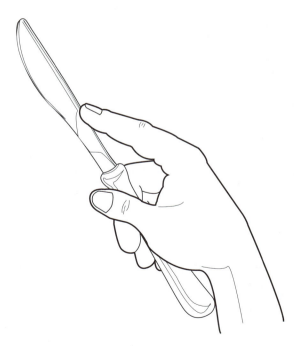

Figure 17.3 The stable position lends support for downward pressure needed to cut with a knife.

- Play "Spider on the Mirror," pressing all finger pulps and thumb pulps together with all fingers in their fully extended position, then alternate adducting and abducting the MP joints of the two hands.
- Rotate two Chinese balls (or marbles, magnetic balls, or wooden beads) around each other within the palm of each hand. This requires activation of all three arches.

At the level of the transverse metacarpal arch, the child should develop full flexion and extension, abduction and adduction and the third degree of freedom (rotation and counter rotation) at the metacarpal phalangeal (MP) joints of all fingers. This rotary movement allows diametric positioning of the thumb pulp against the index pulp for secure holding of tiny objects such as strings or straws. It also facilitates shaping therapy putty or clay within the thumb and finger pulps into tiny round balls. The MP joint of the dominant hand typically develops more rotation and counter rotation than the recessive hand's MP because it has been manipulating toys and small objects. MP arching and rotation of the digits creates a separation between the index and long finger when a pencil is held in the tripod (thumb, index, and middle finger) digits. Rotation at the MP level is used in writing when rounding over the tops of letters. Without arching and rotation at the index MP joint, separation between the two digits will restrict mobility. The pencil grip will remain static rather than advancing to a dynamic grip.

Motoric Separation of the Two Sides of the Hand

Capener (1956) found that refinement of skill with the radial side of the hand (thumb, index, and long finger) is best achieved when the ulnar side of the hand (ring and little finger) is stationary and provides support to the MP arch. Stability at the MP arch level is achieved when ulnar digits are flexed against the palm or postured in extension combined with abduction of the little finger. Either stabilizing posture of the MP arch will shift more isolated control to the radial digits. Motoric separation allows for a division of labor within one hand for activities such as cutting with scissors, tying shoe laces, writing with a pencil, or holding a tube of toothpaste while turning the cap. Development of this skill division was studied extensively by Exner (1997) as it relates to finger-to-palm and palm-to-finger translation movements with stabilization of the ring and little fingers. Practicing the following activities will promote development of this skill: (a) picking up three, four, and then five small objects and moving them into and out of the palm one at a time, (b) snapping the thumb and long finger using a lateral motion while holding the ring and little fingers flexed, and (c) rolling tiny round balls of therapy putty between the pulps of the index finger and thumb.

UPPER EXTREMITY SUPPORT FOR WRITING

Despite meeting early intervention goals in foundation motor skills, most children with DCD encounter serious problems with writing. Difficulties arise in developing speed, rhythm, slant, and consistency of letter formations. The child's efforts to write often fail even though he or she is devoting an inordinate amount of mental and physical energy to the task. Observing every joint of the upper extremities as the student is working with a pencil can be helpful in preliminary planning of teaching or remedial strategies for this complex motor skill.

Shoulders

Shoulder stability may or may not be a significant factor in penmanship training depending on the writer's technique for distal stabilization of the hand. When the mid-portion of the forearm proximal to the ulnar border of the hand is properly stabilized on the desk surface and rotated at 50–65 degrees from its pronated position, the writer should achieve adequate stability to control the elbow, wrist, thumb, and fingers for writing. When the recessive hand cooperates in controlling the paper, the shoulder girdle can be kept in a more consistent and balanced posture.

Elbow

The ability to integrate the subtle adjustments of the elbow with the hand will be lacking if the elbow does not move fluidly into supination (palm-up posture). Limited ROM at the elbow often slows or inhibits distal rounding of strokes over the tops of cursive letters such as "a" and "c" and capitals "B" and "P."

Conversely, when the elbow joint lacks stability, the writer will often grasp the muscle mass just distal to the elbow to lend support to the joint. Without complementary use of the recessive hand, management of the paper will become a challenge. Additional proximal joint stability is required to maintain distal control as the writing hand moves away from the body midline. In order to gain more stability, some right handers externally rotate their shoulder joint to adduct the humerus against the rib cage. This will increase elbow supination and the progressive tilting of letters in a clockwise direction as the writing hand moves toward the right margin.

Wrist/Hand

Bushnell (1970) stated that the wrist and hand function as a single physiological unit in the interplay of flexion and extension as the hands are being used. Since no other joint can compensate for wrist limitations, a functional evaluation of the wrist should be included in all handwriting evaluations. Limited ROM and/or stabilization of the wrist in extension will compromise abduction and rotation of the thumb at the carpometacarpal (CMC) joint. The thumb metacarpal can be functionally stabilized for skilled use when the joint is fully abducted and rotated for distal holding. This dynamic thumb position allows for intrinsic muscle manipulation of a pencil by the skilled digits.

Dominant/Recessive Hand Partnership

Guiard (1987) states that the significant question about dominance is how the two hands interact or complement each other's action in any given task. Each hand's role is essential in high level skills. In writing, the recessive hand "frames" the movement for the dominant hand by setting and confining the spatial context in which skilled movement will take place. The framing and stabilizing activity begins in the recessive hand before the action of the dominant hand is initiated. Dominant hand movements are built upon recessive hand movements. The dominant hand's movements are micrometric (lower in excursion and faster in repetition rate), rehearsed, and internally driven or preprogrammed. The recessive hand is macrometric (higher in excursion and slower in repetition), improvisational, and externally driven. Each hand must assume its role for skill to develop to its highest level in a complex and lateralized motor task.

ANALYSES OF COMMON GRIPS

A distal digital pencil grip will be of greater value to the child with a coordination disorder than to his or her peers. The skin of the finger pulps has the highest density of mechanoreceptors needed to control a writing tool. Johansson and Westling (1987) report that afferent inputs from the finger pulps are involved in precise motor control and have a facilitating effect on finger movements, particularly flexion. Distal holding with curved digits naturally positions the interphalangeal (IP) joints to move freely while providing the greatest amount of sensory information to the nervous system for motor execution and correction. Moberg (1958) found that tactile input from an adducted thumb shaft and the lateral border of the index finger provides significantly less sensory input for motor control and correction than that provided by the thumb and index pulps. Long, Conrad, Hall, and Furler (1970) used electromyography to confirm that, when the hand is in a power configuration (a closed thumb web), proprioceptive input from the lumbricales for regulating axial force is compromised. Distal holding allows the easiest manipulation of the pencil in a proximal-distal axis because the skilled digits flex and extend in a simple synergy at the interphalangeal IP joints.

In the following pages, pencil grips most commonly seen in classrooms will be analyzed for stability, mobility, and sensory motor control. Limiting and facilitating factors of each grip will be discussed along with orthopedic problems that their persistent use may cause. When a child has adopted a pencil grip that is inefficient or harmful to his or her joints, it is wise to intervene as early as possible. A later section of this chapter will present strategies for intervention. There are multiple variations within each grip analyzed, but the grips generally fit the following categories.

Index Grip

Both IP joints of the index finger are partially flexed to cradle the upper shaft of the pencil and stabilize it proximally (Figure 17.4). The partially opposed thumb, positioned opposite the pulps of long and ring fingers, clutches the mid shaft of the pencil. The distal end of the pencil is braced against the posterior surface and/or fingernail of the little finger. The wrist assumes between 45 and 55 degrees of flexion and is stabilized on the ulnar styloid process against the desk surface. This grip position does allow the child to visually monitor his hand while writing, but tactile

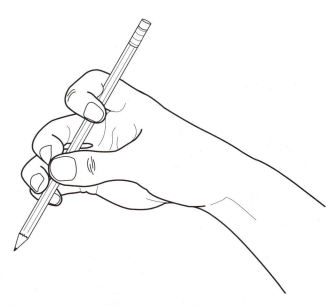

Figure 17.4 The index grip is often used by children who are expected to write before establishing dominance.

and proprioceptive inputs from the digits are compromised. The elbow is rotated beyond its mid-range position so its use is limited in the writing process. In writing with this grip, the three skilled digits function primarily to stabilize rather than mobilize the pencil. The flexed wrist is not in a position to work reciprocally with the digits. Down-stroking is accomplished by a combination of wrist and thumb flexion in combination with flexion of digits III and IV. The little finger, serving as the distal stabilizer of the pencil, is passively pushed into flexion by the distal shaft of the pencil when the hand is down stroking letters. The little finger extends and combines with incomplete extension of the MP and IP thumb joints and wrist extensors for ascending strokes. Wrist extension and ulnar deviation and thumb hyper-extension combine with extension of the little finger for rotation over the tops of letters. This inefficient index grip often is adopted by a child who has not settled into a secure handedness at the time written work becomes a demanding part the school curriculum. An index grip rarely is satisfactory for the child once written work moves beyond circling the correct response or filling in blanks.

"Locked" Grip with Thumb Wrap

The pencil is pressed against the radial side of the third digit above or below the distal interphalangeal (DIP) joint (Figure 17.5). The index finger pulp is firmly pressed by the thumb downward on the shaft of the pencil. The heavy pressure on the shaft of the pencil forces the proximal interphalangeal joint (PIP) of the index

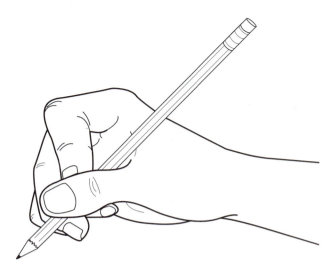

Figure 17.5   Thumb wrap grip.

finger into hyperflexion. This allows hyperextension at the DIP joint, commonly called "white knuckle grip." The transverse metacarpal arch is fairly flat. The thumb is adducted with supination and locked over the index finger, and sometimes over the middle finger as well. Digits IV and V are flexed to stabilize the MP arch and support the middle finger; they flex and extend to manipulate the writing motions. The wrist is straight or slightly extended and the forearm slightly rotated from a fully pronated position. This "locked" grip mechanically restricts digital manipulation of the pencil along its proximal-distal axis. With persistent use of the strong adductor and flexor to stabilize and mobilize the pencil, the MP joint structures of the thumb will be outwardly stressed. This may cause pain and degenerative disease over time. If the ligaments of the hands are very lax and the adductor of the thumb rotates the thumb metacarpal into full supination, the combined stress may partially tear the ulnar collateral ligament at the MP joint of the thumb.

"Locked" Grip with Thumb Tuck

The pencil is pressed against the radial side of the third or fourth digit above or below the DIP joint (Figure 17.6). The index and/or middle finger pulps firmly press downward on the tucked thumb as it holds the pencil. The transverse metacarpal arch is fairly flat. The thumb is adducted with supination and locked under the index finger and/or middle finger. Digit V is flexed to stabilize the MP arch to support the writing finger. The wrist is straight or slightly extended. This "locked" grip mechanically restricts digital manipulation of the pencil along its proximal-distal axis. With persistent use of the strong adductor and flexor to

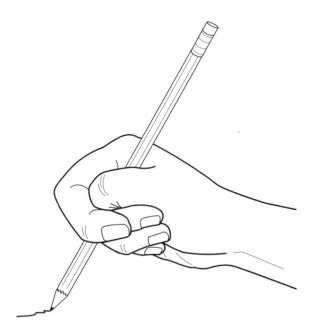

Figure 17.6 Thumb tuck grip.

stabilize and mobilize the pencil, the MP joint structures of the thumb will be outwardly stressed and cause pain and possibly degenerative disease over time.

Lateral Pinch Grip

The proximal phalanx or the thumb pulp is adducted to stabilize the pencil shaft against the lateral border of the index finger (Figure 17.7). The thumb-index web space is partially closed. Four fingers are adducted and loosely flexed into the palm. The transverse metacarpal arch is fairly flat. The forearm is firmly stabilized in a pronated position on the desk surface. The pencil is mobilized by thumb flexion combined with flexion and extension at the joints of either the two radial digits or all four fingers working as a unit. Firmly stabilized against the index finger, the pencil will mechanically block rotation at the index MP joint and impede the rounding of strokes over the tops of letters. In analyzing Graphograms (computerized printouts) of the effect of pencil grip on writing speed, pressure, and pause, Meeks (cited by Benbow, 1995) found a significant break in rhythm and slowing of motion whenever a proximal joint was recruited to round a stroke. The pronated posture of the forearm restricts the subtle involvement of the elbow in coordination with distal digital movements. Joint problems at the MP joint of the thumb may be caused when the thumb adductor is primarily used for stabilizing rather than manipulating the pencil.

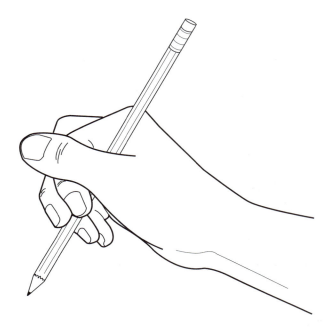

Figure 17.7   Lateral pinch grip.

Quadrupod Grip: Static to Dynamic

The pencil is stabilized against the radial side of the fourth finger by the thumb pulp (Figure 17.8). The little finger is flexed to stabilize the MP arch and support the other three fingers. The pulps of the thumb and two digits hold the pencil in a secure lateral posture. The wrist is extended 25–35 degrees, allowing subtle flexion/extension interplay with the four active digits. The forearm is rotated 50–60 degrees from pronation, allowing elbow rotation to combine with the digits for rounding over the tops of letters. The pencil, held in the open index-thumb web space, is in position to become more dynamic as the child is required to print in reduced ruled spaces. Additionally this grip will allow lateral deviation of the fingers for rounding over the tops of letters without having to recruit more proximal, less accurate, and slower joints. If the grip remains static all strokes will have to be done by proximal upper extremity joints. This will significantly reduce writing speed and refinement. However, the quadrupod grip usually becomes dynamic. It is considered an efficient grip because it allows translation movements with the four digits. Benbow (1990) found, during timed writing contests, that third grade children writing on ³⁄₈-inch ruled paper using a dynamic quadrupod grip were as fast and accurate as children who used a dynamic tripod grip.

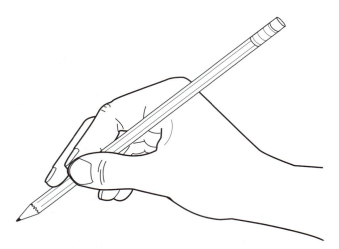

Figure 17.8 Quadrupod grip: static to dynamic.

Tripod Grip: Static to Dynamic

The pencil is stabilized against the radial side of the middle finger by the thumb pulp (Figure 17.9). The two ulnar digits are flexed to stabilize the MP arch, support the third finger and shift control to the skilled side of the hand. The MP arch is fully curved so that a separation is created between the index and long finger for an active and balanced three digit grip. All IP joints of the thumb, index, and long

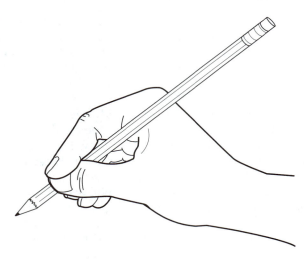

Figure 17.9 Tripod grip: static to dynamic.

finger are partially flexed. This posture allows the high density mechanoreceptors of the three digit pulps to regulate just enough pressure to prevent slippage of the pencil and to manipulate the pencil in the most efficient manner. The thumb-index web is fully expanded and in a position to become dynamic when the ruled space is reduced. The wrist is stabilized in about 20 degrees of extension, allowing the subtle interplay of wrist and digit movement. Occasionally, when the grip remains static all strokes will have to be produced by proximal upper extremity joints, which will significantly reduce writing speed. However, the three-digit hold usually becomes dynamic and is considered the most efficient grip because it naturally and comfortably allows the longest, freest translation movements toward and away from the palm with the three skilled digits.

Adapted Tripod Grip

The pencil is stabilized within the index and long finger web space (Figure 17.10). The distal end of the pencil is stabilized distally by the thumb pulp against the radial aspect of the long finger. The shaft of the pencil wedges a separation between the index and long finger for tripod positioning. All joints of the index, long finger, and thumb are rounded and hold the pencil distally. The two ulnar digits are flexed to stabilize the MP arch, support the third finger and shift control to the skilled side of the hand. The wrist is stabilized in about 20 degrees extension allowing the subtle interplay of wrist and finger movement. This grip allows maximum input from mechanoreceptors of the three digit pulps to regulate pencil pressure and write in a more efficient manner. This is the adaptation of choice when the acquired pencil grip is not motorically efficient or is stressful to the

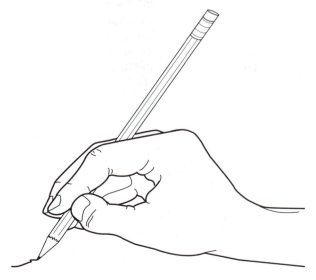

Figure 17.10   Adapted tripod grip.

thumb and finger joints. The narrower web space between the index and long finger provides a secure point of stability from which to control the pencil. The muscles used to produce the writing strokes are the same as those used when the dynamic tripod grip is positioned within the thumb-index web space.

Process for Altering an Inefficient Grip

The following sequence can make the transition to the adapted grip less stressful and more successful. The instructor demonstrates how to position a pencil between the index and long fingers and makes large random patterns on the paper using shoulder and elbow movements. The child imitates the instructor and positions the pencil between the same digits to makes some large free flowing marks (no finger movements and no letters). After the child adjusts to the feel of the pencil in the new position, he or she should be encouraged to draw anything he or she wants to draw. When the grip feels more natural to him or her, the child should attempt to write numbers or letters. Whenever the new grip becomes annoying, the child should be encouraged to temporarily shift back to his or her old grip. As soon as he or she feels ready, the child should return to the new grip. When a child understands the reason for adopting a new pencil grip, is encouraged to alternate between the new grip and the old grip, and can control the timing of the alternating scheme, he or she will gradually gain more comfort and control with the adapted grip and use it consistently.

Several positioning devices (Figure 17.11) may be used to guide writers in better placement of their fingers while holding a pencil. Although the use of positioning devices is more effective in developing an efficient grip, rather than correcting an inefficient one, they can provide some comfort and positional benefit. The Pencil Pal (Figure 17.12) was designed to reduce hyperextension of the distal interphalangeal joint (DIP) of the index finger by stabilizing the pencil at the level of the index MP joint rather than deep within the thumb web space. This shift in the angle of the pencil reduces "white knuckle" discomfort in many children, allowing dynamic control of the pencil with the skilled digits.

Levine (1987), Schneck (1991), Ziviani (1987), and Benbow (1990) have reported that reduced tactile sensitivity is common in children with inefficient pencil grips. Benbow (1995) experimented with applying a narrow strip of stretchy tape over the

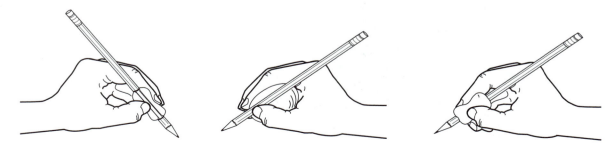

Figure 17.11   Finger placement devices to aid pencil holding.

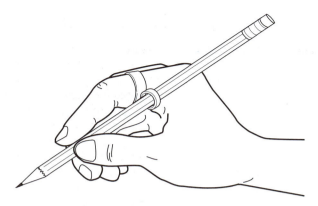

Figure 17.12   The Pencil Pal provides a higher point of stability for the pencil, which reduced DIP hyperextension.

dorsal aspect of the writing digits to increase the flow of afferent impulses from the slightest movement of the digits. The tape is gently stretched over the middle dorsal aspects of all three finger joints and affixed over the metacarpal bone (Figure 17.13). Taping over the two thumb joints may be helpful as well. Children say that the tape helps them to feel their fingers better so they can write better.

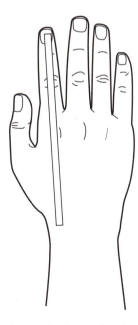

Figure 17.13   Tape ($\frac{1}{3}$-inch wide) applied to index finger to increase tactile input. Thumb taping also may be indicated.

GRAPHIC TRAINING FOR CHILDREN WITH DCD

Handwriting is the most complex and utilized motor skill required in education, yet little attention is paid to how, when, or where pencil practice best enhances the development of this skill. Connolly (1973) says that adults seem to assume that children will somehow know the best way to hold a pencil or that they will acquire the skill through incidental experience. He states that, in the course of development of the child's motor skills, there is evidence of transfer between different forms of action. For example, once a precision grip is mastered with a spoon, it begins to be used in drawing with a pencil or painting with a brush. Experience has taught therapists that the child with DCD does not automatically make this transfer. The static distal holding of a fork and spoon typically precedes holding and manipulating a pencil. Correcting silverware holding does make positioning and holding writing implements less awkward and more efficient to develop.

A pencil is such a mundane tool that it does not receive the respect it deserves. As an extension of the hand, the pencil must be held in a manner that provides both stability and mobility. Speed, axial force and control, pausing, and endurance while writing can be influenced by the way the writer grips his or her pencil. Rosenbloom and Horton (1971) found that some children adopt a pencil grip as early as 2½ years of age. With repeated use, an early grip may be kinesthetically reinforced long before the child enters first grade. Some children, usually girls, spend vast amounts of time "writing" before they have developed adequate stability in their hands, established a dominant hand, or learned the names of the letters they are trying to copy. Through trial and error experience with markers, crayons, and pencils, some grips will become very efficient, but others will become very inefficient. Benbow (1987) and Schneck (1991) found more inefficient grips among typically developing girls than boys in public schools in the Boston area.

SELECTION OF AN APPROPRIATE WRITING SYSTEM FOR A CHILD WITH DCD

The expectation that a primary school child with disordered motor control should learn two graphic systems (printing and cursive writing) should receive evaluation from professionals knowledgeable in motor control and learning before any formal training is initiated. Perceptual and motor coordination skill requirements differ considerably in the many graphic programs currently available.

Printing is highly dependent on the child's potential in the following visual motor integration skills: (a) part-to-whole analysis and synthesis (the ability to mentally separate letters into their line segments and then reposition them to form letters), (b) controlled starting and stopping at an intended point, (c) visual motor integration of the diagonal (the hardest line orientation to produce and used frequently in printed formations), (d) the ability to space letters within a word and between words in a meaningful way, and (e) the ability to produce written work at a functional speed above second grade level.

Most printing is practiced with the paper positioned square to the edge of the desk, rather than on a slant, which matches the angle of wrist flexion for efficient down stroking. This paper position requires rotation of the forearm into additional pronation to make each vertical stroke. Repositioning the paper to an accommodating slant when cursive writing is introduced creates great distress in children who are insecure and frustrated by their continuing lack of success with printing. Children with spatial difficulties, known to be more rigid in their learning style, have a disconcerting task in shifting to a second writing system. Most of these children, despite their struggles, will not have reached a functional level in printing during the first two or three years of school. Making an abrupt shift to cursive style in mid-second or third grade is often beyond their tolerance. When demands for written work increases, these students often revert to the less efficient but more practiced skill of printing. Mixing letters from the two-letter systems often becomes an added problem.

Second grade seems to be an optimal time for most children to learn cursive handwriting. Student interest is high, and students have not yet acquired faulty habits of "inventive cursive" before formal instruction begins. A writing curriculum with instructional techniques to accommodate for perceptual and motor learning deficits should enable nearly all students to advance to cursive writing at a time when less written output is required. Training activities of combining letters into simple two- and three-letter words to practice letter formations and connector units are at a more appropriate cognitive level for second graders. Initiating cursive writing instruction at the beginning of second grade allows a full year for students to stabilize this motor learning and be prepared for the higher volume and cognitive level of written work expected in third grade.

Cursive writing is favored because (a) the movement patterns lend themselves to more automatic or kinesthetic motor learning, (b) reversals and transpositions are less likely to occur, (c) the connected line enables learning words as units, and (d) production is faster because the multiple starts and stops and reorientations of line segments are eliminated for each letter. The greatest obstacle in learning cursive script for a child with coordination difficulties is the distorted sequence of movements most evident in producing repetitive movements of a reciprocal nature.

Clough (1999) designed a pre-cursive program for the cursive program Loops and Other Groups (Benbow, 1990) when she found slowing the pace of the standard progression was not an effective adaptation for the more challenged students. In her pre-cursive program students learned, internalized, and mastered the four basic strokes aided by additional visual and verbal cues to develop consistency and good form. The strokes were taught kinesthetically in the manner recommended by Benbow in the Loops program. Teaching the students to connect the four strokes in various patterns was addressed before letter learning; as a result they were able to learn fluidity in cursive writing.

Later, when a student is consistently coached to visualize the letter form as it relates to some common object in his or her environment and to verbalize the motor plan while paying attention to the feel of the movement, any letter form will begin to feel familiar to him or her with consistent repetition. The motor patterns for letters and frequently used words will be established in the child's kinesthetic memory with extended practice. Once letters are fixed in kinesthetic memory, he or she will gradually be able to increase writing speed without a reduction in quality. This learning will be preferable to remaining dependent on visual motor guidance of the writing hand to control the printed output.

Speed of handwriting will probably be the most serious deterrent for a student with DCD to acquire functional skill in handwriting. When the quality of the student's handwriting is acceptable but the quantity below grade expectation, adjustment in the length of assignments should be made. The instructor should carefully evaluate which segments of an assignment will cover the pertinent material to be learned and expect the child to complete those parts fully with care.

Once a child has developed isolated finger skills, usually about the beginning of third grade for children with DCD, keyboard skills should be introduced. This skill usually is best learned on a typewriter which provides more movement feedback for learning correct finger use. Hunt-and-peck method should be avoided. Children are extremely resistant to giving it up because they have to slow down to learn functional keyboard skill. By the age of 8 or 9, most students can learn this demanding skill in a way that will allow them to produce satisfactory written material using a typewriter or computer.

LEARNING HANDWRITING

Remember the old saying, "Practice makes perfect, so be careful what you practice." Writing, unless practiced correctly, does not make perfect. It makes permanent! If the child's practice is erratic and disorganized he or she will not receive appropriate feedback to establish and keep refining the motor patterns. Graphic training for a child with a motor disorder will require the most precise teaching and copious supervision while the child is practicing to prevent faulty habits and incorrect letter formations from being reinforced. Repairing handwriting is a great deal more difficult, frustrating, and time consuming than teaching it thoroughly and reinforcing skill mastery to the automatic level during the initial training period.

Fitts and Posner (1967) have described the progression of learning a new motor skill through three phases of learning. The three phases are (a) cognitive, (b) associative, and (c) autonomous. The phases are most apparent in analyzing the processes of learning to write. During the cognitive phase the child is guided in analyzing the letter forms and developing strategies to perform the necessary movement patterns. Cognitive and visual analysis are necessary for planning the motor progression. These, coupled with eye hand control, are of primary importance during the initial learning phase. This is followed by the associative phase. Practice, instructional support, and the development of self-monitoring strategies will be needed to establish consistent skill development. Once the child has learned the basic letter forms, he or she will need to adjust and refine his or her newly learned motor skills. Visual feedback should decline as proprioceptive feedback becomes the primary control system. As the associative stage progresses, the child will be able to give attention to the mechanics of spacing words meaningfully, filling vertical line spaces, and developing a consistent slant. During the final or autonomous stage, the child will be able to write with progressive reduction in attention to the motor demands of the writing process. This will free the child to focus his or her attention on the higher cognitive skills, since knowledge of the subject, word retrieval, grammar, punctuation, syntax, and spelling all need to be performed simultaneously.

THE LEARNING SETTING

- Every student should face the chalkboard where letter analysis and demonstration will be guided by the instructor. Facing forward will reduce directional and positional confusion for the novice writers.
- Chair height should allow firm contact of the child's heels on the floor for weight shifting as the writing arm moves horizontally away from the midline. Knees and hips should be flexed at 90 degrees. Weight should be evenly distributed on both hips. Children who are unable to shift weight through the lower extremities and rotate through the trunk will lower their weight forward onto the non-writing arm and maintain balance through forearm rotation and lateral tilting of the trunk. This will severely limit the complementary use of the hands in the writing task.
- Desk height should be 2 inches above the writer's bent elbow when the child is seated on a properly fitted chair. If the desk is too high, the upper arms will be too widely abducted for maximum control of the hands. If the desk height is too low, the child will be inclined into a flexed position and may use his or her recessive hand to support his or her head rather than stabilize and adjust the paper. The distance between the chair and desk should be just enough to allow for trunk rotation as the writing hands moves horizontally away from his or her midline.

STUDENT PREPARATION FOR HANDWRITING TRAINING

- Every teaching session should begin with each child assuming a symmetrical position to write. Children who lack postural sensitivity often fail to make the adjustments to counterbalance themselves as weight shifts during writing. Maintaining the head, trunk, and arms in a balanced and comfortable posture is crucial for learning to write kinesthetically. Many children with coordination disabilities do not keep readjusting their posture so the instructor should cue them to shift their weight for better balance.
- Functional visual problems are typically the reason that a child shifts his or her eyes and/or head into a posture that is too close or tilted excessively in order to visually guide the writing hand with one eye. If the child's eye and head position interferes with normal postural control in writing, he or she should be referred for a thorough evaluation of visual function.
- The slant of the paper should run parallel to the line of the writing arm when the hands are relaxed and together at midline on the desktop. A piece of masking tape can serve as a positional jig until paper alignment is automatically assumed. The lower corner of the paper should be placed about 2 inches toward the dominant side of the child's midline.

- Advancing the paper upward on the desk as the writing progresses downward on the page should be stressed. The writing hand should remain below the writing line so that the wrist is in a functional position to work reciprocally with finger movements. Upward adjusting of the paper will prevent the need for the eyes to move closer and closer to the paper in order to monitor what is being written at the bottom of the page.

TERMINOLOGY

Lines

Demonstrate and define the spatial terms as they relate to the writing line. Highlight the writing line to reduce confusion about where to start letters. The dotted middle marker above the writing line indicates the highest level for half-space letters. The dotted middle marker below the writing line indicates the lowest level loops should descend below the writing line. The top or head line indicates where whole space letters reach above the writing line. In order to learn the "feel" of the vertical proportion of each letter, the student should completely fill the indicated spaces.

Lead-In Stroke

In the curriculum Loops and Other Groups, the lead-ins for the four-letter groups climb, slant, loop, or follow an overhand curve according to their group placement. The lead-in stroke determines the group assignment of each letter. All lead-in strokes for the 26 lower case letters begin on the writing line to the left of the space where the letter will be written. Naming the group helps the child visualize the lead-in stroke as it relates to a clock, a kite string, a stunt plane making loops, or hills and valleys. All lead-in strokes and single line segments are easier to control when moving the pencil quickly; children should be coached to speed up when writing these components. A quick-flowing stroke is easier to produce and will enhance kinesthetic learning.

Retrace Strokes

These are line segments where the initial line is traced over in order to move to a new position before changing direction to continue the letter. For example, one retraces the clockwise lead-in stroke that climbs over the top of the letter "a" to the 1 o'clock position by moving counterclockwise between the 1 o'clock and 9 o'clock position before separating and rounding down to the writing line. Twenty-two lower case letters have retrace units. Initially, a retraced segment requires close visual guidance to make a clean retrace. Children should be coached to slow down while retracing.

Release or Lead-Out Stroke

Twenty-two lower case letters must return to the writing line before curving upward to be continued as the lead-in for the following letter. Right-hand line segments at the completion of a letter should be returned to the writing line for accuracy and easier reading. Release strokes typically are the fastest written segment of a letter.

INSTRUCTOR'S GUIDE FOR TEACHING

The instructor draws a 15-inch model of the letter on the chalkboard. Special attention is given to the letter's position between the three vertically divided spaces of the line. This large model is used to teach the following:

a. Indicate the starting point to the left of the letter position on the writing line.
b. Identify lead-in groups to reinforce visualization of the initial movement.
c. Mark all the locations where the letter touches the writing line, the middle marker above or below the writing line, and the head line. Triangular shapes made by the letter and the writing line should be colored in to show the negative shapes formed by the letter.
d. Rehearse the verbalized motor plan (or "talk to your hand") using consistent terminology during the tracing of the entire movement pattern. Many children need an additional reminder: "Say what you are doing and do what you are saying." As soon as the child is writing a letter on paper accurately and faster than he or she is subvocalizing the motor plan, the child should discontinue the verbal support. If the child needs to cue him- or herself at a later time, this technique can be reemployed.

As additional rules are required for subsequent letters, they should be taught with the motor plan of the new letter. For example, when a letter contains two parallel ascending lines such as "u" or two parallel descending lines such as "n," the child should be taught to look back at the first line and not let the opening get wider.

Momentary stopping points are included in the instructions for children who have difficulty shifting direction in a continuous flow pattern. These stops will allow for the visual motor reorganizing required for the child to continue in a new direction.

STUDENT'S MOTOR LEARNING SEQUENCE

Students extend their index and long fingers while holding down digits IV and V with the thumb (separating the two sides) of their writing hand. Using isolated shoulder movements, the instructor and class rehearse the entire motor plan while they "trace" the chalkboard model letter in the air.

While tracing the letter in the air, the students should be encouraged to simultaneously picture the letter shape and stroke progression in their heads while shifting their attention to the "feel" of the shoulder movements.

When a student is confident that he or she has mastered the motor plan, the child should close his or her eyes to visualize the letter, rest an elbow on his or her desk, and verbalize the motor plan while tracing the letter in the air using elbow and wrist movements. The instructor should verify the child's verbalized motor plan before the child is allowed to write the letter on paper. In order to reduce stress, children should omit writing their name on practice papers during the beginning practice of this complex motor skill. Before attempting the first letter on paper, it is wise to reassure the students that some of their letters will look pretty good, some not so good, and others might be just awful. This is to be expected, and with practice, all the letters will look fine.

Half-inch divided-line practice paper should be cut vertically into 4-inch widths. The narrow strip of paper will keep the writing hand closer to the midline where the child has more stability and better control during the initial learning period. Writing lines should be highlighted to avoid confusion about where to start all lead-in strokes.

While continually subvocalizing the motor plan, each child writes the letter to be learned 10 times. During practice sessions, he or she should draw a line through any letter he or she feels is incorrect, rather than erasing, which is a waste of practice time. Children enjoy being detectives of their own graphic evidence. Finding specific errors will help the child deduce strategies for self correction. On completion of the tenth letter, the child should evaluate his or her own work by looking for line touches, clean retraces, and triangular shapes (Figure 17.14). Being made aware of these details helps the child to avoid reinforcing incorrect patterns when practicing on his or her own. The child should circle all the letters that are correct. Of the circled letters, the child should mark the very best one. After this is verified by the instructor, he or she repeats writing the letter 15 more times guided by his or her own kinesthetic model. The initial letter of each of the four groups must be over-learned to the automatic kinesthetic level so it can be modified for the remaining letters in the group. Visualizing while verbalizing letters within groups will reinforce motor learning of the entire group. This makes kinesthetic memory learning most efficient.

When a letter is reliably and consistently written, the student should learn to connect it in double letter combinations or short words. Before advancing to the following letter in any group, the child must be able to write the new letter without looking. Successfully using his or her kinesthetic sense to write a letter builds confidence, and the child will be motivated to try the next letter. Each letter will come more easily and naturally because the major part of the letter has been kinesthetically mastered.

At this stage in the learning process, it is imperative for the child to understand that the brain learns to write faster than the hand. The hand will need multiple

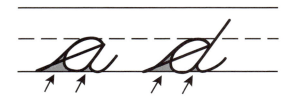

Figure 17.14a Arrows indicate negative shapes created between the writing line and letter strokes.

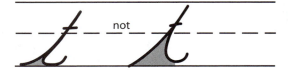

Figure 17.14b Knowing that the triangle should be tiny prevents premature release of down stroke. *Used with permission from* Loops and Other Groups *by Mary Benbow, copyright 1990 by Therapy Skill Builders, a division of Communication Skill Builders, Inc., P.O. Box 42050, Tucson, AZ.*

repetitions before it will be able to operate on "automatic pilot" while he or she is thinking about what he or she wants to communicate. However, when the child attains this level of motor skill, he or she will gradually increase his or her writing speed while maintaining quality.

"Mystery Writing" is a relaxing technique that can powerfully reinforce kinesthesia and motor learning. It can be taught once students have learned a few letters. The novice writer stands beside the instructor at the chalkboard. The child holds a piece of chalk in his or her dominant hand and closes his or her eyes. The instructor moves the child's hand holding the chalk to write a letter or short word on the chalkboard. The child must visualize the letter from the motor input and identify the letter or word before checking the evidence. The instructor and students should alternate leadership roles in this activity. When the activity is understood by the children, they can pair off to play.

INTERVENTION WITH OLDER STUDENTS

When a middle or high school aged student feels defeated by his or her inability to produce written work, intervention requires therapeutic wisdom, sound knowledge, and respect. If the student has established very poor motor habits in his or her struggle with printing over several years, introducing the child to cursive writing can offer the child a chance to establish more productive habits. Enlisting his or her cooperation to join a team to work against this obstacle in his or her school career can lead to a practical solution. What frequently seems agreeable to a defeated student is this: "You do not have a problem. We have a problem. My goal is to discover what will work well in the least amount of time; yours is to give it your best try so we can decide which techniques will work best for you."

Demystify the Problem

The student/instructor team evaluates and discusses the student's difficulties with writing. The following areas should be considered: (a) hand, paper, and sitting posture, (b) the pencil grip when writing words, compared to the pencil grip while drawing something of the child's own choosing, and (c) the child's potential to duplicate motor patterns.

"Production Consistency Observation Sheet" (Figure 17.15) requires repeating 20 half-inch shapes (a square, circle, triangle and the cursive form of capital "A") using free-hand strokes. The first 15 drawings of the shape should be positioned in three evenly spaced rows with five figures across on a half sheet of unlined paper. On completion of the 15th shape, the student closes his or her eyes or averts his or her gaze and completes a fourth row of 5 additional shapes that correspond to the three rows he or she has just drawn above. The quality seen in the first three rows indicates the student's visual motor control in repeating a shape with consistency in form, size, and spacing. The last row is a graphic demonstration of the student's kinesthetic learning potential for both configuring and spacing. Quality of output on this task is a good indication of a student's potential for learning cursive writing (Benbow, 1999).

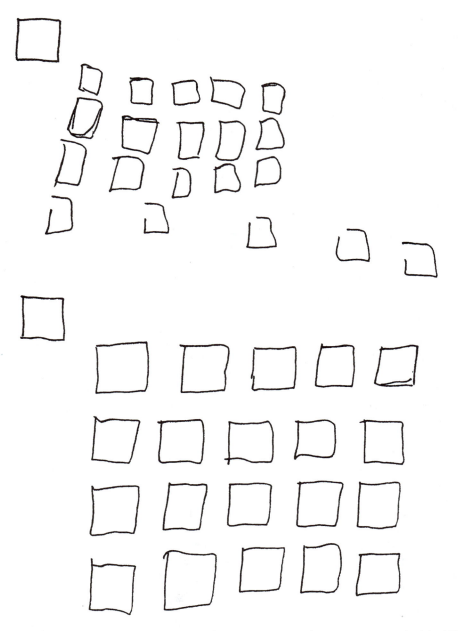

Figure 17.15 Production consistency of a poor writer at the top, compared with skill of a peer who learned to write efficiently.

The width of the line should be compatible with the bluntness of the writing implement and/or the student's grip excursion with a writing tool. Lines over a half inch wide naturally elicit the use of more proximal, less skilled joints. Regardless of age, when fine motor muscles are trained for graphic skills, the letter or number size must be within the reach of the digits that manipulate the pencil. Writing flows more naturally and shows better control when the student uses a compatibly ruled paper. Many students with coordination problems and motorically inefficient grips produce their best quality writing within ¼-inch ruled paper and prefer it to the ⅜- or ½-inch ruled paper. A graphic way to evaluate the most compatible rule of writing paper is to ask a student to draw, using a continuous stroke, within the variously sized circles on a "Distal Control Sheet" (Figure 17.16). If the student shows

Distal Finger Control

Rest side of hand on desk. Use one stroke to circle
left from top around to top within the donut.

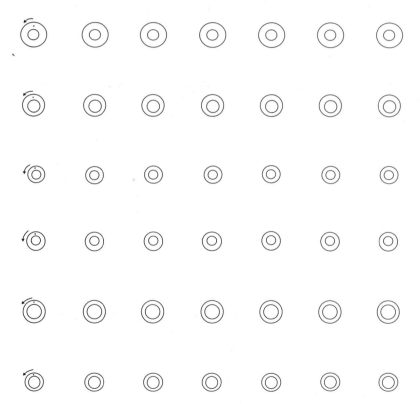

Figure 17.16 Skill in continuous circling can determine a comfortable line rule for his or her writing paper. *Used with permission from* Loops and Other Groups *by Mary Benbow, copyright 1990 by Therapy Skill Builders, a division of Communication Skill Builders, Inc., P.O. Box 42050, Tucson, AZ.*

better control and is more comfortable circling within the smallest circles, he or she will probably prefer and write better on narrow ruled paper. This is usually the case for a student with a restricted pencil grip.

If the student is able and willing to attempt some cursive letters, he or she should write a connected cursive alphabet. This alphabet sample should be followed by the student's writing another alphabet with eyes closed. Like letters from the two samples should be evaluated for similarities to determine which ones have been learned kinesthetically and will require no further work.

A time-limited but realistic intervention schedule should be established. Timed teaching and practice sessions, with coaching to avoid inaccurate or ineffective performance, should enable the student to gain functional skill and confidence. During the academic year, scheduling is difficult, but daily training over a period of six weeks is usually the most effective way to schedule. A summer recess period when academic demands are removed from daily routines is a better time for intensive help.

Errors made in cursive formations tend to cluster. For example, if the over-the-top lead-in stroke does not continue to the one o'clock position or the retraced stroke does not return to the writing line before the release stroke in the letter "a," the same error will usually occur in "d," "g," and "q."

Overall appearance of the student's writing can often be significantly improved by gaining control of the 10 letters that descend below the writing line to the middle marker below. Loops that descend a half space below the writing line can be difficult for youngsters who have coordination problems, especially if coupled with visual convergence insufficiency. Kinesthetically developing the "feel" for the distance to drop the stroke below the writing line should improve the appearance and readability of seven lower case and three capital letters. A momentary stop at the middle marker below the writing line helps to control the enlargement of the loops and prevents interference with the words on the line below.

Lower case letters account for 95–98% of letter use. Therefore, more time, effort, and attention should be allotted to the kinesthetic mastery of the 26 lower case letters. Clearly writing the capital letters used in the student's signature and address should be a definite goal. Many upper case block letters are acceptable substitutes for cursive letters. Having to pause and motor plan a few capital letters will not seriously impede overall writing efficiency.

Once the student is able to form the 26 letters correctly, he or she will need to develop speed for writing to be a functional skill. To determine which letters need to be brought up to speed, have the student write a connected cursive alphabet with eyes open and another with eyes closed. Identify the "think breaks" or pauses in both samples (Figure 17.17). Pauses are the darker interruptions (graphite lumps) seen in the connector stroke preceding the letters where the student had to pause to recall the motor plan. He or she should reinforce these letter motor plans until they become automatic.

"Mystery Writing" is an enjoyable exercise that will powerfully reinforce kinesthesia and motor learning with a student of any age. For techniques used in this activity with beginning students in cursive instruction, see the description above.

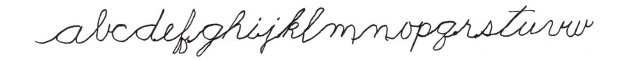

Figure 17.17   Think breaks or pauses allow the writer to motor plan the subsequent letter.

SUMMARY AND CONCLUSIONS

The development of hand and writing skills involves a complex interplay among the musculo-skeletal, visual, proprioceptive, cognitive, and motor elements for the production of efficient hand skills, especially in children with DCD. Kinesthesis is an important key to understanding handwriting problems and for preventing or remediating them. When a motor skill is barely taught and haphazardly practiced and reinforced to the automatic level of performance, this kinesthetic learning can last a lifetime, blocking effective and efficient performance of the skill and frustrating any attempt to modify it. For the child with DCD, early intervention can replace this negative learning with a positive experience. When any complex motor skill is analyzed to determine the underlying causes of the problems, compensation and teaching techniques are properly sequenced, and the skill practiced to the automatic level of performance, kinesthesia is a life-long blessing in the performance of that skill.

APPENDIX

Accommodations to Functional Settings for Children with Developmental Coordination Disorder

Teresa May-Benson, Peg Ingolia, and Jane Koomar

In addition to providing intervention that helps remediate areas of difficulty for children with developmental coordination disorder (DCD), it is critical to structure their environments for success. This is true in the home and school settings, as it helps to lend the consistency and predictability that have been identified as important to children's success in completing daily living tasks. Below are samples of suggestions and strategies from experts who work with children who have DCD.

IN THE CLASSROOM SETTING

- Give simple step-by-step directions for the student with difficulty in motor planning. Help the child identify the steps needed to accomplish the task. Demonstrate or ask another student to model the motor activity and then ask the student to try.
- Use a consistent approach to teaching the child a new skill. Allow time for practice. It may take a child with motor planning delays much more time to learn and "polish" a new skill.

- Present directions for new activities in the child's best modality—visual, auditory, or multisensory—in order to facilitate learning. Use modeling, demonstration, and repetition as necessary. Monitor the child to be sure the information is understood and the task initiated.
- Help the student plan out a task by asking questions such as, "What materials do you need?" or "What do you do first?"
- Provide several suggestions or create a brainstorming session in a peer group for the child who has difficulty formulating ideas for projects or assignments.
- Set up a variety of activities in an obstacle course format. Begin simply and increase the complexity as the student is able to handle the tasks. "Simon Says" or sequencing games are good for motor planning.
- A carpet square on the floor can help the child find and remain in "his own space" during group or discussion times.
- A child with motor planning difficulties may need assistance to recognize and improve work that is not yet accurate.
- To prepare the child for transitions, use a timer or inform him or her ahead of time to identify when it is time to change activities.
- Using pictures or a list written on the blackboard to order the day's activities can help the child with sequencing difficulties organize the day for smoother transitions.
- Help the child develop organizational skills by having a consistent place to store materials once he or she has completed a task.
- To help the student stay organized and focused on challenging academic work you can:
  a. Have the children use a finger or file card under lines to keep place in reading or math.
  b. Use graph paper for math work.
  c. Keep the amount of visual information presented on a page to a minimum.
  d. Cover an area of the page to expose only one or two problems at a time.
- To provide additional structure, give the student letter and number guides from which to copy. Tape them to the desk if needed.
- Touching base with homeroom teachers can help ensure that all the books and papers for homework actually make it into the child's backpack.

(Suggestions from OTA–Watertown, P.C. Classroom Accommodations Checklist, Watertown, MA.)

- Give short assignments so that the child can feel instant success in completing a task. Document the length of time a child can focus on one task and structure the assignment so that it can be completed in that amount of time.
- Provide a system for checking off the steps in a task when they are accomplished.
- Give one direction at a time. After one direction is successfully completed, add another direction. For example: "Stand on the line." PAUSE. Wait until the class is on the line. "We are going to . . . (one direction)" PAUSE "and . . . (a second direction)."
- Help the child physically move through an action in order to learn it.

- Mark the boundaries of games, for example, rope, yarn, masking tape, or chalk can be used to mark a game circle, or the start and finish lines.
- Stop the action between children's turns in order to get everyone's attention.
- Give students different assignments within games, for example one child can jump the rope while another runs through the turning rope; size and distance of targets can be varied for each child.
- Schedule a calming familiar backup game if the structure of a new game fails. Before the new game is discarded, try to alter the structure for future success.

(Suggestions from the Sensory Motor Handbook—A Guide for Implementing and Modifying Activities, *by Julie Bissell, Jean Fisher, Carol Owens, and Patricia Polcyn, SII, 1988.)*

- Students should learn to underline key ideas while they read. What they have underlined might then be reread or skimmed. A cycle of read, underline, and summarize must be an established practice that is integrated with writing.
- The skills involved in maintaining a neat notebook may be very hard for children with organizational problems. Help should be provided in this area.
- Specific instructions about maintaining an assignment pad need to be given and coordinated between home and school. Parents and teachers should review periodically.
- Divide tasks into stages, and allocate sufficient time to each stage.
- The "home office" should be set up effectively. If at all possible, children should not work in their bedrooms, which are distracting and associated with sleep rather than sustained attention to detail. There should be a predictable site for work at home and a quiet time for cognitive pursuits. There should be no distraction by television, loud discussion, or other competing stimuli (with the possible exception of music as white noise).
- If a student has no particular homework, time should still be predictably set aside for productive efforts in cognitive areas (crosswords, workbooks, and writing).

(Suggestions from Developmental Variations and Learning Disorders, *by Melvin D. Levine, 1987.)*

IN THE HOME SETTING

Many of the suggestions outlined above are also helpful in the home environment. In addition, the following are often helpful:

- Set clothing out on the bed in a row to help with dressing. Have the child take articles from left to right.
- Label drawers and rearrange them top to bottom in order of first to last items needed.
- Help the child get prepared the night before. Ask, "What do you need for tomorrow?"
- Model the thinking process by verbalizing steps aloud to help the child incorporate this process into his/her routine.

- Use labeled bins or drawers to teach the child that toys have a place.
- Have him or her clean up one activity before beginning another.
- Give the child the option of time-out or quiet time alone when he or she feels overstimulated or overwhelmed.

(Suggestions from OTA–Watertown, P.C. Home Accommodations Checklist, Watertown, MA.)

- Color code the child's room to keep belongings separate and to assist in putting things away.
- Especially for toddlers and preschoolers, establish large bins with a few of their favorite toys, so that they can keep tidy and the bins can be moved to different play areas.
- Group similar toys together and keep them in the areas in which they are most often used, to help in organizing and keeping home areas organized.
- Use sketches or a catalog picture taped to boxes to identify items that belong in the boxes.
- Make a game of clean-up time. Ask, "Can you pick up all the stuffed animals and put them back before I finish with the blocks?"
- Involve older children in your organizing efforts. For example, take them shopping for organizing items with you. Let them help choose the colors and styles.
- Assign a special shelf or drawer in the bathroom for the child's belongings.
- Have your child establish a color-coding system for homework folders (by subject).
- Teach your child how to label notebooks and arrange desk supplies.
- When you first see your child after school, ask about homework and discuss what the assignments are and about how long they should take. You can help set up a time management system. If necessary, you can establish a reward such as, "After you finish you can watch a half hour of television."

(Suggestions from Organize Yourself, *by Ronnie Eisenberg, Macmillan Publishing Co., New York, 1986.)*

References

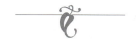

CHAPTER 1

Abbie, M. H., Douglas, H. M., & Ross, K. E. (1978). The clumsy child: Observations in cases referred to the gymnasium of the Adelaide children's hospital over a three-year period. *Medical Journal of Australia, 1,* 65–69.

Ahern, K. (1995). *Family systems factors and the diagnostic process of movement difficulties in children.* Unpublished doctoral dissertation, University of Western Australia, Perth.

American Psychiatric Association (1987). *Diagnostic and statistical manual of mental disorders* (3rd ed. revised). Washington, DC: Author.

American Psychiatric Association (1994). *Diagnostic and statistical manual of mental disorders* (4th ed.). Washington, DC: Author.

Anderson, B. J., Alcantara, A. A., & Greenough, W. T. (1997). Motor-skill learning: Changes in synaptic organization of the rat cerebellar cortex. *Neurobiology of Learning & Memory, 66*(2), 221–229.

Annell, A. (1949). School problems in children of average or superior intelligence: A preliminary report. *Journal of Mental Science, XCV,* 901–909.

Arnheim, D. D., & Sinclair, W. A. (1975). *The clumsy child: A program of motor therapy.* St Louis: Mosby.

Ayres, A. J. (1960). Occupational therapy for motor disorders resulting from impairment of the central nervous system. *Rehabilitation Literature, 21,* 302–310.

Ayres, A. J. (1965). Patterns of perceptual-motor dysfunction in children: A factor analytic study. *Perceptual and Motor Skills, 20,* 335–358.

Ayres, A. J. (1972a). *Sensory integration and learning disorders.* Los Angeles: Western Psychological Services.

Ayres, A. J. (1972b). Types of sensory integrative dysfunction among disabled learners. *American Journal of Occupational Therapy, 26*(1), 13–18.

Ayres, A. J. (1977). Cluster analyses of measures of sensory integration. *American Journal of Occupational Therapy, 31,* 362–366.

Ayres, A. J. (1980). *Sensory integration and learning disorders.* Los Angeles: Western Psychological Corporation.

Ayres, A. J. (1985). *Developmental dyspraxia and adult onset apraxia.* Torrance, CA: Sensory Integration International.

Ayres, A. J. (1989). *The Sensory Integration and Praxis Tests.* Los Angeles: Western Psychological Services.

Ayres, A. J., Mailloux, Z. K., & Wendler, C. L. W. (1987). Developmental dyspraxia: Is it a unitary function? *Occupational Therapy Journal of Research, 7*(2), 93–110.

Bagley, W. C. (1900/01). On the correlation of mental and motor ability in school children. *Journal of American Psychology, 12,* 193–205.

Barnett, A. L., Kooistra, L., & Henderson, S. E. (1998). "Clumsiness" as syndrome and symptom. *Human Movement Science, 17,* 435–447.

Benbow, M. (1995). Principles and practices of teaching handwriting. In A. Henderson & C. Pehoski (Eds.), *Hand function in the child* (pp. 255–281). St Louis: Mosby.

Beyer, R. (1993). *Motor proficiency of males with attention deficit hyperactive disorder and males with learning disabilities.* Ann Arbor, MI: UMI.

Bouffard, M., Watkinson, E. J., Thompson, L. P., Causgrove Dunn, J. L., & Romanow, S. K. E. (1996). A test of the activity deficit hypothesis with children with movement difficulties. *Adapted Physical Activity Quarterly, 13,* 61–73.

Brenner, M. W., Gillman, S., Zangwill, O. L., & Farrell, M. (1967). Visuo-motor disability in schoolchildren. *British Medical Journal, 4,* 259–262.

Broer, M. (1955). Evaluation of a basic skills curriculum for women students of low motor ability at the University of Washington. *Research Quarterly, 26,* 15–27.

Bundy, A. (1991). Play theory and sensory integration. In A. G. Fisher, E. A. Murray, & A. C. Bundy (Eds.), *Sensory integration: Theory and practice* (pp. 46–68). Philadelphia: F. A. Davis.

Cantell, M. H., Smyth, M. M., & Ahonen, T. P. (1994). Clumsiness in adolescence: Educational, motor, and social outcomes of motor delay detected at 5 years. *Adapted Physical Activity Quarterly, 11,* 115–129.

Cermak, S. (1985). Developmental dyspraxia. In E. A. Roy (Ed.), *Neuropsychological studies of apraxia and related disorders* (pp. 225–248). Amsterdam: North-Holland.

Cermak, S. (1991). Somatodyspraxia. In A. G. Fisher, E. A. Murray, & A. C. Bundy (Eds.), *Sensory integration: Theory and practice* (pp. 137–165). Philadelphia: F. A. Davis.

Cermak, S. (in press). Developmental dyspraxia and clumsiness in children. In D. Tupper (Ed.), *Developmental neuropsychology and soft neurological signs: An update.* Special issue of *Developmental Neuropsychology.*

Clements, S. D. (1966). *Minimal brain dysfunction in children: Terminology and identification. NINBD Monograph 3.* Washington, DC: U. S. Government.

Conrad, K., Cermak, S., & Drake, C. (1983). Differentiation of praxis among children. *American Journal of Occupational Therapy, 37,* 466–473.

Cooke, R. W. I., & Abernethy, L. J. (1999). Cranial magnetic resonance imaging and school performance in very low birth weight infants in adolescence. *Archives of Disease in Childhood Fetal Neonatal Edition, 81,* F11-F121.

Cratty, B. J. (1975). *Remedial motor activity for children.* Philadelphia: Lea & Febiger.

Cratty, B. J. (1994). *Clumsy child syndromes: Descriptions, evaluation and remediation.* Chur, Switzerland: Harwood.

Cratty, B. J., Ikeda, N., Martin, M. M., Jennett, C., & Morris, M. (1970). *Movement activities, motor ability and the education of children.* Springfield, IL: Charles C. Thomas.

De Ajuriaguerra, J., & Stambak, M. (1969). Developmental dyspraxia and psychomotor disorders. In P. J. Vinken & G. W. Bruyn (Eds.), *Handbook of clinical neurology. Vol. 4. Disorders of speech perception and symbolic behavior* (pp. 443–464). Amsterdam: North-Holland.

Dellen, T. van, Vaessen, W., & Schoemaker, M. (1990). Clumsiness: Definition and selection of subjects. In A. F. Kalverboer (Ed.), *Developmental biopsychology* (pp. 135–152). Ann Arbor, MI: University of Michigan Press.

Denckla, M. B. (1984). Developmental dyspraxia: The clumsy child. In M. D. Levine & P. Satz (Eds.), *Middle childhood: Development and dysfunction,* (pp. 245–260). Baltimore: University Park.

Denckla, M. B., & Roeltgen, D. P. (1992). Disorders of motor function and control. In I. Rapin & S. J. Segalowitz (Eds.), *Handbook of neuropsychology. Vol. 6. Child neuropsychology* (pp. 455–476). Amsterdam: Elsevier Science.

Denckla, M. B., Rudel, R. G., Chapman, C., & Krieger, J. (1985). Motor proficiency in dyslexic children with and without attentional disorders. *Archives of Neurology, 42,* 228–231.

Dewey, D. (1995). What is developmental dyspraxia? *Brain & Cognition, 29,* 254–274.

Drillien, C., & Drummond, M. (1983). *Developmental screening and the child with special needs: A population study of 5000 children. Clinics in Developmental Medicine No. 86.* London: Heinemann.

Dyspraxia Foundation (1998). <http://www. emmbrook. demon. co. uk/dysprax/ pupilsup. htm>.

Dyspraxia Parent Website. <http://www. emmbrook. demon. co. uk/dysprax/ report. htm>.

Ford, F. R. (1960). *Diseases of the nervous system in infancy, childhood and adolescence* (4th ed.). Springfield, IL: Charles C. Thomas.

Fox, A. M., & Lent, B. (1996). Clumsy children primer on developmental coordination disorder. *Canadian Family Physician, 42,* 1965–1971.

Frostig, M. (1968). Sensory-motor development. *Special Education, 57*(2), 18–20.

Geuze, R. H., & Kalverboer, A. F. (1990). Inconsistency and adaptation in timing of clumsy children. *Journal of Human Movement Studies, 13,* 421–432.

Gillberg, I. C., & Gillberg, C. (1989). Children with preschool minor neurodevelopmental disorders. IV. Behaviour and school achievement at age 13. *Developmental Medicine and Child Neurology, 31,* 3–13.

Gillberg, I. C., Gillberg C., & Groth, J. (1989). Children with preschool minor neurodevelopmental disorders. V. Neurodevelopmental profiles at age 13. *Developmental Medicine and Child Neurology, 31,* 14–24.

Gottlieb, G. (1998). Normally occurring environmental and behavioral influences on gene activity: From central dogma to probabilistic epigenesis. *Psychological Review, 105,* 792–802.

Gubbay, S. S. (1975). *The clumsy child: A study in developmental apraxic and agnosic ataxia.* London: W. B. Saunders.

Gubbay, S. S. (1978). The management of developmental apraxia. *Developmental Medicine and Child Neurology, 20,* 643–646.

Gubbay, S. S. (1985). Clumsiness. In J. A. M. Frederiks (Ed.), *Handbook of clinical neurology. Vol. 2. Neurobehavioral disorders* (pp. 159–167). Amsterdam: Elsevier.

Gubbay, S. S., Ellis, E., Walton, J. N., & Court, S. D. M. (1965). Clumsy children: A study of apraxic and agnosic defects in 21 children. *Brain, 88,* 295–312.

Hall, D. (1988). Clumsy children. *British Medical Journal, 296,* 375–376.

Hart, H. (1999). Terminology to benefit children. *Developmental Medicine and Child Neurology, 41,* 651.

Harvey, W. J., & Reid, G. (1997). Motor performance of children with attention-deficit hyperactivity disorder: A preliminary investigation. *Adapted Physical Activity Quarterly, 14,* 189–202.

Henderson, L., Rose, P., & Henderson, S. (1992). Reaction time and movement time in children with developmental coordination disorder. *Journal of Child Psychology and Psychiatry, 33,* 895–905.

Henderson, S. E. (1994). Editorial. *Adapted Physical Activity Quarterly, 11,* 111–114.

Henderson, S. E., & Barnett, A. L. (1998). The classification of specific motor coordination disorders in children: Some problems to be resolved. *Human Movement Science, 17,* 449–469.

Henderson, S. E., & Hall, D. (1982). Concomitants of clumsiness in young school children. *Developmental Medicine and Child Neurology, 24,* 448–460.

Henderson, S. E., & Sugden, D. A. (1992). *Movement Assessment Battery for Children manual.* Sidcup, Kent: The Psychological Corporation.

Hoare, D. (1991). *Classification of movement dysfunctions in children: Descriptive and statistical approaches.* Unpublished doctoral dissertation, University of Western Australia, Nedlands, Australia.

Hoare, D. (1994). Subtypes of developmental coordination disorder. *Adapted Physical Activity Quarterly, 11,* 158–169.

Illingworth, R. S. (1963). The clumsy child. In M. Bax & R. Mac Keith (Eds.), *Minimal cerebral dysfunction. Little Club Clinics in Developmental Medicine No. 10* (pp. 26–27). London: Heinemann Medical.

Illingworth, R. S. (1968). Delayed motor development. *Pediatric Clinics of North America, 15,* 569–580.

Johnson, G. B. (1932). Physical skill tests for sectioning classes into homogeneous units. *Research Quarterly of the American Physical Education Association, 3*(1), 128–136.

Johnston, O., Short, H., & Crawford, J. (1987). Poorly coordinated children: A survey of 95 cases. *Child: Care, Health and Development, 13,* 361–376.

Jongmans, M. J., Henderson, S. E., de Vries, L., & Dubowitz, L. (1993). Duration of periventricular densities in preterm infants and neurological outcome at six years of age. *Archives of Disease in Childhood, 69,* 9–13.

Jongmans, M. J., Mercuri, E., Dubowitz, L. M. S., & Henderson, S. E. (1998). Perceptual-motor difficulties and their concomitants in six-year-old children born prematurely. *Human Movement Science, 17,* 629–653.

Kadesjo, B., & Gillberg, C. (1999). Developmental coordination disorder in Swedish 7-year-old children. *Journal of the American Academy of Child & Adolescent Psychiatry, 38*(7), 820–828.

Kaplan, B. J., Wilson, B., Dewey, D., & Crawford, S. (1994, October). *The genetic basis of clumsiness, and its overlap with other disorders.* Paper presented at the conference Children and Clumsiness Public Forum, London, Canada.

Kaplan, B. J., Wilson, B., Dewey, D., & Crawford, S. (1998). DCD may not be a discrete disorder. *Human Movement Science, 17,* 471–490.

Keogh, J. F. (1968). Incidence and severity of awkwardness among regular school boys and educationally subnormal boys. *Research Quarterly, 39,* 806–808.

Keogh, J. F., Sugden, D., Reynard, C. L., & Calkins, J. (1979). Identification of clumsy children: Comparisons and comments. *Journal of Human Movement Studies, 5,* 32–41.

Kephart, N. C. (1960). *The slow learner in the classroom.* Columbus, OH: Merrill Books.

Kleim, J. A., Swain, R. A., Armstrong, K. A., Napper, R. M. A., Jones, T. A., & Greenough, W. T. (1998). Selective synaptic plasticity with the cerebellar cortex following complex motor skill learning. *Neurobiology of Learning & Memory, 69*(3), 274–289.

Knuckey, N. W., Apsimon, T. T., & Gubbay, S. S. (1983). Computerized axial tomography in clumsy children with developmental apraxia and agnosia. *Brain and Development, 5*(1), 14–20.

Kolb, B. (1999). Synaptic plasticity and the organization of behavior after early and late brain injury. *Canadian Journal of Experimental Psychology, 53,* 62–75.

Kong, E. (1963). Minimal cerebral palsy: The importance of its recognition. In M. Bax & R. Mac Keith (Eds.), *Minimal cerebral dysfunction. Little Club Clinics in Developmental Medicine No. 10* (pp. 29–31). London: Heinemann Medical.

Lafuze, M. (1951). A study of the learning of fundamental skills by college freshman women of low motor ability. *Research Quarterly, 22,* 149–157.

Larkin, D., & Hoare, D. (1992). The movement approach: A window to understanding the clumsy child. In J. J. Summers (Ed.), *Approaches to the study of motor control and learning* (pp. 413–439). Amsterdam: Elsevier Science.

Laszlo, J., & Bairstow, P. (1983). Kinaesthesis: Its measurement, training and relationship to motor control. *Quarterly Journal of Experimental Psychology, 35,* 411–421.

Levene, M. I., Dowling, S., Graham, M., Fogelman, K., Galton, M., & Phillips, M. (1992). Impaired motor function (clumsiness) in five-year-old children: Correlation with neonatal ultrasound scans. *Archives of Diseases in Childhood, 67,* 687–690.

Levine, M. D., Oberklaid, F., & Meltzer, L. (1981). Developmental output failure: A study of low productivity in school-aged children. *Pediatrics, 67*(1), 18–25.

Liepert, J., Miltner, W. H. R., Bauder, H., Sommer, M., Dettmers, C., Taub, E., & Weiller, C. (1998). Motor cortex plasticity during constraint-induced movement therapy in stroke patients. *Neuroscience Letters, 250*(1), 5–8.

Lippitt, L. C. (1926). *A manual of corrective gymnastics.* New York: Macmillan.

Lord, R., & Hulme, C. (1988). Visual perception and drawing ability in clumsy and normal children. *British Journal of Developmental Psychology, 6,* 1–9.

Lundy-Ekman, L., Ivry, R., Keele, S., & Woollacott, M. (1991). Timing and force control deficits in clumsy children. *Journal of Cognitive Neuroscience, 3,* 370–377.

Mæland, A. F. (1992). Identification of children with motor coordination problems. *Adapted Physical Activity Quarterly, 9,* 330–342.

Marlow, N., Roberts, B. L., & Cooke, R. W. I. (1993). Outcome at 8 years for children of birthweights of 1250 g or less. *Archives of Disease in Childhood, 68,* 286–290.

McHale, K., & Cermak, S. A. (1992). Fine motor activities in elementary school: Preliminary findings and provisional implications for children with fine motor problems. *American Journal of Occupational Therapy, 46,* 898–903.

McKinlay, I. (1988). Children with motor learning difficulties: Not so much a syndrome—More a way of life. *Physiotherapy, 73,* 635–638.

Mervis, C. B., Robinson, B. F., & Pani, J. R. (1999). Visuospatial construction. *American Journal of Human Genetics, 65,* 1222–1229.

Michelsson, K., & Lindahl, E. (1993). Relationship between perinatal risk factors and motor development at the ages of 5 and 9 years. In A. F. Kalverboer, B. Hopkins, & R. Geuze (Eds.), *Motor development in early and later childhood: Longitudinal approaches* (pp. 266–285). Cambridge: Cambridge University Press.

Missiuna, C. (1994). Motor skill acquisition in children with developmental coordination disorder. *Adapted Physical Activity Quarterly, 11,* 214–235.

Missiuna, C., & Polatajko, H. J. (1995). Developmental dyspraxia by any other name. *American Journal of Occupational Therapy, 49,* 619–628.

Miyahara, M. (1994). Subtypes of students with learning disabilities based upon gross motor functions. *Adapted Physical Activity Quarterly, 11,* 368–382.

Miyahara, M., & Mobs, I. (1995). Developmental dyspraxia and developmental coordination disorder. *Neuropsychology Review, 5,* 245–268.

Mon-Williams, M. A., Wann, J. P., & Pascal, E. (1999). Visual-proprioceptive mapping in children with developmental coordination disorder. *Developmental Medicine and Child Neurology, 41,* 247–254.

Morris, P. R., & Whiting, H. T. A. (1971). *Motor impairment and compensatory education.* London: G. Bell & Sons.

Norrelgen, F., Lacerda, F., & Forssberg, H. (1999). Speech discrimination and phonological working memory in children with ADHD. *Developmental Medicine and Child Neurology, 41,* 335–339.

Oliver, J., & Keogh, J. F. (1967). Helping the physically awkward. *Special Education, 56*(1), 22–25.

Orton, S. T. (1937). *Reading, writing and speech problems in children.* New York: Norton.

Ozols, E. J., & Rourke, B. P. (1985). Dimensions of social sensitivity in two types of learning-disabled children. In B. P. Rourke (Ed.), *Neuropsychology of learning disabilities: Essentials of subtype analysis* (pp. 281–301). New York: Guilford Press.

Pinto-Martin, J. A., Whitaker, A. H., Feldman, J. F., Van Rossem, R., & Paneth, N. (1999). Relation of cranial ultrasound abnormalities in low-birthweight infants to motor or cognitive performance at ages 2, 6, and 9 years. *Developmental Medicine and Child Neurology, 41,* 826–833.

Polatajko. H. J. (1999). Developmental coordination disorder (DCD): Alias the clumsy child syndrome. In K. Whitmore, H. Hart, & G. Willems (Eds.), *A neurodevelopmental approach to specific learning disorders. Clinics in Developmental Medicine, no. 45* (pp. 119–133). London: Mac Keith Press.

Polatajko, H. J., Fox, A. M., & Missiuna, C. (1995). An international consensus on children with developmental coordination disorder. *Canadian Journal of Occupational Therapy, 62*(1), 3–6.

Prechtl, H. F. R., & Stemmer, C. J. (1962). The choreiform syndrome in children. *Developmental Medicine and Child Neurology, 4,* 119–127.

Primeau, L. (1992). *Game playing behavior in children with developmental dyspraxia.* Unpublished master's dissertation, University of Southern California, Los Angeles, California.

Rarick, G. L., & McKee, R. (1949). A study of twenty third-grade children exhibiting extreme levels of achievement on tests of motor proficiency. *Research Quarterly, 20,* 142–152.

Rarick, G. L., Dobbins, D. A., & Broadhead, G. D. (1976). *The motor domain and its correlates in educationally handicapped children.* Englewood Cliffs, NJ: Prentice Hall.

Rasmussen, P., Gillberg, C., Waldenstrom, E., & Svenson, B. (1983). Perceptual, motor and attentional deficits in seven-year-old children: Neurological and neurodevelopmental aspects. *Developmental Medicine and Child Neurology, 25,* 315–333.

Revie, G., & Larkin, D. (1993). Looking at movement: Problems with teacher identification of poorly coordinated children. *ACHPER National Journal, 40*(4), 4–9.

Rispens, J., & van Yperen, T. A. (1997). How specific are "Specific Developmental Disorders"? The relevance of the concepts of specific developmental disorders for the classification of childhood developmental disorders. *Journal of Child Psychology and Psychiatry, 38,* 351–363.

Rizzolatti, G., Luppino, G., & Matelli, M. (1998). The organization of the cortical motor system: New concepts. *Electroencephalography and Clinical Neurophysiology, 106,* 283–296.

Rose, B., Larkin, D., & Berger, B. (1994). Perceptions of social support in children of low, moderate and high levels of coordination. *ACHPER Healthy Lifestyles Journal, 41*(4), 18–21.

Rose, B., Larkin, D., & Berger, B. (1997). Coordination and gender influences on the perceived competence of children. *Adapted Physical Activity Quarterly, 14,* 210–221.

Rourke, B. P. (1989). *Nonverbal learning disabilities: The syndrome and the model.* New York: Guilford.

Rowe, J. B., & Frackowiak, R. S. J. (1999). The impact of brain imaging technology on our understanding of motor function and dysfunction. *Current Opinion in Neurobiology, 9,* 728–734.

Schoemaker, M. M., & Kalverboer, A. F. (1994). Social and affective problems of children who are clumsy: How early do they begin? *Adapted Physical Activity Quarterly, 11,* 130–140.

Schoemaker, M. M., Hijlkema, M. G. J., & Kalverboer, A. F. (1994). Physiotherapy for clumsy children—An evaluation study. *Developmental Medicine and Child Neurology, 36,* 143–155.

Shaw, L., Levine, M. D., & Belfer, M. (1982). Developmental double jeopardy: A study of clumsiness and self-esteem in children with learning problems. *Developmental and Behavioral Pediatrics, 3*(4), 191–196.

Short, H., & Crawford, J. (1984, February). Last to be chosen: The awkward child. *Pivot, 2,* 32–36.

Smyth, M. M., & Mason, U. C. (1997). Planning and execution of action in children with and without developmental coordination disorder. *Journal of Child Psychology and Psychiatry, 38,* 1023–1037.

Smyth, T. R. (1992). Impaired motor skill (clumsiness) in otherwise normal children: A review. *Child: Care, Health and Development, 18,* 283–300.

Smyth, T. R., & Glencross, D. (1986). Information processing deficits in clumsy children. *Australian Journal of Psychology, 38,* 13–22.

Sövik, N., & Mæland, A. F. (1986). Children with motor problems (clumsy children). *Scandinavian Journal of Educational Research, 30,* 39–53.

Sprinkle, J., & Hammond, J. (1997). Family, health, and developmental background of children with developmental coordination disorder. *Australian Educational and Developmental Psychologist, 14*(1), 55–62.

Stephenson, E., McKay, C., & Chesson, R. (1990). An investigative study of early developmental factors in children with motor/learning difficulties. *British Journal of Occupational Therapy, 53*(1), 4–6.

Stordy, B. J. (2000). Dark adaptation, motor skills, docosahexaenoic acid, and dyslexia. *American Journal of Clinical Nutrition, 71*(1 Suppl S), 323S-326S.

Strang, J., & Rourke, B. P. (1985). Adaptive behavior of children who exhibit specific arithmetic disabilities and associated neuropsychological abilities and deficits. In B. P. Rourke (Ed.), *Neuropsychology of learning disabilities: Essentials of subtype analysis* (pp. 302–328). New York: Guilford.

Sugden, D., & Keogh, J. (1990). *Problems in movement skill development.* Columbia, SC: University of South Carolina Press.

Symes, K. (1972). Clumsiness and the sociometric status of intellectually gifted boys. *Bulletin of Physical Education, 9,* 35–40.

Szklut, S., Cermak, S., & Henderson, A. (1995). Learning disabilities. In D. Umphred (Ed.), *Neurological rehabilitation* (3rd ed., pp. 312–359). St. Louis: Mosby.

Tan, S. K., Parker, H. E., & Larkin, D. (2001). Concurrent validity of motor tests used to identify children with motor impairment. *Adapted Physical Activity Quarterly, 18*(2), 168–182.

Taylor, M. J. (1990). Marker variables for early identification of physically awkward children. In G. Doll-Tepper, C. Dahms, B. Doll, & H. von Selzam (Eds.), *Adapted physical activity* (pp. 379–386). Berlin: Springer-Verlag.

Touwen, B. C. L. (1990). Variability and stereotypy of spontaneous motility as a predictor of neurological development of preterm infants. *Developmental Medicine and Child Neurology, 32,* 501–508.

Visser, J., Geuze, R. H., & Kalverboer, A. F. (1998). The relationship between physical growth, the level of activity and the development of motor skills in adolescence: Differences between children with DCD and controls. *Human Movement Science, 17,* 573–608.

Wall, A. E. (1982). Physically awkward children: A motor development perspective. In J. P. Das, R. F. Mulcahy, & A. E. Wall (Eds.), *Theory and research in learning disabilities* (pp. 253–268). New York: Plenum Press.

Wall, A. E., Reid, G., & Paton, J. (1990). The syndrome of physical awkwardness. In G. Reid (Ed.), *Problems in movement control* (pp. 283–316). Amsterdam: Elsevier Science.

Walton, J. N., Ellis, E., & Court, S. D. M. (1962). Clumsy children: Developmental apraxia and agnosia. *Brain, 85,* 603–612.

Watkins, K. E., Gadian, D. G., & Vargha-Khadem, F. (1999). Functional and structural brain abnormalities associated with a genetic disorder of speech and language. *American Journal of Human Genetics, 65,* 1215–1221.

Weingarten, G. (1980). The contribution of athletic and physical variables to social status in Israeli boys. *International Journal of Physical Education, 17,* 23–26.

Wigglesworth, R. (1963). The importance of recognising minimal cerebral dysfunction in paediatric practice. In M. Bax & R. Mac Keith (Eds.), *Minimal cerebral dysfunction. Little Club Clinics in developmental Medicine no. 10* (pp. 34–38). London: Heinemann Medical.

Williams, H., Woollacott, M., & Ivry, R. (1992). Timing and motor control in clumsy children. *Journal of Motor Behavior, 24,* 165–172.

Willingham, D. B. (1998). A neuropsychological theory of motor skill learning. *Psychological Bulletin, 105,* 558–584.

Wilson, P., & McKenzie, B. E. (1998). Information processing deficits associated with developmental coordination disorder: A meta-analysis of research findings. *Journal of Child Psychology and Psychiatry, 39,* 829–840.

Wolff, P. H., Melngailis, I., Obregon, M., & Bedrosian, M. (1995). Family patterns of developmental dyslexia. Part II: Behavioral phenotypes. *American Journal of Medical Genetics (Neuropsychiatric Genetics), 60,* 494–505.

World Health Organisation (1996). *Multiaxial classification of child and adolescent psychiatric disorders.* Cambridge: Cambridge University Press.

Wright, H., & Sugden, D. (1996). A two-step procedure for the identification of children with developmental co-ordination disorder in Singapore. *Developmental Medicine and Child Neurology, 38,* 1099–1105.

Yarmolenko, A. (1933). The motor sphere of school-age children. *Journal of Genetic Psychology, 42,* 298–318.

CHAPTER 2

Ahonen, T. (1990). *Developmental coordination disorders in children. A developmental neuropsychological follow-up study. Jyväskylä studies in education, psychology & social research, 78:* Jyväskylä, Finland: University of Jyväskylän.

American Psychiatric Association. (1994). *Diagnostic and statistical manual of mental disorders* (4th ed.). Washington, DC: Author.

Barton, E. J., & Ascione, F. R. (1984). Direct observation. In T. H. Ollendick & M. Hersen (Eds.), *Child behaviour assessment.* New York: Pergamon Press.

Cantell, M. (1998). *Developmental coordination disorder in adolescence: Perceptual motor, academic and social outcomes of early motor delay. Research reports on sport & health, 112.* LIKES-Research Centre for Sport & Health Science: Jyväskylä, Finland.

Cantell, M. H., Smyth, M. M., & Ahonen, T. K. (1994). Clumsiness in adolescence: Educational, motor and social outcomes. *Adapted Physical Activity Quarterly, 11,* 115–129.

Cantell, M. H., Smyth, M. M., & Ahonen, T. K. (2001). *Developmental coordination disorder in 17-year-old adolescents: Perceptual motor outcome of early motor delay.* Manuscript submitted for publication.

Cantell, M. H., Smyth, M. M., & Ahonen, T. K. (2001). *Developmental coordination disorder in 17-year-old adolescents: Academic and social outcomes of early motor delay.* Manuscript in preparation.

Connolly, K. J., & Forssberg, H. (1997). *Neurophysiology and neuropsychology of motor development.* London: Mac Keith Press.

Damon, W., & Hart, D. (1988). *Self-understanding in childhood and adolescence.* Cambridge: Cambridge University Press.

Dent-Read, C., & Zukow-Goldring, P. (1997). Introduction: Ecological realism, dynamic systems, and epigenetic systems approaches to development. In C. Dent-Read & P. Zukow-Goldring, *Evolving explanations of development* (pp. 1–22). Washington, DC: American Psychiatric Association.

Duncan, T. E., Duncan, S. C., Strycker, L. A., Li, F., & Alpert, A. (1999). *An introduction to latent variable growth curve modeling: Concepts, issues, and applications.* Mahwah, NJ: Erlbaum.

Erhardt, P., McKinlay, I. A., & Bradley, G. (1987). Coordination screening for children with and without moderate learning difficulties: Further experience with Gubbay's tests. *Developmental Medicine and Child Neurology, 29,* 666–673.

Gallahue, D. L., & Ozmun, J. C. (1995). *Understanding motor development* (3rd ed.). Madison, WI: Brown & Benchmark.

Geuze, R., & Börger, H. (1993). Children who are clumsy: Five years later. *Adapted Physical Activity Quarterly, 10,* 10–21.

Gillberg, I. C. (1985). Children with minor neurodevelopmental disorders. III: Neurological and neurodevelopmental problems at age 10. *Developmental Medicine and Child Neurology, 27,* 3–16.

Gillberg, C. (1998). Hyperactivity, inattention and motor control problems—prevalence, comorbidity and background factors. *Folia Phoniatrica et Logopaedia, 50*(3), 107–117.

Gillberg, I. C., Carlström, G., Svenson, B., & Waldenström, E. (1982). Perceptual, motor and attentional deficits in seven-year-old children: Epidemiological aspects. *Journal of Child Psychology and Psychiatry, 23,* 131–144.

Gillberg, I. C., & Gillberg, C. (1989). Children with preschool minor neurodevelopmental disorders. IV: Behaviour and school achievement at age 13. *Developmental Medicine and Child Neurology, 31,* 3–13.

Gillberg, I. C., Gillberg, C., & Groth, J. (1989). Children with preschool minor neurodevelopmental disorders. V: Neurodevelopmental profiles at age 13. *Developmental Medicine and Child Neurology, 31,* 14–24.

Goldberg, D. (1981). *The General Health Questionnaire.* Windsor, England: NFER-Nelson Publishing Company.

Hadders-Algra, M., Huisjes, H. J., & Touwen, B. C. L. (1988). Perinatal correlates of major and minor neurological dysfunction at school age: A multivariate analysis. *Developmental Medicine and Child Neurology, 30,* 472–481.

Hall, D. (1988). Clumsy children. *British Medical Journal, 296,* 375–376.

Harter, S. (1982). *Manual for the self-perception profile for children.* Denver, CO: University of Denver.

Harter, S. (1987). The determinants and mediational role of global self-worth in children. In N. Eisenberg (Ed.), *Contemporary issues in developmental psychology* (pp. 219–242). New York: Wiley.

Harter, S. (1988). *Manual for the self-perception profile for adolescents.* Denver, CO: University of Denver.

Hellgren, L., Gillberg, C., Gillberg, I. C., & Enerskog, I. (1993). Children with deficits in attention, motor control and perception (DAMP) almost grown up: General health at 16 years. *Developmental Medicine and Child Neurology, 35,* 881–892.

Hellgren, L., Gillberg, I. C., Bagenholm, A., & Gillberg, C. (1994). Children with deficits in attention, motor control and perception (DAMP) almost grown up: Psychiatric and personality disorders at age 16 years. *Journal of Child Psychology and Psychiatry, 35,* 1255–1271.

Henderson, S. (1993). Motor development and minor handicap. In A. F. Kalverboer, B. Hopkins, & R. H. Geuze (Eds.), *Motor development in early and later childhood: Longitudinal approaches* (pp. 286–306). Cambridge: Cambridge University Press.

Henderson, S. E., & Hall, D. (1982). Concomitants of clumsiness in young schoolchildren. *Developmental Medicine and Child Neurology, 24,* 448–460.

Henderson, S., May, M., & Umney, D. S. (1989). An exploratory study of goal-setting behaviour, self-concept and locus of control in children with movement difficulties. *European Journal of Special Needs Education, 4*(1), 1–15.

Henderson, S. E., & Sugden, D. A. (1992). *Movement Assessment Battery for Children manual.* Sidcup, Kent: The Psychological Corporation.

Kalverboer, A. F. (1988). Follow-up of biological high-risk groups. In M. Rutter (Ed.), *Studies of psychosocial risk: The power of longitudinal data* (pp. 114–137). Cambridge: Cambridge University Press.

Kalverboer, A. F. De Vries, H. J., & van Dellen, T. (1990). Social behaviour in clumsy children as rated by parents and teachers. In A. F. Kalverboer (Ed.), *Developmental biopsychology. Experimental and observational studies in children at risk* (pp. 257–269). Ann Arbor: University of Michigan Press.

Kirby, A., & Drew, S. (1999, October). *Is DCD a diagnosis that we should be using for adults? Is clumsiness the issue in adults and adolescents?* Paper presented at the 4th Biennial workshop on children with Developmental Coordination Disorder: From Research to Diagnostics and Intervention. Groningen, The Netherlands.

Knuckey, N. W., & Gubbay, S. S. (1983). Clumsy children: A prognostic study. *Australian Pediatric Journal, 19,* 9–13.

Larkin, D., & Parker H. E. (1999). Physical activity profiles of adolescents who experienced motor learning difficulties. In D. Drouin, C. Lepine, & C. Simard (Eds.), *Proceedings of the 11th International Symposium for Adapted Physical Activity* (pp. 175–181) Quebec, Canada.

Larkin, D., & Parker, H. (1997, May). *Physical self-perceptions of adolescents with a history of developmental coordination disorder.* Poster presentation at NASPSPA, Denver, USA.

Latash, M. L., & Anson, J. G. (1996). What are "normal movements" in atypical populations? *Behavioral and Brain Sciences, 19,* 55–106.

Losse, A., Henderson, S. E., Elliman, D., Hall, D., Knight, E., & Jongmans, M. (1991). Clumsiness in children—Do they grow out of it? A 10-year follow-up study. *Developmental Medicine and Child Neurology, 33,* 55–68.

Lunsing, R. J., Hadders-Algra, M., Huisjes, H. J., & Touwen, B. C. L, (1992). Minor neurological dysfunction from birth to 12 years. I: Increase during late school age. *Developmental Medicine and Child Neurology, 34,* 399–403.

Lyytinen, H. & Ahonen, T. (1989). Motor precursors of learning disabilities. In D. J. Bakker & H. van der Vlugt (Eds.), *Learning disabilities: Vol. 1. Neuropsychological correlates and treatment* (pp. 35–43). Amsterdam: Swets & Zeitlinger.

Mæland, A. F. (1992). Self-esteem in children with and without motor coordination problems. *Scandinavian Journal of Educational Research, 36,* 313–321.

Marsh, H. W., Richards, G. E., Johnson, S., Roche, L., & Tremayne, P. (1994). Physical self-description questionnaire: Psychometric properties and a multitrait-multimethod analysis of relations to existing instruments. *Journal of Sport and Exercise Psychology, 16,* 270–305.

Mulderij, K. J. (1996). Research into the lifeworld of physically disabled children. *Child: Care, Health and Development, 22*(5), 311–322.

Novicki, S., & Strickland, B. R. (1973). A locus of control scale for children. *Journal of Consulting and Clinical Psychology, 40,* 148–154.

Piek, J., Dworcan, M., Barrett, N. C., & Coleman, R. (2000). Determinants of self worth in children with and without developmental coordination disorder. *International Journal of Disability, Development and Education, 47*(3), 259–272.

Rasmussen, P., Gillberg, E., Waldenstrom, E., & Svenson, B. (1983). Perceptual, motor and attentional deficits in 7-year-old children: Neurological and neurodevelopmental aspects. *Developmental Medicine and Child Neurology, 25,* 315–333.

Rutter, M. (1998). Foreword. In J. Rispens, T. A. van Yperen, & W. Yule (Eds.), *Perspectives on the classification of specific developmental disorders.* Dordrecht: Kluwer Academic Publishers.

Schoemaker, M. M., & Kalverboer, A. F. (1994). Social and affective problems of children who are clumsy: How early do they begin? *Adapted Physical Activity Quarterly, 11,* 130–140.

Shafer, S. Q., Shaffer, D., O'Connor, P. A., & Stokman, C. J. (1986). Hard thoughts on neurological soft signs (pp. 133–143). In M. Rutter (Ed.), *Developmental neuropsychiatry.* Edinburgh: Churchill Livingstone.

Shaffer, D., Schonfield, I., O'Connor, P. A., Stokman, C., Trautman, P., Shafer, S., & Ng, S. (1985). Neurological soft signs and their relationship to psychiatric disorder and intelligence in childhood and adolescence. *Archives of General Psychiatry, 42,* 343–351.

Smyth, M. M., & Anderson, H. I. (1999, October). *Coping with clumsiness in the school ground: Social and physical play in children with coordination impairments.* Paper presented at the 4th Biennial workshop on children with Developmental Coordination Disorder: From Research to Diagnostics and Intervention. Groningen, The Netherlands.

Soorani-Lunsing, R. J., Hadders-Algra, M., Olinga, A. A., & Huisjes, H. J. (1993). Is minor neurological dysfunction at 12 years related to behaviour and cognition. *Developmental Medicine and Child Neurology, 35,* 321–330.

Soorani-Lunsing, R. J., Hadders-Algra, M., Huisjes, H. J., & Touwen, B. C. L. (1994). Neurobehavioural relationships after the onset of puberty. *Developmental Medicine and Child Neurology, 36,* 334–343.

Sövik, N., & Mæland, A. (1986). Children with motor problems (clumsy children). *Scandinavian Journal of Educational Research, 30,* 39–53.

Spreen, O. (1988). *Learning disabled children growing up: A follow-up into adulthood.* Oxford: Oxford University Press.

Spreen, O. (1989). Long-term sequelae of learning disability: A review of outcome studies. In D. J. Bakker & H. van der Vlugt (Eds.), *Learning disabilities, Vol 1: Neurological correlates and treatment* (pp. 55–70). Amsterdam: Swets & Zeitlinger.

Stokman, C. J., Shafer, S. Q., Shaffer, D., Ng, S., O'Connor, P. A., & Wolff, R. W. (1986). Assessment of neurological soft signs in adolescents: Reliability studies. *Developmental Medicine and Child Neurology, 28,* 428–439.

Stott, D. H., Moyes, F. A., & Henderson, S. E. (1984). *The Test of Motor Impairment.* San Antonio, TX: Psychological Corporation.

Sugden, D., & Wright, S. (1998). *Motor coordination disorders.* Developmental clinical psychology and psychiatry series, 39. Thousand Oaks, CA: Sage.

Touwen, B. C. L. (1979). *The examination of the child with minor neurological dysfunction. Clinics in developmental medicine, No 71.* London: S. I. M. P. with Heinemann Medical.

Van Dellen, T., Vaessen, W., & Schoemaker, M. M. (1990). Clumsiness: Definitions and selection of subjects. In A. F. Kalverboer (Ed.), *Developmental biopsychology. Experimental and observational studies in children at risk* (pp. 135–152). Ann Arbor: University of Michigan Press.

Van Manen, M. (1990). *Researching lived experience.* Boston: Althouse Press.

Visser, J., Geuze, R. H., & Kalverboer, A. F. (1998). The relationship between physical growth, level of activity and the development of motor skills in adolescence: Differences between children with DCD and controls. *Human Movement Science, 17,* 573–608.

World Health Organisation. (1996). *Multiaxial classification of child and adolescent psychiatric disorders.* Cambridge: Cambridge University Press.

CHAPTER 3

Ahonen, T. (1990). *Developmental coordination disorders in children: A developmental neuropsychological follow-up study. Jyvaskyla studies in education, psychology, and social research, 78.* Jyvaskyla, Finland: University of Jyvaskyla.

American Psychiatric Association. (1994). *Diagnostic and statistical manual of mental disorders* (4th ed.). Washington, DC: Author.

Ayres, A. J. (1985). *Developmental apraxia and adult onset apraxia.* Torrance, CA: Sensory Integration International.

Ayres, A. J., Mailloux, Z. K., & Wendler, C. L. (1987). Developmental dyspraxia: Is it a unitary function? *Occupational Therapy Journal of Research, 7,* 93–110.

Ayres, J. A. (1972). *Sensory integration and learning disorders.* Los Angeles: Western Psychological Services.

Bairstow, P. J., & Laszlo, J. I. (1981). Kinaesthetic sensitivity to passive movements in children and adults, and its relationship to motor development and motor control. *Developmental Medicine and Child Neurology, 23,* 606–616.

Bergstrom, K., & Bille, B. (1978). Computed tomography of the brain in children with minimal brain damage: A preliminary study of 46 children. *Neuropadiatrie, 9*, 378–384.

Biederman, J., Faraone, S. V., Keenan, K., Steingard, R., & Tsuang, M. T. (1991). Familial association between attention deficit disorder and anxiety disorders. *American Journal of Psychiatry, 18*, 251–256.

Biederman, J., Newcorn, J., & Sprich, S. E. (1991). Comorbidity of attention deficit hyperactivity disorder with conduct, depressive, anxiety, and other disorders. *American Journal of Psychiatry, 148*, 564–577.

Brenner, M. W., & Gillman, S. (1966). Visuo-motor ability in school children—A survey. *Developmental Medicine and Child Neurology, 8*, 686–703.

Brenner, M. W., & Gillman, S. (1968). Verbal intelligence, visuomotor ability and school achievement. *British Journal of Educational Psychology, 38*, 75–78.

Brenner, M. W., Gillman, S., & Farrell, M. F. (1968). Clinical study of eight children with visual dysfunction and educational problems. *Journal of Neurological Sciences, 6*, 45–61.

Brenner, M. W., Gillman, S., Zangwill, O. L., & Farrell, M. (1967). Visuo-motor disability in schoolchildren. *British Medical Journal, 4*, 259–262.

Bruininks, R. H. (1978). *Bruininks-Oseretsky Test of Motor Proficiency: Examiner's manual.* Circle Pines, MN: American Guidance Service.

Cantell, M. H., Smyth, M. M., & Ahonen, T. P. (1994). Clumsiness in adolescence: Educational, motor and social outcomes of motor delay detected at 5 years. *Adapted Physical Activity Quarterly, 11*, 115–129.

Cantwell, D. P., & Baker, L. (1991). Association between attention deficit-hyperactivity disorder and learning disorders. *Journal of Learning Disabilities, 24*, 88–95.

Cermak, S. A. (1985). Developmental dyspraxia. In E. A. Roy (Ed.), *Neuropsychological studies of apraxia and related disorders* (pp. 225–248). Amsterdam: North Holland.

Cermak, S. A. (1991). Somatodyspraxia. In A. G. Fisher, E. A. Murray, & A. C. Bundy (Eds.), *Sensory integration: Theory and practice* (pp. 137–170). Philadelphia: F. A. Davis.

Cermak, S. A., Coster, W., & Drake, C. (1980). Representational and non-representational gestures in boys with learning disabilities. *American Journal of Occupational Therapy, 34*, 19–26.

Cermak, S. A., Trimble, H., Coryell, J., & Drake, C. (1990). Bilateral motor coordination in adolescents with and without learning disabilities. *Physical and Occupational Therapy in Pediatrics, 10*, 5–18.

Chase, C. H., Rosen, G. D., & Sherman, G. F. (1996). *Developmental dyslexia: Neural, cognitive, and genetic mechanisms.* Baltimore: York Press.

Clements, S. G., & Peters, J. E. (1962). Minimal brain dysfunctions in the school-age child. *Archives of General Psychiatry, 6*, 185–197.

Conrad, K., Cermak, S. A., & Drake, C. (1983). Differentiation of praxis among children. *American Journal of Occupational Therapy, 37*, 466–473.

Cratty, B. J. (1994). *Clumsy child syndromes: Descriptions, evaluation and remediation.* Chur, Switzerland: Harwood Academic Publishers.

De Ajuriaguerra, J., & Stambak, M. (1969). Developmental dyspraxia and psychomotor disorders. In P. J. Vinken & G. W. Bruyn (Eds.), *Handbook of clinical neurology. Vol. 4: Disorders of speech perception and symbolic behavior.* Amsterdam: North-Holland.

Dewey, D. (1991). Praxis and sequencing skills in children with sensorimotor dysfunction. *Developmental Neuropsychology, 7,* 197–206.

Dewey, D. (1993). Error analysis of limb and orofacial praxis in children with developmental motor deficits. *Brain and Cognition, 23,* 203–221.

Dewey, D., & Kaplan, B. J. (1992). Analysis of praxis task demands in the assessment of children with developmental motor deficits. *Developmental Neuropsychology, 8,* 367–379.

Dewey, D., & Kaplan, B. J. (1994). Subtyping of developmental motor deficits. *Developmental Neuropsychology, 10,* 265–284.

Dewey, D., Kaplan, B. J., Wilson, B. N., & Crawford, S. G. (1999). *Developmental coordination disorder and developmental dyspraxia: Are we talking about the same thing?* Paper presented at the International Neuropsychology Society 27th Annual Meeting, Boston.

Dewey, D., & Wall, K. (1997). Praxis and memory deficits in language impaired children. *Developmental Neuropsychology, 13,* 507–512.

Dykman, R. A., & Ackerman, P. T. (1991). Attention deficit disorder and specific reading disability: Separate but often overlapping disorders. *Journal of Learning Disabilities, 24,* 95–103.

Erhardt, P., McKinlay, I. A., & Bradley, G. (1987). Coordination screening for children with and without moderate learning difficulties: Further experience with Gubbay's tests. *Developmental Medicine and Child Neurology, 29,* 666–673.

Fletcher, J. M., & Satz, P. (1985). Cluster analysis and the search for learning disability subtypes. In B. P. Rourke (Ed.), *Neuropsychology of learning disabilities: Essentials of subtype analysis* (pp. 40–64). New York: Guilford Press.

Fox, M. (1995). Management issues. In H. P. Polatajko & A. M. Fox (Eds.), *Final report on the Conference Children and Clumsiness: A Disability in Search of Definition.* London, Ontario: International Consensus Meeting.

Fox, M. A., & Lent, B. (1996). Clumsy children: Primer on developmental coordination disorder. *Canadian Family Physician, 42,* 1965–1971.

Frostig, M. (1963). Visual perception in the brain-injured child. *American Journal of Orthopsychiatry, 33,* 665–671.

Geuze, R., & Borger, H. (1993). Children who are clumsy: Five years later. *Adapted Physical Activity Quarterly, 10,* 10–21.

Geuze, R., & Kalverboer, A. F. (1987). Inconsistency and adaptation in timing of clumsy children. *Journal of Human Movement Studies, 13,* 421–432.

Gilger, J. W., & Kaplan, B. J. (1999). *Learning disabilities are manifestations of atypical brain development.* Manuscript submitted for publication.

Gordon, N., & McKinlay, I. (1980). *Helping clumsy children.* New York: Churchill Livingstone.

Gubbay, S. S. (1975a). *The clumsy child.* London: W. B. Saunders.

Gubbay, S. S. (1975b). Clumsy children in normal schools. *Medical Journal of Australia, 1,* 233–236.

Gubbay, S. S., Ellis, E., Walton, J. N., & Court, S. D. M. (1965). Clumsy children: A study of apraxic and agnosic defects in 21 children. *Brain, 88,* 295–312.

Hall, D. M. B. (1988). Clumsy children. *British Medical Journal, 296,* 375–376.

Henderson, S. E., & Barnett, A. L. (1998). The classification of specific motor coordination disorders in children: Some problems to be solved. *Human Movement Science, 17,* 449–470.

Henderson, S. E., & Hall, D. (1982). Concomitants of clumsiness in young school children. *Developmental Medicine and Child Neurology, 24,* 448–460.

Henderson, S. E., & Sugden, D. A. (1992). *Movement Assessment Battery for Children.* Kent: The Psychological Corporation.

Hill, E. L., Bishop, D. V. M., & Nimmo-Smith, I. (1998). Representational gestures in developmental coordination disorder and specific language impairment: Error-types and the reliability of ratings. *Human Movement Science, 17,* 655–678.

Hoare, D. (1994). Subtypes of developmental coordination disorder. *Adapted Physical Activity Quarterly, 11,* 158–169.

Hooper, S. R., & Willis, W. G. (1989). *Learning disability subtyping.* New York: Springer-Verlag.

Horak, F. B., Shumway-Cook, A., Crowe, T. K., & Black, F. O. (1988). Vestibular function and motor proficiency of children with impaired hearing or with learning disability and motor impairment. *Developmental Medicine and Child Neurology, 30,* 64–79.

Hulme, C., Biggerstaff, A., Moran, G., & McKinlay, I. (1982). Visual, kinaesthetic and cross-modal judgements of length by normal and clumsy children. *Developmental Medicine and Child Neurology, 24,* 461–471.

Hulme, C., & Lord, R. (1986). Clumsy children—A review of recent research. *Child: Care, Health and Development, 12,* 257–269.

Hulme, C., Smart, A., & Moran, G. (1982). Visual perceptual deficits in clumsy children. *Neuropsychologia, 20,* 475–481.

Hulme, C., Smart, A., Moran, G., & McKinlay, I. (1984). Visual kinaesthetic and cross-modal judgements of length by clumsy children: A comparison with young normal children. *Child: Care, Health and Development, 10,* 117–125.

Iloeje, S. O. (1987). Developmental apraxia among Nigerian children in Enugor, Nigeria. *Developmental Medicine and Child Neurology, 29,* 502–507.

Johnston, O., Short, H., & Crawford, J. (1987). Poorly coordinated children: A survey of 95 cases. *Child: Care, Health and Development, 13,* 361–376.

Kadesjo, B., & Gillberg, C. (1998). Attention deficits and clumsiness in Swedish 7-year-old children. *Developmental Medicine and Child Neurology, 40,* 796–804.

Kalverboer, A. F., de Vries, H. J., & van Dellen, T. (1990). Social behavior in clumsy children as rated by parents and teachers. In A. F. Kalverboer (Ed.), *Developmental biopsychology: Experimental and observational studies in children at risk* (pp. 257–269). Ann Arbor: University of Michigan Press.

Kaplan, B. J., Wilson, B. N., Dewey, D. M., & Crawford, S. G. (1997). *DCD is simply one manifestation of atypical brain development.* Paper presented at the Developmental Coordination Disorder III, Cardiff, Wales.

Kaplan, B. J., Wilson, B. N., Dewey, D. M., & Crawford, S. G. (1998). DCD may not be a discrete disorder. *Human Movement Science, 17,* 471–490.

Kavale, K. A., & Nye, C. (1985–86). Parameters of learning disabilities in achievement, linguistic, neuropsychological, and social/behavioral domains. *Journal of Special Education, 19*, 443–458.

Knuckey, N. W., Apsimon, T. T., & Gubbay, S. S. (1983). Computerized axial tomography in clumsy children with developmental apraxia and agnosia. *Brain and Development, 5*, 14–19.

Laszlo, J. I., & Bairstow, P. J. (1983). Kinaesthesis: Its measurement training and relationship to motor control. *Quarterly Journal of Experimental Psychology, 35*, 411–421.

Laszlo, J. I., Bairstow, P. J., Bartrip, J., & Rolfe, U. T. (1988). Clumsiness or perceptuo-motor dysfunction? In A. M. Colley & J. R. Beech (Eds.), *Cognition and action in skilled behavior* (pp. 293–308) Amsterdam: Elsevier Science.

Lee, D. N., & Aronson, E. (1974). Visual proprioceptive control of stance. *Journal of Human Movement Studies, 1*, 87–95.

Lennox, L., Cermak, S. A., & Koomar, J. (1988). Praxis and gesture comprehension in 4-, 5-, and 6-year-olds. *American Journal of Occupational Therapy, 42*, 99–104.

Lord, R., & Hulme, C. (1987a). Kinaesthetic sensitivity of normal and clumsy children. *Developmental Medicine and Child Neurology, 29*, 720–725.

Lord, R., & Hulme, C. (1987b). Perceptual judgements of normal and clumsy children. *Developmental Medicine and Child Neurology, 29*, 250–257.

Lord, R., & Hulme, C. (1988a). Patterns of rotary pursuit performance in clumsy and normal children. *Journal of Child Psychology and Psychiatry, 29*, 691–701.

Lord, R., & Hulme, C. (1988b). Visual perception and drawing ability in clumsy and normal children. *British Journal of Developmental Psychology, 6*, 1–9.

Losse, A., Henderson, S. A., Elliman, D., Hall, D., Knight, E., & Jongmans, M. (1991). Clumsiness in children: Do they grow out of it? A 10-year follow-up study. *Developmental Medicine and Child Neurology, 33*, 55–68.

Lundy-Ekman, L., Ivry, R., Keele, S. W., & Woollacott, M. (1991). Timing and force control deficits in clumsy children. *Journal of Cognitive Neuroscience, 3*, 367–376.

Macnab, J. L., Miller, L. T., & Polatajko, H. J. (1999). The search of subtypes of developmental coordination disorder: Revising Hoare's solution. Manuscript submitted for publication.

Milligan, G. W., & Cooper, M. C. (1987). Methodology review: Clustering methods. *Applied Psychological Measurement, 11*, 329–354.

Missiuna, C. (1994). Motor skill acquisition in children with developmental coordination disorder. *Adapted Physical Activity Quarterly, 11*, 214–235.

Missiuna, C., & Polatajko, H. (1995). Developmental dyspraxia by any other name: Are they all just clumsy children? *American Journal of Occupational Therapy, 49*(7), 619–627.

Miyahara, M. (1994). Subtypes of students with learning disabilities based upon gross motor functions. *Adapted Physical Activity Quarterly, 11*, 368–382.

Morris, R., Blashfield, R., & Satz, P. (1981). Neuropsychology and cluster analysis: Problems and pitfalls. *Journal of Clinical Neuropsychology, 3*, 79–99.

Murphy, J. B., & Gliner, J. A. (1988). Visual and motor sequencing in normal and clumsy children. *Occupational Therapy Journal of Research, 8*, 89–103.

O'Brien, V., Cermak, S. A., & Murray, E. (1988). The relationship between visual-perceptual motor abilities and clumsiness in children with and without learning disabilities. *American Journal of Occupational Therapy, 42,* 359–363.

Orton, S. T. (1937). *Reading, writing and speech problems in children.* New York: Norton.

Piek, J. P., & Skinner, R. A. (1999). Timing and force control during a sequential tapping task in children with and without motor coordination problems. *Journal of the International Neuropsychological Society, 5,* 320–329.

Polatajko, H. J., Fox, A. M., & Missiuna, C. (1995). An international consensus on children with developmental coordination disorder. *Canadian Journal of Occupational Therapy, 62,* 3–6.

Powell, R. P., & Bishop, D. V. M. (1992). Clumsiness and perceptual problems in children with specific language impairment. *Developmental Medicine and Child Neurology, 34,* 755–765.

Riccio, C. A., & Hynd, G. W. (1996). Neuroanatomical and neurophysiological aspects of dyslexia. *Topics in Language Disorders, 16,* 1–13.

Rispens, J., & van Yperen, T. A. (1997). How specific are "Specific Developmental Disorders"? The relevance of the concept of specific developmental disorders for the classification of childhood developmental disorders. *Journal of Child Psychology and Psychiatry, 38,* 351–363.

Rösblad, B., & von Hofsten, C. (1994). Repetitive goal-directed arm movements in children with developmental coordination disorders: Role of visual information. *Adapted Physical Activity Quarterly, 11,* 190–202

Rourke, B., & Tsatsanis, K. D. (1996). Syndrome of nonverbal learning disabilities: Psycholinguistic assets and deficits. *Topics in Language Development, 16,* 30–44.

Roussounis, S. H., Gaussen, T. H., & Stratton, P. (1987). A 2-year follow-up study of children with motor coordination problems identified at school entry age. *Child: Care, Health and Development, 13,* 377–391.

Schoemaker, M. M., & Kalverboer, A. F. (1994). Social and affective problems of children who are clumsy: How early do they begin? *Adapted Physical Activity Quarterly, 11,* 130–140.

Shaywitz, B. A., & Shaywitz, S. E. (1991). Comorbidity: A critical issue in attention deficit disorder. *Journal of Child Neurology, 6*(suppl.), S13-S22.

Silver, L. B. (Ed.). (1992). *The misunderstood child.* Blue Ridge Summit, PA: Tab Books.

Smyth, T. R., & Glencross, D. J. (1986). Information processing deficits in clumsy children. *Australian Journal of Psychology, 38,* 13–22.

Snow, J. H., Blondis, T., & Brady, L. (1988). Motor and sensory abilities with normal and academically at-risk children. *Archives of Clinical Neuropsychology, 3,* 227–238.

Sugden, D., & Keogh, J. (1990). *Problems in movement skill development.* Columbia: University of South Carolina Press.

Sugden, D. A., & Wann, C. (1987). Kinaesthesis and motor impairment in children with moderate learning difficulties. *British Journal of Educational Psychology, 57,* 225–236.

Szatmari, P. (1992). The epidemiology of attention-deficit hyperactivity disorders. In G. Weiss (Ed.), *Attention-deficit hyperactivity disorder* (pp. 361–372). Philadelphia: W. B. Saunders.

Taylor, M. J. (1990). Marker variables for early identification of physically awkward children. In G. Doll-Tepper, C. Dahms, B. Doll, & H. von Selzam (Eds.), *Adapted physical activity* (pp. 379–386). Berlin: Springer-Verlag.

van Dellen, T., & Geuze, K. H. (1988). Motor response programming in clumsy children. *Journal of Child Psychology and Psychiatry, 29,* 489–500.

Walton, J. N., Ellis, E., & Court, S. D. M. (1962). Clumsy children: Developmental apraxia and agnosia. *Brain, 85,* 603–612.

Wann, J. P., Mon-Williams, M., & Rushton, K. (1998). Postural control and coordination disorders: The swinging room revisited. *Human Movement Science, 17,* 491–513.

Williams, H. G., Woollacott, M. H., & Ivry, R. (1992). Timing and motor control in clumsy children. *Journal of Motor Behavior, 24,* 165–172.

Wilson, P. H., & McKenzie, B. E. (1998). Information processing deficits associated with developmental coordination disorder: A meta-analysis of research findings. *Journal of Child Psychology and Psychiatry, 39,* 829–840.

World Health Organization. (1992). *The ICD-10 classification of mental and behavioural disorders: Clinical descriptions and diagnostic guidelines.* Geneva: World Health Organization.

Wright, H. C., & Sugden, D. A. (1996). The nature of developmental coordination disorder: Inter- and intragroup differences. *Adapted Physical Activity Quarterly, 13,* 357–371.

Zangwill, O. L. (1960). Deficiency of spatial perception. In M. Bax, E. Clayton-Jones, & R. Mac Keith (Eds.), *Child neurology and cerebral palsy. Little Club Clinics in Developmental Medicine, No. 2* (pp. 133–136). London: Spastics Society.

CHAPTER 4

American Psychiatric Association. (1994). Diagnostic and statistical manual of mental disorders (4th ed.). Washington, DC: Author.

Annett, M., Eglinton, E., & Smythe, P. (1996). Types of dyslexia and the shift to dextrality. Journal of Child Psychology and Psychiatry and Allied Disciplines, 37, 167–180.

Annett, M., & Turner, A. (1974). Laterality and the growth of intellectual abilities. British Journal of Educational Psychology, 44, 37–46.

Armitage, M., & Larkin, D. (1993). Laterality, motor asymmetry and clumsiness in children. Human Movement Science, 12, 155–177.

Badian, N. A., & Wolff, P. H. (1977). Manual asymmetries of motor sequencing in reading disability. Cortex, 13, 343–349.

Barnett, A., & Henderson, S. E. (1992). Some observations on the figure drawings of clumsy children. British Journal of Educational Psychology, 62, 341–355.

Bishop, D. V. M. (1990). Handedness, clumsiness and developmental language disorders. Neuropsychologia, 28, 681–690.

Bishop, D. V. M., & Edmundson, A. (1987). Specific language impairment as a maturational lag: Evidence from longitudinal data on language and motor development. Developmental Medicine and Child Neurology, 29, 442–459.

Bjørgen, I. A., Undheim, J. O., Nordvik, K. A., & Romslo, I. (1987). Dyslexia and hormone deficiencies. European Journal of Psychology of Education, 2, 283–295.

Bogen, J. E. (1993). The callosal syndromes. In K. M. Heilman & R. Valenstein (Eds.), Clinical neuropsychology (3rd ed., pp. 337–407). New York: Oxford University Press.

Bradford, A., & Dodd, B. (1994). The motor planning abilities of phonologically disordered children. European Journal of Disorders of Communication, 29, 349–369.

Bradford, A., & Dodd, B. (1996). Do all speech-disordered children have motor deficits. Clinical Linguistics and Phonetics, 10, 77–101.

Brenner, M. W., Gillman, S., Zangwill, O. L., & Farrell, M. (1967). Visuo-motor disability in school children. British Medical Journal, 4, 259–262.

Brinton, B., Fujiki, M., Spencer, J. C., & Robinson, L. A. (1997). The ability of children with specific language impairment to access and participate in an ongoing interaction. Journal of Speech Hearing and Language Research, 40, 1011–1025.

Corballis, M. C. (1998). Cerebral asymmetry: Motoring on. Trends in Cognitive Sciences, 2, 152–157.

Deiber, M. P., Passingham, R. E., Cloebatch, J. G., Friston, K. J., Nixon, P. D., & Frackowiak, R. S. J. (1991). Cortical areas and the selection of movement: A study with positron emission tomography. Experimental Brain Research, 84, 393–402.

Denckla, M. B. (1985). Motor co-ordination in dyslexic children: Theoretical and clinical implications. In F. H. Duffy & N. Geschwind (Eds.), Dyslexia: A neuroscientific approach to clinical evaluation (pp. 187–195). Boston: Little, Brown.

Denckla, M. B., Rudel, R. G., & Broman, M. (1980). The development of a spatial orientation skill in normal, learning-disabled, and neurologically impaired children. In D. Caplan (Ed.), Biological studies of mental processes (pp. 44–59). Cambridge, MA: MIT Press.

Dewey, D. (1995). What is developmental dyspraxia? Brain and Cognition, 29, 254–274.

Dewey, D., & Wall, K. (1997). Praxis and memory deficits in language-impaired children. Developmental Neuropsychology, 13, 507–512.

Dow, R. S., & Moruzzi, G. (1958). The physiology and pathology of the cerebellum. Minneapolis: University of Minnesota Press.

Eccles, J. C., Ito, M., & Szentagothai, J. (1967). The cerebellum as a neuronal machine. New York: Springer-Verlag.

Edwards, S., Ellams, J., & Thompson, J. (1976). Language and intelligence in dysphasia: Are they related? British Journal of Disorders of Communication, 11, 83–94.

Fawcett, A. J., & Nicolson, R. I. (1992). Automatisation deficits in balance for dyslexic children. Perceptual and Motor Skills, 75, 507–529.

Fawcett, A. J., & Nicolson, R. I. (1995). Persistent deficits in motor skill of children with dyslexia. Journal of Motor Behavior, 27, 235–240.

Fawcett, A. J., & Nicolson, R. I. (1999). Performance of dyslexic children on cerebellar and cognitive tests. Journal of Motor Behavior, 31, 68–78.

Fawcett, A. J., Nicolson, R. I., & Dean, P. (1996). Impaired performance of children with dyslexia on a range of cerebellar tasks. Annals of Dyslexia, 46, 259–283.

Gaddes, W. H. (1985). Learning disabilities and brain function. A neuropsychological approach (2nd ed.). New York: Springer-Verlag.

Geschwind, N., & Galaburda, A. M. (1985). Cerebral lateralization. Biological mechanisms, associations, and pathology. I: A hypothesis and a program for research. Archives of Neurology, 42, 428–459.

Gjessing, H. J., Nygaard, H. D., & Solheim, R. (1988). Bergen-prosjektet. Utviklingsforløp og læreproblemer hos elever i grunnskolen III. Studier av barn med dysleksi og andre lesevansker [Studies of children with dyslexia and other reading disabilities]. Bergen: Universitetsforlaget.

Galaburda, A., & Livingstone, M. (1993). Evidence for a magnocellular defect in developmental dyslexia. In P. Tallal, M. Galaburda, R. R. Llinas, & C. von Euler (Eds.), Temporal information processing in the nervous system. Special reference to dyslexia and dysphasia. Annals of the New York Academy of Sciences, vol. 682 (pp. 70–82). New York: New York Academy of Sciences.

Gubbay, S. S. (1975). The clumsy child. A study of developmental apraxic and agnosic ataxia. London: W. B. Saunders.

Gubbay, S. S. (1978). The management of developmental apraxia. Developmental Medicine and Child Neurology, 20, 643–646.

Harter, S. (1978). Effectance motivation reconsidered: Toward a developmental model. Human Development, 1, 34–64.

Henderson, S. E. (1977). Finding the clumsy child: Genesis of a test of motor impairment. Journal of Human Movement Studies, 3, 38–48.

Henderson, S. E., & Hall, D. (1982). Concomitants of clumsiness in young schoolchildren. Developmental Medicine and Child Neurology, 24, 448–460.

Henderson, S. E., May, D. S., & Umney, M. (1989). An exploratory study of goal-setting behaviour, self-concept and locus of control in children with movement difficulties. European Journal of Special Needs Education, 4, 1–15.

Hewes, G. W. (1973). Primate communication and the gestural origins of language. Current Anthropology, 14, 5–24.

Hill, E. L. (1998). A dyspraxic deficit in specific language impairment and developmental coordination disorder? Evidence from hand and arm movements. Developmental Medicine and Child Neurology, 40, 388–395.

Hill, E. L., Bishop, D. V. M., & Nimmo-Smith, I. (1998). Representational gestures in developmental coordination disorder and specific language impairment: Error-types and the reliability of ratings. Human Movement Science, 17, 655–678.

Holmes, G. (1917). The symptoms of acute cerebellar injuries due to gunshot injuries. Brain, 40, 461–535.

Holmes, G. (1939). The cerebellum of man. Brain, 62, 1–30.

Ivry, R. (1993). Cerebellar involvement in the explicit representation of temporal information. In P. Tallal, M. Galaburda, R. R. Llinas, & C. von Euler (Eds.), Temporal information processing in the nervous system: Special reference to dyslexia and dysphasia. Annals of the New York Academy of Sciences, vol. 682 (pp. 214–230). New York: New York Academy of Sciences.

Ivry, R. B., & Diener, H. C. (1991). Impaired velocity perception in patients with lesions of the cerebellum. Journal of Cognitive Neuroscience, 3, 355–366.

Ivry, R. B., & Keele, S. W. (1989). Timing functions of the cerebellum. Journal of Cognitive Neuroscience, 1, 134–150.

Jeeves, M. A. (1990). Agenesis of the corpus callosum. In R. D. Nebes & S. Corkin (Eds.), Handbook of neuropsychology, Vol. 4 (pp. 99–114). Amsterdam: Elsevier Science.

Kalliopuska, M., & Karila, I. (1987). Association of motor performance on cognitive, linguistic, and socioemotional factors. Perceptual and Motor Skills, 65, 399–405.

Keele, S., Ivry, R., & Pokorny, D. (1987). Force control and its relation to timing. Journal of Motor Behaviour, 19, 96–114.

Keele, S., Pokorny, R., Corcos, D., & Ivry, R. (1985). Do perception and motor production share common timing mechanisms? Acta Psychologia, 60, 173–193.

Kelso, J. A. S. (1995). Dynamic patterns: The self-organization of brain and behavior. Cambridge, MA: MIT Press.

Kelso, J. A. S., Holt, K. G., Rubin, P., & Kugler, P. N. (1981). Patterns of interlimb coordination emerge from properties of non-linear, limit cycle oscillatory processes: Theory and data. Journal of Motor Behaviour, 13, 226–261.

Kelso, J. A. S., & Tuller, B. (1981). Towards a theory of apractic syndromes. Brain and Language, 13, 224–245.

Keogh, J. F., Sugden, D. A., Reynard, C. L., & Calkins, J. A. (1979). Identification of clumsy children: Comparisons and comments. Journal of Human Movement Studies, 5, 32–41.

Kimura, D. (1982). Left-hemisphere control of oral and brachial movements and their relation to communication. Philosophical Transactions of the Royal Society of London, B298, 135–149.

Kimura, D. (1993). Neuromotor mechanisms in human communication. Oxford psychology series no. 20. New York: Oxford University Press.

Kimura, D., & Archibald, Y. (1974). Motor functions of the left hemisphere. Brain, 97, 337–350.

Kohen-Raz, R. (1981). Postural control and learning disabilities. Early Child Development and Care, 7, 329–352.

Lambe, E. K. (1999). Dyslexia, gender, and brain imaging. Neuropsychologia, 37, 521–536.

Levinson, H. N. (1973). Dysmetric dyslexia and dyspraxia: Hypothesis and study. Journal of American Academy of Child Psychiatry, 12, 690–701.

Levinson, H. N. (1988). The cerebellar-vestibular basis of learning disabilities in children, adolescents and adults: Hypothesis and study. Perceptual and Motor Skills, 67, 983–1006.

Levinson, H. N. (1991). Dramatic favourable responses of children with learning disabilities or dyslexia and attention deficit disorder to antimotion sickness medications: Four case reports. Perceptual and Motor Skills, 73, 723–738.

Liberman, A. M. (1993). In speech perception, time is not what it seems. In P. Tallal, M. Galaburda, R. R. Llinas, & C. von Euler (Eds.), Temporal information processing in the nervous system: Special reference to dyslexia and dysphasia. Annals of the New York Academy of Sciences, vol. 682 (pp. 264–271). New York: New York Academy of Sciences.

Liepmann, H. (1908). Drei Aufsätze aus dem Apraxiegebiet. Berlin: Karger Verlag. [Translated by D. Kimura (1980) as Translations from Liepmann's essays on apraxia. University of Western Ontario, Department of Psychology Research Bulletin, no. 506.]

Losse, A., Henderson, S. E., Elliman, D., Hall, D., Knight, E., & Jongmans, M. (1991). Clumsiness in children—Do they grow out of it? A 10-year follow-up study. Developmental Medicine and Child Neurology, 33, 55–68.

Mæland, A. F. (1992). Identification of children with motor coordination problems. In A. F. Mæland (Ed.), Learning disabilities and motor coordination problems in schoolchildren (pp. 42–58). Trondheim, Norway: Universitetet i Trondheim, Den Allmenvitenskapelige Høyskolen.

Moore, L. H., Brown, W. S., Markee, T. E., Theberge, D. C., & Zvi, J. C. (1996). Callosal transfer of finger localisation information in phonologically dyslexic adults. Cortex, 32, 311–322.

Nickisch, A. (1998). Motorische Störungen bei Kindern mit verzögerter Sprachentwicklung. Folia Phoniatrica, 40, 147–152.

Nicolson, R. I., & Fawcett, A. J. (1990). Automaticity: A new framework for dyslexia research? Cognition, 35, 159–182.

Nicolson, R. I., Fawcett, A. J., Berry, E. L., Jenkins, I. H., Dean, P., & Brooks, D. J. (1999). Association of abnormal cerebellar activation with motor learning difficulties in dyslexic adults. Lancet, 353, 1662–1667.

Njiokiktjien, C., Valk, J., & Ramaekers, G. (1988). Malfunction or damage to the corpus callosum? A clinical and MRI study. Brain & Development, 10, 92–99.

Notherdaeme, M., Amorosa, H., Ploog, M., & Scheimann, G. (1988). Quantitative and qualitative aspects of associated movements in children with specific developmental speech and language disorders and in normal pre-school children. Journal of Human Movement Studies, 15, 151–169.

O'Dwyer, S. (1987). Characteristics of highly and poorly co-ordinated children. Irish Journal of Psychology, 8, 1–8.

Olson, R., Wise, B., Conners, F., Rack, J., & Fulker, D. (1989). Specific deficits in component reading and language skills: Genetic and environmental influences. Journal of Learning Disabilities, 22, 339–348.

Orton, S. T. (1937). Reading, writing, and speech problems in children: A presentation of certain types of disorders in the development of the language faculty. New York: Norton.

Owen, S. E., & McKinlay, I. A. (1997). Motor difficulties in children with developmental disorders of speech and language. Child: Care, Health and Development, 23, 315–325.

Paul, R., Cohen, D. J., & Caparulo, B. K. (1983). A longitudinal study of patients with severe developmental disorders of language learning. Journal of the American Academy of Child Psychiatry, 22, 525–534.

Paulesu, E., Frith, U., Snowling, M., Gallagher, A., Morton, J., Frackowiak, R. S. J., & Frith, C. D. (1996). Is developmental dyslexia a disconnection syndrome? Evidence from a PET scanning. Brain, 119, 143–157.

Plaza, M. (1997). Phonological impairment in dyslexic children with and without early speech-language disorder. European Journal of Disorders of Communication, 32, 277–290.

Powell, R. P., & Bishop, D. V. M. (1992). Clumsiness and perceptual problems in children with specific language impairment. Developmental Medicine and Child Neurology, 34, 755–765.

Preilowski, B. (1972). Possible contribution of the anterior forebrain commisures to bilateral co-ordination. Neuropsychologia, 10, 267–277.

Preilowski, B. (1990). Intermanual transfer, interhemispheric interaction, and handedness in man and monkeys. In C. B. Trevarthen (Ed.), Brain circuits and functions of the mind: Essays in honor of Roger W. Sperry (pp. 168–180). New York: Cambridge University Press.

Preis, S., Bartke, S., Willers, R., & Müller, K. (1995). Motor skills in children with persistent specific grammatical language impairment. Journal of Human Movement Studies, 29, 133–148.

Preis, S., Schittler, P., & Lenard, H. G. (1997). Motor performance and handedness in children with developmental language disorder. Neuropediatrics, 28, 324–327.

Quinn, K., & Geffen, G. (1986). The development of tactile transfer of information. Neuropsychologia, 24, 793–804.

Rintala, P., Pienimäki, K., Ahonen, T., Cantell, M., & Kooistra, L. (1998). The effects of a psychomotor training programme on motor skill development in children with developmental language disorders. Human Movement Science, 17, 721–737.

Rizzolatti, G., & Arbib, A. (1998). Language within our grasp. Trends in Neuroscience, 21, 188–194.

Roland, P. E., Larsen, B., Lassen, N. A., & Skinhoj, E. (1980). Supplementary motor area and other cortical areas in organization of voluntary movement in man. Journal of Neurophysiology, 43, 118–136.

Rutter, M. (1978). Prevalence and types of dyslexia. In A. L. Benton & D. Pearl (Eds.), Dyslexia. An appraisal of current knowledge (pp. 3–28). New York: Oxford University Press.

Rutter, M., Graham, P., & Yule, W. (1970). A neuropsychiatric study in childhood. Clinics in developmental medicine (nos. 35/36). London: SIMP with Heinemann Medical.

Rutter, M., & Yule, W. (1975). The concept of reading retardation. Journal of Child Psychology and Psychiatry, 16, 181–197.

Schlaug, G., Knorr, U., & Seitz, R. J. (1994). Inter-subject variability of cerebral activations in acquiring a motor skill—A study with positron emission tomography. Experimental Brain Research, 98, 523–534.

Schoemaker, M., & Kalverboer, A. F. (1994). Social and affective problems of children who are clumsy: How early do they begin? Adapted Physical Activity Quarterly, 11, 130–140.

Seitz, R. J., Schlaug, G., Knorr, U., Steinmetz, H., Tellmann, L., & Herzog, H. (1996). Neurophysiology of the human supplementary motor area: Positron emission tomography. Advances of Neurology, 70, 167–175.

Shaw, L., Levine, M. D., & Belfer, M. (1982). Developmental double jeopardy: A study of clumsiness and self-esteem in children with learning problems. Developmental and Behavioral Pediatrics, 3, 191–196.

Sigmundsson, H. (1999). Inter-modal matching and bi-manual co-ordination in children with hand-eye co-ordination problems. Nordisk Fysioterapi, 3, 55–64.

Sigmundsson, H., Ingvaldsen, R. P., & Whiting, H. T. A. (1997a). Inter- and intra-sensory modality matching in children with hand-eye co-ordination problems. Experimental Brain Research, 114, 492–499.

Sigmundsson, H., Ingvaldsen, R. P., & Whiting, H. T. A. (1997b). Inter- and intra-sensory modality matching in children with hand-eye co-ordination problems: Exploring the developmental lag hypothesis. Developmental Medicine and Child Neurology, 12, 790–796.

Sigmundsson, H., Whiting, H. T. A., & Ingvaldsen, R. P. (1999). "Putting your foot in it"! A window into clumsy behaviour. Behavioural Brain Research, 102, 131–138.

Silva, P. A., McGee, R., & Williams, S. (1985). Some characteristics of 9-year-old boys with general reading backwardness or specific reading retardation. Journal of Clinical Psychology and Psychiatry, 26, 407–421.

Stein, J. F. (1993). Dyslexia- impaired temporal information processing? In P. Tallal, M. Galaburda, R. R. Llinas, & C. von Euler (Eds.), Temporal information processing in the nervous system: Special reference to dyslexia and dysphasia. Annals of the New York Academy of Sciences, vol. 682 (pp. 83–86). New York: New York Academy of Sciences.

Stein, J. F. (1994). Developmental dyslexia, neural timing and hemispheric lateralization. International Journal of Psychophysiology, 18, 241–249.

Stein, J. F., & Glickstein, M. (1992). Role of the cerebellum in visual guidance of movement. Physiological Reviews, 72, 967–1017.

Stevenson, J. (1984). Predictive value of speech and language screening. Developmental Medicine and Child Neurology, 26, 528–538.

Tallal, P. (1980). Auditory temporal perception, phonics, and reading disabilities in children. Brain and Language, 9, 182–198.

Tallal, P., Curtiss, S., & Kaplan, R. (1988). The San Diego longitudinal study: Evaluating the outcomes of preschool impairment in language development. In S. E. Gerber & G. T. Mencher (Eds.), International perspectives on communication disorders (pp. 86–126). Washington, DC: Gallaudet University Press.

Tallal, P., Stark, R., Kallman, C., & Mellits, D. (1981). A reexamination of some non-verbal perceptual abilities of language-impaired and normal children as a function of age and sensory modality. Journal of Speech and Hearing Research, 24, 351–357.

Tamas, L. B., Schibasaki, T., Horikoshi, S., & Ohye, C. (1993). General activation of cerebral metabolism with speech: A PET study. International Journal of Psychophysiology, 14, 199–208.

Van Rossum, J. H. A., & Vermeer, A. (1990). Perceived competence: A validation study in the field of motoric remedial teaching. International Journal of Disability, Development and Education, 37, 71–91.

Wolf, M. (1982). The word retrieval process and reading in children and aphasics. In K. E. Nelson (Ed.), Children's language. Vol. 3 (pp. 437–493). Hillsdale, NJ: Lawrence Erlbaum.

Wolff, P. H. (1993). Impaired temporal resolution in developmental dyslexia. In P. Tallal, M. Galaburda, R. R. Llinas, & C. von Euler (Eds.), Temporal information processing in the nervous system: Special reference to dyslexia and dysphasia. Annals of the New York Academy of Sciences, vol. 682 (pp. 87–103). New York: New York Academy of Sciences.

Wolff, P. H., Cohen, C., & Drake, C. (1984). Impaired motor timing control in specific reading retardation. Neuropsychologia, 22, 587–600.

Wolff, P. H., Melngailis, I., Obregon, M., & Bedrosian, M. (1995). Family patterns of developmental dyslexia. Part II. Behavioral phenotypes. American Journal of Medical Genetics (Neuropsychiatric Genetics), 60, 494–505.

Wolff, P. H., Michel, G. F., & Ovrut, M. (1990). The timing of syllable repetitions in developmental dyslexia. Journal of Speech and Hearing Research, 33, 281–289.

Wolff, P. H., Michel, G. F., Ovrut, M., & Drake C. (1990). Rate and timing precision of motor coordination in developmental dyslexia. Developmental Psychology, 26, 349–359.

World Health Organization. (1980). International classification of impairments, disabilities and handicaps—A manual of classification relating to the consequences of disease. Geneva: Author.

World Health Organization. (1997). International classification of impairments, activities and participation (ICIDH-2). A manual of dimensions of disablement and functioning. Geneva: Author.

CHAPTER 5

American Psychiatric Association. (1987). *Diagnostic and Statistical Manual of Mental Disorders* (3rd ed., revised). Washington, DC: Author.

Armitage, M., & Larkin, D. (1993). Laterality, motor asymmetry and clumsiness. *Human Movement Science, 12,* 155–177.

Bairstow, P. J., & Laszlo, J. I. (1981). Kinaesthetic sensitivity to passive movements in children and adults, and its relationship to motor development and motor control. *Developmental Medicine and Child Neurology, 23,* 606–616.

Bairstow, P. J., & Laszlo, J. I. (1989). Deficits in the planning, control and recall of hand movements, in children with perceptuo-motor dysfunction. *British Journal of Developmental Psychology, 7,* 251–273.

Banich, M. T. (1995). Interhemispheric processing: Theoretical considerations and empirical approaches. In R. J. Davidson & K. Hugdahl (Eds.), *Brain asymmetry* (pp. 427–450). Cambridge, MA: MIT Press.

Barnett, A., & Henderson, S. E. (1992). Some observations on the figure drawings of clumsy children. *British Journal of Educational Psychology, 62,* 341–355.

Beech, J. R., & Harding, L. M. (1984). Phonemic processing and the poor reader from a developmental lag viewpoint. *Reading Research Quarterly, 3,* 357–366.

Berk, L. (1997). *Child development.* Boston: Allyn and Bacon.

Bogen, J. E. (1990). Parietal hemispheric independence with the neocommissures intact. In C. Trevarthen (Ed.), *Brain circuits and functions of the mind* (pp. 215–230). New York: Cambridge University Press.

Bogen, J. E. (1993). The callosal syndromes. In K. M. Heilman & R. Valenstein (Eds.), *Clinical neuropsychology* (3rd ed., pp. 337–407). New York: Oxford University Press.

Brenner, M. W., Gillman, S., Zangwill, O. L., & Farrell, M. (1967). Visuo-motor disability in schoolchildren. *British Medical Journal, 4,* 259–262.

Dare, M. T., & Gordon, N. (1970). Clumsy children: A disorder of perception and motor organisation. *Developmental Medicine and Child Neurology, 12,* 178–185.

Denckla, M. B. (1984). Developmental dyspraxia. The clumsy child. In M. D. Levine & P. Satz (Eds.), *Middle childhood: Development and dysfunction* (pp. 245–260). Baltimore: University Park Press.

Doyle, A. J. R., Elliott, J. M., & Connolly, K. J. (1986). Measurement of kinaesthetic sensitivity. *Developmental Medicine and Child Neurology, 30,* 80–92.

Dunn, H. G. (1986). *Sequelae of low birthweight: The Vancouver study. Clinics in Developmental Medicine, nos. 95/96.* London: Mac Keith Press with Blackwell Scientific.

Elliott, J. M., Connolly, K. J., & Doyle, A. J. R. (1988). Development of kinaesthetic sensitivity and motor performance in children. *Developmental Medicine and Child Neurology, 30,* 80–92.

Faglioni, P., & Basso, A. (1985). Historical perspectives on neuroanatomical correlates of limb apraxia. In E. A. Roy (Ed.), *Neuropsychological studies of apraxia and related disorders* (pp. 3–44). Amsterdam: Elsevier Science.

Fleishman, E. A. (1966). Human abilities and the acquisition of skill. In E. A. Bilodeau (Ed.), *Acquisition of skill* (pp. 147–167). New York: Academic Press.

Galin, D., Diamond, R., & Herron, J. (1977). Development of crossed and uncrossed tactile localisation on the fingers. *Brain and Language, 4,* 588–590.

Geffen, G., Nilsson, J., & Quinn, K. (1985). The effect of lesions of the corpus callosum on finger localisation. *Neuropsychologia, 4,* 497–514.

Geschwind, N. (1975). The apraxias: Neural mechanisms of disorders of learned movement. *American Scientist, 63,* 188–195.

Gibson, J. J. (1966). *The senses considered as perceptual systems.* Boston: Houghton Mifflin.

Gordon, N., & McKinlay, I. (1980). *Helping clumsy children.* Edinburgh: Churchill Livingstone.

Gubbay, S. S. (1975). *The clumsy child: A study of developmental apraxia and agnosic ataxia.* London: Saunders.

Gubbay, S. S., Ellis, T., Walton, J. N., & Court, S. D. M. (1965). Clumsy children: A study of apraxic and agnosic defects in 21 children. *Brain, 88,* 295–312.

Haywood, K. M. (1993). *Life span motor development.* Champaign, IL: Human Kinetics.

Heilman, K. M., & Rothi, L. J. G. (1993). Apraxia. In K. M. Heilman & R. Valenstein (Eds.), *Clinical neuropsychology* (3rd ed., pp. 141–163). New York: Oxford University Press.

Henderson, L., Rose, P., & Henderson, S. E. (1992). Reaction time and movement time in children with a developmental coordination disorder. *Journal of Child Psychology and Psychiatry, 33,* 895–905.

Henderson, S. E. (1992). Clumsiness or developmental coordination disorder: A neglected handicap. *Current Paediatrics, 2*, 158–162.

Henderson, S. E. (1993). Motor development and minor handicap. In A. F. Kalverboer, B. Hopkins, & R. Geuze (Eds.), *Motor development in early and later childhood: Longitudinal approaches* (pp. 286–306). Cambridge: Cambridge University Press.

Henderson, S. E., Barnett, A., & Henderson, L. (1994). Visuospatial difficulties and clumsiness: On the interpretation of conjoined deficits. *Journal of Child Psychology and Psychiatry, 35*, 961–969.

Henderson, S. E., & Hall, D. (1982). Concomitants of clumsiness in young schoolchildren. *Developmental Medicine and Child Neurology, 24*, 448–460.

Henderson, S. E., & Sugden, D. (1992). *The Movement Assessment Battery for Children*. Kent, U. K.: The Psychological Corporation.

Hofsten, C. von, & Rösblad, B. (1988). The integration of sensory information in the development of precise manual pointing. *Neuropsychologia, 26*, 805–821.

Hulme, C. (1981). *Reading retardation and multi-sensory teaching*. London: Routledge & Kegan Paul.

Hulme, C., Biggerstaff, A., Moran, G., & McKinlay, I. (1982). Visual, kinaesthetic and cross-modal judgements of length by normal and clumsy children. *Developmental Medicine and Child Neurology, 24*, 461–471.

Hulme, C., Smart, A., & Moran, G. (1982). Visual perceptual deficits in clumsy children. *Neuropsychologia, 20*, 475–481.

Hulme, C., Smart, A., Moran, G., & McKinlay, I. (1984). Visual, kinaesthetic and cross-modal judgements of length by clumsy children: A comparison with young normal children. *Child: Care, Health and Development, 10*, 117–125.

Jeannerod, M. (1988). *The neural and behavioural organisation of goal-directed movements*. New York: Oxford University Press.

Jeeves, M. A. (1990). Agenesis of the corpus callosum. In R. D. Nebes & S. Corkin (Eds.), *Handbook of neuropsychology* (pp. 99–114). Amsterdam: Elsevier Science.

Jongmans, M. (1989). *The relationship between perception and action in manual control of children with specific movement difficulties*. Unpublished study. Faculty of Human Movement Sciences. Free University Amsterdam.

Kalat, J. W. (1995). *Biological psychology*. Florence, KY: Brooks/Cole Publishing Company.

Kolb, B., & Whishaw, I. Q. (1996). *Fundamentals of human neuropsychology*. New York: W. H. Freeman and Company.

Laszlo, J. I. (1990). Child perceptuo-motor development: Normal and abnormal development of skilled behaviour. In C. A. Hauert (Ed.), *Developmental psychology: Cognitive, perceptuo-motor and neurophysiological perspective. Advances in psychology, 64* (pp. 273–308). Amsterdam: North-Holland.

Laszlo, J. I., & Bairstow, P. J. (1980). The measurement of kinaesthetic sensitivity in children and adults. *Development Medicine and Child Neurology, 22*, 454–464.

Laszlo, J. I., & Bairstow, P. J. (1985). *Perceptual-motor behaviour: Developmental assessment and therapy*. London: Holt, Rinehart and Winston.

Laszlo, J. I., Bairstow, P. J., Bartrip, J., & Rolfe., U. T. (1988). Clumsiness or perceptuo-motor dysfunction. In A. M. Colley & J. R. Beech (Eds.), *Cognition and action in skilled behaviour* (pp. 293–309). Amsterdam: Elsevier Science.

Laszlo, J. I., & Sainsbury, K. M. (1993). Perceptual-motor development and prevention of clumsiness. *Psychological Research, 55,* 167–174.

Lee, D. N., Daniel, B. M., Turnbull, J., & Cook, M. L. (1990). Basic perceptuo-motor dysfunctions in cerebral palsy. In M. Jeannerod (Ed.), *Attention and performance. XIII: Motor representation and control* (pp. 593–603). Hillsdale, NJ: Erlbaum.

Lee, D. N., Hofsten, C. von, & Cotton, E. (1997). Perception in action approach to cerebral palsy. In K. J. Connolly & H. Forssberg (Eds.), *Neurophysiology and neuropsychology of motor development* (pp. 257–285). London: Mac Keith Press.

Lord, R., & Hulme, C. (1987). Kinaesthetic sensitivity of normal and clumsy children. *Developmental Medicine and Child Neurology, 29,* 720–725.

Losse, A., Henderson, S. E., Elliman, D., Hall, D., Knight, E., & Jongmans, M. (1991). Clumsiness in children. Do they grow out of it? A 10-year follow-up study. *Developmental Medicine and Child Neurology, 33,* 55–68.

Mæland, A. F. (1992). Identification of children with motor coordination problems. *Adapted Physical Activity Quarterly, 9,* 330–342.

Mima, T., Sadato, N., Yazawa, S., Hanakawa, T., Fukuyama, H., Yonekura, Y., & Shibasaki, H. (1999). Brain structures related to active and passive finger movements in man. *Brain, 122,* 1989–1997.

Mishkin, M., Ungerleider, L. G., & Macho, K. A. (1983). Object vision and spatial vision: Two cortical pathways. *Trends in Neurosciences, 6,* 414–417.

Morris, P. R., & Whiting, H. T. A. (1971). *Motor impairment and compensatory education.* Philadelphia: G. Bell.

Mountcastle, V. B., Lynch, J. C., Georgopoulos, A., Sakata, H., & Acuna, C. J. (1975). Posterior parietal association cortex of the monkey: Command functions for operations within extrapersonal space. *Journal of Neurophysiology, 38,* 871–908.

Murphy, J. B., & Gliner, J. A. (1988). Visual and motor sequencing in normal and clumsy children. *Occupational Therapy Journal of Research, 8,* 89–101.

Njiokiktjien, C., de Sonneville, L., & Vaal, J. (1994). Callosal size in children with learning disabilities. *Behavioural Brain Research, 64,* 213–218.

O'Leary, D. S. (1980). A developmental study of interhemispheric transfer in children aged five to ten. *Child Development, 51,* 743–750.

Orton, S. T. (1937). *Reading, writing and speech problems in children.* New York: Norton.

Paulesu, E., Frith, U., Snowling, M., Gallagher, A., Morton, J., Frackowiak, R. S. J., & Frith, C. D. (1996). Is developmental dyslexia a disconnection syndrome? Evidence from a PET scanning. *Brain, 119,* 143–157.

Powell, R. P., & Bishop, D. V. M. (1992). Clumsiness and perceptual problems in children with specific language impairment. *Developmental Medicine and Child Neurology, 34,* 755–765.

Preilowski, B. (1972). Possible contribution of the anterior forebrain commissures to bilateral co-ordination. *Neuropsychologia, 10,* 267–277.

Preilowski, B. (1990). Intermanual transfer, interhemispheric interaction, and handedness in man and monkeys. In C. Trevarthen (Ed.), *Brain circuits and functions of the mind* (pp. 160–180). New York: Cambridge University Press.

Quinn, K., & Geffen, G. (1986). The development of tactile transfer of information. *Neuropsychologia, 24,* 793–804.

Robinson, D. L., Goldberg, M. E., & Stanton, G. B. (1978). Parietal association cortex in the primate: Sensory mechanisms and behavioural modulations. *Journal of Neurophysiology, 41,* 910–932.

Rösblad, B., & Hofsten, C. von. (1992). Perceptual control of manual pointing in children with motor impairments. *Physiotherapy Theory and Practice, 8,* 223–233.

Rutter, M. (1984). Issues and prospects in developmental neuropsychiatry. In M. Rutter (Ed.), *Developmental neuropsychiatry.* Edinburgh: Churchill Livingstone.

Sandström, C. I. (1953). Sex differences in localisation and orientation. *Acta Psychologica, 9,* 82–96.

Sandström, C. I., & Lundberg, I. (1956). A genetic approach to sex differences in localisation. *Acta Psychologica, 12,* 247–253.

Shafer, D. D. (1993). Patterns of handedness: Comparative study of nursery school children and captive gorillas. In J. P. Ward & W. D. Hopkins (Eds.), *Primate laterality: Current behavioural evidence of primate asymmetries* (pp. 267–283). New York: Springer Verlag.

Sherrington, C. S. (1906). *The integrative action of the nervous system.* New Haven: Yale University Press.

Sigmundsson, H. (1999). Inter-modal matching and bi-manual co-ordination in children with hand-eye co-ordination problems. *Nordisk Fysioterapi, 3,* 55–64.

Sigmundsson, H., Ingvaldsen, R. P., & Whiting, H. T. A. (1997a). Inter- and intra-sensory modality matching in children with hand-eye co-ordination problems. *Experimental Brain Research, 114,* 492–499.

Sigmundsson, H., Ingvaldsen, R. P., & Whiting, H. T. A. (1997b). Inter- and intra-sensory modality matching in children with hand-eye co-ordination problems: Exploring the developmental lag hypothesis. *Developmental Medicine and Child Neurology, 39,* 790–796.

Sigmundsson, H., Pedersen, A. V., Whiting, H. T. A., & Ingvaldsen, R. P. (1998). We can cure your child's clumsiness! A review of intervention methods. *Scandinavian Journal of Rehabilitation Medicine, 30,* 101–106.

Sigmundsson, H., Whiting, H. T. A., & Ingvaldsen, R. P. (1999). Putting your foot in it! A window into clumsy behaviour. *Behavioural Brain Research, 102,* 131–138.

Smyth, T. R. (1991). Abnormal clumsiness in children: A programming defect? *Child: Care, Health and Development, 17,* 283–294.

Smyth, T. R. (1992). Impaired motor skill (clumsiness) in otherwise normal children: A review. *Child: Care, Health and Development, 18,* 283–300.

Smyth, T. R. (1994). Clumsiness in children: A defect of kinaesthetic perception? *Child: Care, Health and Development, 20,* 27–36.

Sövik, N., & Mæland, A. F. (1986). Children with motor problems ("clumsy children"). *Scandinavian Journal of Educational Research, 30,* 39–53.

Sperry, R. W. (1974). Lateral specialisation in the surgically separated hemispheres. In F. O. Schmitt & F. G. Worden (Eds.), *The neurosciences: Third study program* (pp. 5–19). Cambridge, MA: MIT Press.

Stark, R. E., Mellits, E. D., & Tallal, P. (1983). Behavioural attributes of speech and language disorders. In C. L. Ludlow & J. A. Cooper (Eds.), *Genetic aspects of speech and language disorders.* New York: Academic Press.

Sugden, D., & Wann, C. (1988). Kinaesthesis and motor impairment in children with moderate learning difficulties. *British Journal of Educational Psychology, 57,* 225–236.

Trevarthen, C. (1974). Cerebral embryology and the split brain. In M. Kinsbourne & W. L. Smith (Eds.), *Hemispheric disconnection and cerebral function* (pp. 208–236). Springfield, IL: Charles C Thomas.

Yakolev, P. I., & Lecours, A. R. (1967). The myelogenetic cycles of regional maturation of the brain. In A. Minkowski (Ed.), *Regional development of the brain in early life* (pp. 3–70). Oxford: Blackwell Science.

Walton, J. N., Ellis, E., & Court, S. (1962). Clumsy children: Developmental apraxia and agnosia. *Brain, 85,* 603–612.

Williams, H. G., Woollacott, M. H., & Ivry, R. (1992). Timing and motor control in clumsy children. *Journal of Motor Behaviour, 24,* 165–172.

CHAPTER 6

American Alliance for Health, Physical Education, Recreation & Dance (AAHPERD). (1980). *Testing for impaired, disabled and handicapped individuals.* Reston, VA: Authors.

Arnheim, D., & Sinclair, W. A. (1979). *The clumsy child: A program of motor therapy (2nd ed.).* St Louis: Mosby.

Ayres, A. J. (1965). Patterns of perceptual-motor dysfunction in children: A factor analytic study. *Perceptual and Motor Skills, 20,* 335–368.

Ayres, A. J. (1989). *The Sensory Integration and Praxis Tests.* Los Angeles: Western Psychological Services.

Barnett, A., & Henderson, S. E. (1998). The classification of specific motor coordination disorders in children: Some problems to be solved. *Human Movement Science, 17,* 449–469.

Beery, K. E. (1997). *Developmental test of visual-motor integration* (4th ed., revised). Los Angeles: Western Psychological Services.

Blackman, J., Levine, M., & Markowitz, M. (1986). *Pediatric Examination at Three (PEET).* Cambridge, MA: Educators Publishing Service.

Brace, D. K. (1927). *Measuring motor ability.* New York: A. S. Barnes.

Bernstein, N. (1967). *The co-ordination and regulation of movement.* Oxford: Pergamon Press.

Bruininks, R. H. (1978). *Bruininks-Oseretsky Test of Motor Proficiency examiners manual.* Circle Pines, MI: American Guidance Service.

Burton, A. W., & Miller, D. E. (1998). *Movement skill assessment.* Champaign, IL: Human Kinetics.

Carpenter, A. (1942). The measurement of general motor capacity and general motor ability in the first three grades. *Research Quarterly, 13,* 444–465.

Case-Smith, J. (1994). The relationships among sensorimotor components, fine motor skill, and functional performance in preschool children. *American Journal of Occupational Therapy, 49,* 645–652.

Cintas, H. L. (1995). Cross-cultural similarities and differences in development and the impact of parental expectations on motor behavior. *Pediatric Physical Therapy, 7,* 103–111.

Cratty, B. J. (1969). *Perceptual-motor behavior and educational processes.* Springfield, IL: Charles C. Thomas.

Davis, W. E. (1984). Motor ability assessment of populations with handicapping conditions: Challenging basic assumptions. *Adapted Physical Activity Quarterly, 1,* 125–140.

Dellen, T. van. (1986). *Response processing and movement organization in clumsy children: An experimental approach.* Groningen, Netherlands: Rijksuniversiteit te Groningen.

Department of Education, Victoria. (1996). *Fundamental motor skills: A manual for classroom teachers.* Melbourne, Australia: Author.

Denckla, M. B. (1974). Development of motor co-ordination in normal children. *Developmental Medicine and Child Neurology, 16,* 729–741.

Dwyer, C. A. (1996). Cut scores and testing: Statistics, judgement, truth, and error. *Psychological Assessment, 8,* 360–362.

Easley, A. M. (1996). Dynamic assessment for infants and toddlers: The relationship between assessment and the environment. *Pediatric Physical Therapy, 8,* 62–69.

Fleishman, E. A., & Ellison, G. D. (1962). A factor analysis of fine manipulative tests. *Journal of Applied Psychology, 46,* 96–105.

Folio, R., & Fewell, R. (2000). *Peabody Developmental Motor Skills—2.* Chicago, IL: The Riverside Publishing Company.

Gardner, M. R. (1995). *Test of Visual Motor Skills—revised.* Hydesville, CA: Psychogical and Educational Publications.

Gentile, A. M. (1987). Skill acquisition: Action, movement, and neuromotor processes. In J. H. Carr, R. B. Shepherd, J. Gordon, A. M. Gentile, & J. M. Held (Eds.), *Movement science foundations for physical therapy in rehabilitation* (pp. 93–154). London: Heinemann.

Gentile, A. M., Higgins, J. R., Miller, E. A., & Rosen, B. M. (1975). The structure of motor tasks. *Mouvement, Actes du 7 Symposium en Appretissage Psycho-motor du Sport* (pp. 11–28). Quebec.

Gutteridge, M. V. (1939). A study of motor achievements of young children. *Archives of Psychology, 244,* 3–178.

Gubbay, S. S. (1975). *The clumsy child: A study of developmental apraxic and agnosic ataxia.* London: W. B. Saunders.

Hammill, D. D., Pearson, N. A., & Voress, J. K. (1993). *Developmental Test of Visual Perception II.* Austin, TX: Pro-ed.

Hands, B., Sheridan, B., & Larkin, D. (1999). Creating categories of performance from continuous motor skill data using a Rasch measurement model. *Journal of Outcome Measurement, 3,* 216–232.

Hempel, W. E., & Fleishman, E. A. (1955). A factor analysis of physical proficiency and manipulative skill. *Journal of Applied Psychology, 39,* 12–16.

Henderson, S. E. (1987). The assessment of "clumsy" children: Old and new approaches. *Journal of Child Psychology and Psychiatry, 28,* 511–527.

Henderson, S. E., & Hall, D. (1982). Concomitants of clumsiness in young school children. *Developmental Medicine and Child Neurology, 24,* 448–460.

Henderson, S. E., & Sugden, D. A. (1992). *Movement Assessment Battery for Children manual.* Sidcup, Kent: The Psychological Corporation.

Higgins, J. (1977). *Human movement: An integrated approach.* St. Louis: Mosby.

Hoare, D. (1991). *Classification of movement dysfunctions in children: Descriptive and statistical approaches.* Unpublished doctoral dissertation, The University of Western Australia, Nedlands, WA, Australia.

Hoare, D. (1994). Subtypes of developmental coordination disorder. *Adapted Physical Activity Quarterly, 11,* 158–169.

Hoare, D., & Larkin, D. (1991). Kinesthetic abilities of clumsy children. *Developmental Medicine and Child Neurology, 33,* 671–678.

Johnston, O., Crawford, J., Short, H., Smyth, T. R., & Moller, J. (1987). Poor coordination in 5 year olds: A screening test for use in schools. *Australian Pediatric Journal, 23,* 157–161.

Kadesjo, B., & Gillberg, C. (1999). Developmental coordination disorder in Swedish 7-year-old children. *Journal of the American Academy of Child and Adolescent Psychiatry, 38,* 820–828.

Kemal, C. (1928). Contribution a l'étude des tests de développement moteur d'Ozeretzky. *Archives de Psychologie, 21,* 93–99.

Keogh, J. F., Sugden, D. A., Reynard, C. L., & Calkins, J. A. (1979). Identification of clumsy children: Comparisons and comments. *Journal of Human Movement Studies, 5,* 32–41.

Knudson, D. V., & Morrison, C. S. (1997). *Qualitative analysis of human movement.* Champaign, IL: Human Kinetics.

Koppitz, E. M. (1963). *Bender Gestalt Test for Young Children.* New York: Grune & Stratton.

Lafayette Instrument Co. (1997). *The Grooved Pegboard Tests.* Lafayette, IN: Lafayette Instrument Company.

Larkin, D., & Parker, H. E. (1998). Teaching landing to children with and without developmental coordination disorder. *Pediatric Exercise Science, 10,* 123–136.

Larkin, D., & Revie, G. (1994). *Stay in step: A gross motor screening test for children K–2.* Sydney, Australia: Author.

Larkin, D., & Rose, B. (1999). *Use of the McCarron Assessment of Neuromuscular Development for DCD identification.* Paper presented at the 4th Biennial Workshop on Children with a Developmental Coordination Disorder, Groningen, The Netherlands.

Lassner, R. (1948). Annotated bibliography on the Oseretsky Tests of Motor Proficiency. *Journal of Consulting Psychology, 12,* 37–47.

Laszlo, J., & Bairstow, P. J. (1985a). *Perceptual-motor behaviour: Developmental assessment and therapy.* London: Holt, Rinehart & Winston.

Laszlo, J., & Bairstow, P. J. (1985b). *Test of kinesthetic sensitivity.* Eastbourne, England: Holt, Rinehart & Winston.

Levine, M. (1996). *Pediatric Examination of Educational Readiness at Middle Childhood 2 (PEERAMID 2).* Cambridge, MA: Educators Publishing Service.

Levine, M. (1996). *Pediatric Early Elementary Examination 2 (PEEX 2).* Cambridge, MA: Educators Publishing Service.

Levine, M., & Schneider, E. (1996). *Pediatric Examination of Educational Readiness (PEER).* Cambridge, MA: Educators Publishing Service.

Mæland, A. F. (1992). Identification of children with motor coordination problems. *Adapted Physical Activity Quarterly, 9,* 330–342.

McCarron, L. T. (1982). *MAND McCarron Assessment of Neuromuscular Development: Fine and gross motor abilities* (rev. ed.). Dallas, TX: Common Market Press.

McCloy, C. H. (1934). The measurement of general motor capacity and general motor ability. *Research Quarterly, 5*(1, Suppl.), 46–61.

Miller, L. (1993). *First Step.* San Antonio, TX: Psychological Corporation.

Miller, L. (1988). *Miller Assessment for Preschoolers (MAP).* San Antonio, TX: Psychological Corporation.

Miller, L., & Roid, G. (1994). *The Toddler and Infant Motor Evaluation T. I. M. E.* San Antonio, TX: Psychological Corporation.

Miyahara, M. (1996). A meta-analysis of intervention studies on children with developmental coordination disorder. *Corpus, Psyche et Societas, 3,* 11–18.

Miyahara, M, Tsujii, M., Hanai, T., Jongmans, M., Barnett, A., Henderson, S. E., Hori, M., Nakanishi, K., & Kageyama, H. (1998). The Movement Assessment Battery for children: A preliminary investigation of its usefulness in Japan. *Human Movement Science, 17,* 679–697.

Morris, M. (1997). Developmental dyspraxia. In L. J. Gonzales Rothi & K. M. Heilman (Eds.), *Apraxia: The neuropsychology of action* (pp. 245–268). Hove, UK: Psychology Press.

Mutti, M., Sterling, H., & Spalding, N. (1993). *Quick Neurological Screening Test II* (2nd revised ed.) Novato, CA: Academic Therapy Publications.

Nichols, P. L., & Chen, T. (1981). *Minimal brain dysfunction.* Hillsdale, NJ: Erlbaum.

Pless, M., Persson, K., Holmback, J., Malm, E., & Soderback, E. (1999). Inter-rater reliability in the Swedish translation of the Movement ABC Checklist. *Nordisk Fysioterapi, 3,* 50–54.

Polatajko, H. J. (1999). Developmental coordination disorder (DCD): Alias the clumsy child syndrome. In K. Whitmore, H. Hart, & G. Willems (Eds.), *A neurodevelopmental approach to specific learning disorders* (pp. 119–133). London: Mac Keith Press.

Pryde, K. M., & Roy, E. A. (1999). Mechanisms of developmental coordination disorders: Individual analyses and disparate findings. *Brain & Cognition, 40,* 230–234.

Puderbaugh, J. K., & Fisher, A. G. (1992). Assessment of motor and process skills in normal young children and children with dyspraxia. *Occupational Therapy Journal of Research, 12,* 195–216.

Rassmussen, P., Gillberg, C., Waldenstrom, E., & Svenson, B. (1983). Perceptual, motor and attentional deficits in seven-year-old children: Neurological and neurodevelopmental aspects. *Developmental Medicine and Child Neurology, 25,* 315–333.

Revie, G., & Larkin, D. (1993). Looking at movement: Problems with teacher identification of poorly coordinated children. *ACHPER National Journal, 40*(4), 4–9.

Riggen, K. J., Ulrich, D., & Ozman, J. C. (1990). Reliability and concurrent validity of the Test of Motor Impairment—Henderson revision. *Adapted Physical Activity Quarterly, 7,* 249–258.

Roach, E. G., & Kephart, N. C. (1966). *The Purdue Perceptual-Motor Survey.* Columbus OH: Merrill.

Rösblad, B., & Gard, L. (1998). The assessment of children with developmental coordination disorders in Sweden: A preliminary investigation of the suitability of the Movement ABC. *Human Movement Science, 17,* 711–719.

Sigmundsson, H., Pedersen, A. V., Whiting, H. T. A., & Ingvaldsen, R. P. (1998). We can cure your child's clumsiness! A review of intervention methods. *Scandinavian Journal of Rehabilitation Medicine, 30,* 101–106.

Sloan, W. (1955). The Lincoln-Oseretsky Motor Development Scale. *Genetic Psychology Monographs, 51,* 183–252.

Smits-Engelsman, S. E., Henderson, S. E., & Michels, C. G. J. (1998). The assessment of children with Developmental Coordination Disorder in the Netherlands: The relationship between the Movement Assessment Battery for Children and the Korperkoordinations Test fur Kinder. *Human Movement Science, 17,* 699–709.

Stott, D. H., Moyes, F. A., & Henderson, S. E. (1972). *The Test of Motor Impairment.* Ontario: Brook Educational Publishing.

Stott, D. H., Moyes, F. A., & Henderson, S. E. (1984). *The Test of Motor Impairment— Henderson revision.* Guelph, Ontario: Brook Educational Publishing.

Sugden, D., & Chambers, M. E. (1998). Intervention approaches and children with developmental coordination disorder. *Pediatric Rehabilitation, 2*(4), 139–147.

Sugden, D., & Sugden, L. (1991). The assessment of movement skill problems in 7- and 9-year-old children. *British Journal of Educational Psychology, 61,* 329–345.

Tabatabainia, M. M., Ziviani, J., & Maas, F. (1995). Construct validity of the Bruininks-Oseretsky Test of Motor Proficiency and the Peabody Developmental Motor Scales. *Australian Occupational Therapy Journal, 42,* 3–13.

Tan, S. K., Parker, H. E., & Larkin, D. (2001) Concurrent validity of motor tests used to identify children with motor impairment. *Adapted Physical Activity Quarterly, 18(2),* 168–182.

Thomas, J. R., & French, K. E. (1985). Gender differences across age in motor performance: A meta-analysis. *Psychological Bulletin, 98,* 260–282.

Tiffin, J. (1960). *Purdue Pegboard.* Lafayette, IN: Lafayette Instrument Company.

Touwen, B. C. L. (1979). *Examination of the child with minor neurological dysfunction* (2nd ed.). London: William Heinemann Medical.

Touwen, B. C. L., & Prechtl, H. F. R. (1970). *The neurological examination of the child with minor nervous dysfunction. Clinics in developmental medicine no. 38.* London: William Heinemann Medical.

Ulrich, D. A. (2000). *TGMD-2 Test of Gross Motor Development second edition examiners manual.* Austin, TX: Pro-ed.

Vandenberg, S. G. (1964). Factor studies of the Lincoln Oseretsky Test of Motor Proficiency. *Perceptual and Motor Skills, 19,* 23–41.

Volman, M. J. M., & Geuze, R. H. (1998). Relative phase stability of bimanual and visuomanual rhythmic coordination patterns in children with a developmental coordination disorder. *Human Movement Science, 17,* 541–572.

Wann, J. P., Mon-Williams, M., & Rushton, K. (1998). Postural control and coordination disorders: The swinging room revisited. *Human Movement Science, 17,* 491–513.

Wilson, B., Dewey, D., & Campbell, A. (1998). *The Developmental Coordination Disorder Questionnaire.* Calgary, Canada: Author.

Wilson, B., Kaplan, B. J., Crawford, S. J., Campbell, A., & Dewey, D. (2000). Reliability and validity of a parent questionnaire on childhood motor skills. *American Journal of Occupational Therapy, 54,* 484–493.

Wilson, B. N., Kaplan, B. J., Crawford, S. G., & Dewey, D. (2000). Interrater reliability of the Bruininks-Oseretsky Test of Motor Proficiency—Long Form. *Adapted Physical Activity Quarterly, 17,* 95–110.

Wilson, B. N., Pollack, N., Kaplan, B. J., & Law, M. (1994). *Clinical Observation of Motor and Postural Skills.* Tucson, AZ: Therapy Skill Builders.

World Health Organisation. (1996). *Multiaxial classification of child and adolescent psychiatric disorders.* Cambridge: Cambridge University Press.

Wright, H. C., & Sugden, D. A. (1996). The nature of developmental coordination disorder: Inter- and intragroup differences. *Adapted Physical Activity Quarterly, 13,* 357–371.

Wright, H. C., Sugden, D. A., Ng, R., & Tan, J. (1994). Identification of children with movement problems in Singapore: Usefulness of the movement ABC checklist. *Adapted Physical Activity Quarterly, 11,* 150–157.

Yarmolenko, A. (1933). The motor sphere of school-age children. *Journal of General Psychology, 42,* 298–318.

Zhu, W. (2000). Score equivalence is at the heart of international measures of physical activity. *Research Quarterly for Exercise and Sport, 71,* 121–128.

CHAPTER 7

Barnett, A., & Henderson, S. E. (1992). Some observations on the figure drawings of clumsy children. *British Journal of Educational Psychology, 62,* 341–355.

Bertenthal, B. I. (1996). Origins and early development of perception, action and representation. *Annual Review of Psychology, 47,* 431–459.

Dwyer, C., & McKenzie, B. E. (1994). Visual memory impairment in clumsy children. *Adapted Physical Activity Quarterly, 11,* 179–189.

Eliasson, A. C. (1995). Sensorimotor integration of normal and impaired development of precision movement of the hand. In A. Henderson & C. Pehoski, (Eds.), *Hand function in the child: Foundations for remediation* (pp. 40–54). St. Louis: Mosby.

Forssberg, H. (1998). The neurophysiology of manual skill development. In: K. J. Connolly (Ed.), *The psychobiology of the hand* (pp. 97–122). Cambridge: Mac Keith Press.

Forsström, A., & von Hofsten, C. (1982). Visually directed reaching of children with motor impairments. *Developmental Medicine and Child Neurology, 24,* 653–661.

Gibson, J. J. (1979). *The ecological approach to visual perception.* Boston: Houghton-Mifflin.

Gillberg, C., & Rasmusson, P. (1982). Perceptual, motor and attentional deficits in seven-year-old children: Background factors. *Developmental Medicine and Child Neurology, 24,* 752–770.

Gillberg, C., Carlström, G., & Rasmusson, P. (1983). Hyperkinetic disorders in seven-year-old children with perceptual, motor and attentional deficits. *Journal of Child Psychology and Psychiatry, 24,* 233–246.

Gillberg, I. C., Winnergard, I., & Gillberg, C. (1993). Screening methods, epidemiology and evaluation of intervention in DAMP in preschool children. *European Journal of Child and Adolescent Psychiatry, 2,* 121–135.

Goodale, M. A., Jakobson, L. S., & Servos, P. (1996). The visual pathways mediating perception and prehension. In A. M. Wing & P. Haggard (Eds.), *Hand and brain: The neurophysiology and psychology of hand movements* (pp. 15–31). San Diego: Academic Press.

Goodale, M. A., & Milner, A. D. (1992). Separate visual pathways for perception and action. *Trends in Neuroscience, 15,* 20–25.

Henderson, S. E., & Hall, D. (1982). Concomitants of clumsiness in young children. *Developmental Medicine and Child Neurology, 24,* 448–460.

Henderson, L., Rose, P., & Henderson, S. (1992). Reaction time and movement time in children with a developmental coordination disorder. *Journal of Child Psychology and Psychiatry, 33,* 895–905.

Henderson, S. E., Barnett, A., & Henderson, L. (1994). Visuospatial difficulties and clumsiness: On the interpretation of conjoined deficits. *Journal of Child Psychology and Psychiatry, 35,* 961–969.

Hulme, C., Biggerstaff, A., Moran, G., & McKinlay, I. (1982). Visual, kinaesthetic and cross-modal judgements of length by normal and clumsy children. *Developmental Medicine and Child Neurology, 24,* 461–471.

Hulme, C., & McKinlay, I. (1984). Visual, kinaesthetic and cross-modal judgements of length by clumsy children: A comparison with young normal children. *Child: Care, Health and Development, 10,* 117–125.

Hulme, C., Smart, A., & Moran, G. (1982). Visual perceptual deficits in clumsy children. *Neuropsychologia, 20,* 475–481.

Hulme, C., Smart, A., Moran, G., & Raine, A. (1983). Visual, kinaesthetic and cross-modal development: Relationship to motor skill development. *Perception, 12,* 477–483.

Jeannerod, M. (1984). The timing of natural prehension movements. *Journal of Motor Behavior, 16,* 235–254.

Jeannerod, M., Decety, J., & Michel, F. (1994). Impairment of grasping movements following bilateral parietal lesion. *Neuropsychologia, 32,* 369–380.

Kadesjö, B., & Gillberg, C. (1998). Attention deficits and clumsiness in Swedish 7-year-old children. *Developmental Medicine and Child Neurology, 40,* 796–804.

Landgren, M., Pettersson, R., Kjellman, B., & Gillberg, C. (1996). ADHD, DAMP and other neurodevelopmental/psychiatric disorders in 6-year-old children: Epidemiology and co-morbidity. *Developmental Medicine and Child Neurology, 38,* 891–906.

Langaas, T., Mon-Williams, M., Wann, P., Pascal, E., & Thompson, C. (1998). Eye movements, prematurity and developmental co-ordination disorder. *Vision Research, 38,* 1817–1826.

Lee, D. N (1980). Visuo-motor coordination in space-time. In G. E. Stelmach & J. Requin (Eds.), *Tutorials in motor behavior* (pp. 281–295). Amsterdam: North-Holland.

Lee, D. N., & Aronsson, E. (1974). Visual proprioceptive control of standing in human infants. *Perception and Psychophysics, 15,* 529–532.

Lefebvre, C., & Reid, G. (1998). Prediction in ball catching by children with and without Developmental Coordination Disorders. *Adapted Physical Activity Quarterly, 15,* 299–315.

Lishman, J. R., & Lee, D. N. (1973). The autonomy of visual kinaesthesis. *Perception, 2*, 287–294.

Lord, R., & Hulme, C. (1987). Perceptual judgements of normal and clumsy children. *Developmental Medicine and Child Neurology, 29*, 250–257.

Lord, R., & Hulme, C. (1988). Visual perception and drawing ability in clumsy and normal children. *British Journal of Developmental Psychology, 6*, 1–9.

Mæland, A. F. (1992). Handwriting and perceptual-motor skills in clumsy, dysgraphic, and "normal" children. *Perceptual and Motor Skills, 75*, 1207–1217.

Mason, C., & Kandel, E. R. (1991). Central visual pathways. In E. R. Kandel, J. H. Schwartz, & T. M. Jessell (Eds.), *Principles of neural science* (pp. 420–439). New York: Elsevier.

Milner, A. D., & Goodale, M. A. (1995). *The visual brain in action. Oxford Psychology Series, no. 27*. Oxford: Oxford University Press.

Mon-Williams, M. A., Mackie R. T., McCulloch, D. L., & Pascal, E. (1996). Visual evoked potentials in children with developmental coordination disorder. *Ophthalmic and Physiological Optics, 16*, 178–183.

Mon-Williams, M. A., Pascal, E., & Wann, J. P. (1994). Ophthalmic factors in developmental coordination disorder. *Adapted Physical Activity Quarterly, 11*, 170–178.

Mon-Williams, M. A., Wann, J. P., & Pascal, E. (1999). Visual-proprioceptive mapping in children with developmental coordination disorder. *Developmental Medicine and Child Neurology, 41*, 247–254.

Murray, E. A., Cermak, S. A., & O'Brien, V. (1990). The relationship between form and space perception, constructional abilities, and clumsiness in children. *American Journal of Occupational Therapy, 44*, 623–628.

O'Brien, V., Cermak, S. A., & Murray, E. (1988). The relationship between visual-perceptual motor abilities and clumsiness in children with and without learning disabilities. *American Journal of Occupational Therapy, 42*, 359–363.

Parush, S., Yochman, A., Cohen, D., & Gershon, E. (1998). Relation of visual perception and visual-motor integration for clumsy children. *Perceptual and Motor Skills, 86*, 291–295.

Ross, R. G., Radant, A. D., & Hommer, D. W. (1993). A developmental study of smooth pursuit eye movements in normal children from 7 to 15 years of age. *Journal of the American Academy of Child and Adolescent Psychiatry, 32*, 783–791.

Rösblad, B., & von Hofsten, C. (1994). Repetitive goal-directed arm movements in children with developmental coordination disorder: Role of visual information. *Adapted Physical Activity Quarterly, 11*, 190–202.

Skorji, V., & McKenzie, B. (1997). How do children who are clumsy remember modelled movements? *Developmental Medicine and Child Neurology, 39*, 404–408.

Ungerleider, L. G., & Mishkin, M. (1982). Two cortical visual systems. In D. J. Ingle, M. A. Goodale, & R. J. W. Mansfield (Eds.), *Analysis of visual behavior* (pp. 549–586). Cambridge, MA: MIT Press.

Van der Meulen, J. H. P., Denier van der Gon, J. J., Gielen, C. C. A. M., Gooskens, R. H. J. M., & Willemse, J. (1991a). Visuomotor performance of normal and clumsy children. I: Fast goal-directed arm movements with and without visual feedback. *Developmental Medicine and Child Neurology, 33*, 40–54.

Van der Meulen, J. H. P., Denier van der Gon, J. J., Gielen, C. C. A. M., Gooskens, R. H. J. M., & Willemse, J. (1991b). Visuomotor performance of normal and clumsy children. II: Arm-tracking with and without visual feedback. *Developmental Medicine and Child Neurology, 33,* 118–129.

Von Hofsten, C. (1993). Prospective control: A basic aspect of action development. *Human Development, 36,* 253–270.

Von Hofsten, C., & Rosander, K. (1996). The development of gaze control and predictive tracking in young infants. *Vision Research, 36,* 81–96.

Wann, J. P. (1986). Handwriting disturbances: Developmental trends. In H. T. A. Whiting & M. Wade (Eds.), *Themes in motor development. Proceedings of the NATO ASI on motor skill acquisition in children (1985: Maastricht, Netherlands)* (pp. 207–222). Dordrecht: Martinus Nijhoff.

Wann, J. P., Mon-Williams, M., & Rushton, K. (1998). Postural control and coordination disorders: The swinging room revisited. *Human Movement Science, 17,* 491–513.

Wilson, P. H., & McKenzie, B. E. (1998). Information processing deficits associated with developmental coordination disorders: A meta-analysis of research findings. *Journal of Child Psychology and Psychiatry, 39,* 829–840.

CHAPTER 8

Capaday, C., & Stein, R. (1986). Amplitude modulation of the soleus H-reflex in the human during walking and standing. *Journal of Neuroscience, 6,* 1308–1313.

Capaday, C., & Stein, R. (1987). Difference in the amplitude of the human soleus H-reflex during walking and running. *Journal of Physiology, 392,* 513–522.

Deitz, V., Schmidtbleicher, D., & Noth, J. (1979). Neuronal mechanisms of human locomotion. *Journal of Neurophysiology, 42,* 1212–1222.

Diener, H., Hore, J., Ivry, R., & Dichgans, J. (1993). Cerebellar dysfunction of movement and perception. *Canadian Journal of Neurological Sciences, 20,* 62–69.

Forsstrom, A., & von Hofsten, C. (1982). Visually directed reaching children with motor impairments. *Developmental Medicine and Child Neurology, 24,* 653–661.

Geuze, R., & Kalverboer, A. (1994). Tapping a rhythm: A problem of timing for children who are clumsy and dyslexic. *Adapted Physical Activity Quarterly, 11,* 203–213.

Gorassini, M., Prochazka, A., & Taylor, J. (1993). Cerebellar ataxia and muscle spindle sensitivity. *Journal of Neurophysiology, 70,* 1853–1862.

Gottlieb, G., Corcos, D., & Agarwal, G. (1989). Organizing principles for single-joint movements. I. A speed-insensitive strategy. *Journal of Neurophysiology, 62,* 342–357.

Gottlieb, G., Corcos, D., & Agarwal, G. (1990). Organizing principles for single-joint movements. III. A speed-insensitive strategy as a default. *Journal of Neurophysiology, 63,* 625–636.

Gottlieb, G., Corcos, D., & Agarwal, G. (1992). Organizing principles for single-joint movements. V. Agonist-antagonist interactions. *Journal of Neurophysiology, 67,* 1417–1426.

Hagbarth, K. (1993). Microneurography and applications to issues of motor control: Fifth annual Stuart Reiner Memorial Lecutre. *Muscle and Nerve, 16,* 693–705.

Henderson, L., Rose, P., & Henderson, S. (1992). Reaction time and movement time in children with a developmental coordination disorder. *Journal of Child Psychology and Psychiatry, 33,* 895–905.

Huh, J., Williams, H., & Burke, J. (1998). Development of bilateral motor control in children with developmental coordination disorders. *Developmental Medicine and Child Neurology, 40,* 474–484.

Hulliger, M. (1993). Fusimotor control of proprioceptive feedback during locomotion and balancing: Can simple lessons be learned for artificial control of gait. *Progress in Brain Research, 97,* 173–180.

Ivry, R., & Keele, S. (1989). Timing functions of the cerebellum. *Journal of Cognitive Neuroscience, 1,* 136–152.

Jaric, S., Corcos, M., Agarwal, G., & Gottlieb, G. (1993). Principles for single-joint movements. II. Generalizing a learned behavior. *Experimental Brain Research, 94,* 514–521.

Lee, D. N., & Lishman, J. R. (1975). Visual proprioceptive control of stance. *Journal of Human Movement Studies, 1,* 87–95.

Llewellyn, M., Yang, J., & Prochazka, A. (1990). Human H-reflexes are smaller in difficult beam walking than in normal treadmill walking. *Experimental Brain Research, 83,* 22–28.

Lord, R., & Hulme, C., (1988). Patterns of rotary pursuit performance in clumsy and normal children. *Journal of Child Psychology and Psychiatry, 29,* 691–701.

Lundy-Ekman, L., Ivry, R., Keele, S., & Woollacott, M. (1991). Timing and force control deficits in clumsy children. *Journal of Cognitive Neuroscience, 3,* 367–376.

Nashner, L., & Berthoz, A. (1978). Visual contribution to rapid motor responses during posture control. *Brain Research, 150,* 403–407.

Nashner, L., & Grimm, R. (1977). Analysis of multiloop dyscontrols in standing cerebellar patients. *Progress in Clinical Neurophysiology, 4,* 300–319.

Nashner, L., Shumway-Cook, A., & Marin, O. (1983). Stance posture control in selected groups of children with cerebral palsy: Deficits in sensory organization and muscular coordination. *Experimental Brain Research, 49,* 393–409.

Schellekens, J., Scholten, C., & Kalverboer, A. (1983). Visually guided hand movements in children with minor neurological dysfunction. Response time and movement organization. *Journal of Child Psychology and Psychiatry, 24,* 89–102.

Smyth, T. R., & Glencross, D. J. (1986). Information processing deficits in clumsy children. *Australian Journal of Psychology, 38,* 13–22.

Van der Meulen, J., Denier van der Gon, J., Gielen, C., Gooskens, R., & Willemse, J. (1991). Visuomotor performance of normal and children with developmental coordination disorder: Fast goal-directed arm movements with and without visual feedback. *Developmental Medicine and Child Neurology, 33,* 40–54.

Volman, M., & Geuze, R. (1998). Relative phase stability of bimanual and visuomanual rhythmic coordination patterns in children with a Development Coordination Disorder. *Human Movement Science, 17,* 541–572.

Wann, J., Mon-Williams, M., & Rushton, K. (1998). Postural control and coordination disorders: The swinging room revisited. *Human Movement Science, 17,* 491–513.

Williams, H., & Burke, J. (1995). Conditioned patellar tendon reflex responses in children with developmental coordination disorder. *Adapted Physical Activity Quarterly, 12,* 250–261.

Williams, H., & Castro, A. (1997). Timing and force characteristics of muscle activity: Postural control in children with and without developmental coordination disorders. *Australian Educational and Developmental Psychologist, 14,* 43–54.

Williams, H., Fisher, J., & Tritschler, M. (1983). Descriptive analysis of static postural control in 4-, 6-, and 8-year old motorically awkward children. *American Journal of Physical Medicine, 62,* 12–26.

Williams, H., Huh, J., & Burke, J. (1998). *Planning of unimanual and bimanual responses in children with developmental coordination disorder: A reaction time analysis.* Unpublished data, Motor Development and Control Laboratory, University of South Carolina, Columbia.

Williams, H., & Woollacott, M. (1997). Characteristics of neuromuscular responses underlying posture control in clumsy children. *Motor Development: Research and Reviews, 1,* 8–23.

Williams, H., Woollacott, M., & Ivry, R. (1992). Timing and motor control in clumsy children. *Journal of Motor Behavior, 24,* 165–172.

Wilson, B., & Trombly, C. (1984). Proximal and distal function in children with and without sensory integrative dysfunction: An EMG study. *Canadian Journal of Occupational Therapy, 51,* 11–17.

Wing, A., & Kristofferson, A. (1973). Response delays and the timing of discrete motor responses. *Perception and Psychophysics, 14,* 5–12.

Wolff, P., Michel, G., Ovrut, M., & Drake, C. (1990). Rate and timing precision of motor coordination in developmental dyslexia. *Developmental Psychology, 26,* 349–359.

CHAPTER 9

Adler, H. (1982). Children with problems in physical education in school. II. Physical factors and psychosocial problems. *Acta Paedopsychiatra, 48,* 33–46.

American Occupational Therapy Association. (1994). Uniform terminology for occupational therapy—third edition. *American Journal of Occupational Therapy, 48,* 1047–1054.

American Occupational Therapy Association. (1986). *Play: A skill for life.* Rockville, MD: American Occupational Therapy Association.

American Psychiatric Association. (1994). Category 315.4—Developmental coordination disorder. *Diagnostic and statistical manual of mental disorders* (4th ed.). Washington, DC: Author.

Ayres, A. (1973). *Sensory integration and learning disorders.* Los Angeles: Western Psychological Corporation.

Ayres, A. (1979). *Sensory integration and the child.* Los Angeles: Western Psychological Corporation.

Ayres, A. (1985). *Developmental dyspraxia and adult-onset apraxia.* Torrance, CA: Sensory Integration International.

Bissell, J., Fisher, J., Owens, C., & Polcyn, P. (1993). *Sensory motor handbook*. Torrance, CA: Sensory Integration International.

Cantell, M., Smyth, M., & Ahonen, T. (1994). Clumsiness in adolescence: Educational, motor, and social outcomes of motor delay detected at 5 years. *Adapted Physical Activity Quarterly, 11*, 115–129.

Case-Smith, J. (1995). The relationships among sensorimotor components, fine motor skill, and functional performance in preschool children. *American Journal of Occupational Therapy, 49*, 645–652.

Cermak, S. (1985). Developmental dyspraxia. In E. Roy (Ed.), *Advances in psychology. Vol. 23: Neuropsychological studies of apraxia and related disorders* (pp. 225–248). New York: North-Holland.

Cermak, S. (1991). Somatodyspraxia. In A. Fisher, E. Murray, & A. Bundy (Eds.), *Sensory integration: Theory and practice* (pp. 137–165). Philadelphia: F. A. Davis.

Cermak, S., Trimble, H., Coryell, J., & Drake, C. (1991). The persistence of motor deficits in older students with learning disabilities. *Japanese Journal of Sensory Integration, 2*(1), 17–31.

Chandler, B. (1997). *The essence of play: A child's occupation*. Rockville, MD: American Occupational Therapy Association.

Clifford, L. D. (1985). *A profile of the leisure pursuits of seven physically awkward children*. Unpublished master's thesis, University of Alberta, Edmonton, Canada.

Cohn, E., Miller, L. J., & Tickle-Degnen, L. (2000). Parental hopes for therapy outcomes: Children with sensory modulation disorders. *American Journal of Occupational Therapy, 54*, 36–43.

Coster, W., & Haley, S. (1992). Conceptualization and measurement of disablement in infants and young children. *Infants and Young Children, 4*(4), 11–22.

Dare, M., & Gordon, N. (1970). Clumsy children: A disorder of perception and motor organization. *Developmental Medicine and Child Neurology, 12*, 178–185.

Dawdy, S. (1981). Pediatric neuropsychology: Caring for the developmentally dyspraxic child. *Clinical Neuropsychology, 3*(1), 30–37.

De Ajuriaguerra, J., & Stambak, M. (1969). Developmental dyspraxia and psychomotor disorder. In P. J. Vinken & G. W. Bruyn (Eds.), *Handbook of clinical neurology, Vol. 4: Disorders of speech, perception and symbolic behavior* (pp. 443–464). New York: North-Holland.

Fox, A. M., & Lent, B. (1996). Clumsy children: Primer on developmental coordination disorder. *Canadian Family Physician, 12*, 1965–1971.

Geuze, R., & Borger, H. (1993). Children who are clumsy: Five years later. *Adapted Physical Activity Quarterly, 10*, 10–21.

Gubbay, S. S. (1975). *The clumsy child: A study in developmental apraxic and agnosic ataxia*. London: W. B. Saunders.

Gubbay, S. S. (1978). The management of developmental apraxia. *Developmental Medicine and Child Neurology, 20*, 643–646.

Gubbay, S. S. (1979). The clumsy child. In C. Rose (Ed.), *Paediatric neurology* (pp. 145–160). Oxford: Blackwell Scientific.

Gubbay, S. S. (1985). Clumsiness. In P. Vinken, G. Bruyn, & H. Klawans (Eds.), *Handbook of clinical neurology. Vol. 2 (46): Neurobehavioral disorders* (pp. 159–167). New York: Elsevier Science.

Haines, C. R., Brown, J. B., Grantham, E. B., Rajagopalan, V. S., & Sutcliffe, P. V. (1985). Neurodevelopmental screen in the school entrant medical examination as a predictor of coordination and communication difficulties. *Archives of Disease in Childhood, 60*, 1122–1127.

Hay, J., & Missiuna, C. (1998). Motor proficiency in children reporting low levels of participation in physical activity. *Canadian Journal of Occupational Therapy, 65*, 64–71.

Henderson, S., & Hall, D. (1982). Concomitants of clumsiness in young school-children. *Developmental Medicine Child Neurology, 24*, 448–460.

Hoare, D. (1994). Subtypes of developmental coordination disorder. *Adapted Physical Activity Quarterly, 11*, 158–169.

Hughes, F. (1995). *Children, play & development* (2nd ed.). Boston: Allyn and Bacon.

Ishpanovich-Radoikovich, V. (1993). Postural, motoric and cognitive functions in children with dyspraxia. *Neuroscience and Behavioral Physiology, 23*(1), 97–100.

Jirgal, D., & Bourna, K. (1989). A sensory integration observation guide for children from birth to three years of age. *Sensory Integration Special Interest Section Newsletter, 12*(2), 3.

Johnston, O., Short, H., & Crawford, J. (1987). Poorly coordinated children: A survey of 95 cases. *Child: Care, Health and Development, 13*, 361–376.

Koomar, J. (1996). Vestibular dysfunction is associated with anxiety rather than behavioral inhibition or shyness. Doctoral dissertation, Boston University, 1996. *UMI Dissertation Services.* (UMI Microform No. 9530623).

Koomar, J., & May-Benson, T. (1999, September). *Relationship of praxis to avocational skills in children with dyspraxia.* Paper presented at the Massachusetts Association for Occupational Therapy Conference, Marlboro, MA.

Leipold, E. E., & Bundy, A. C. (2000). Playfulness in children with attention deficit hyperactivity disorder. *Occupational Therapy Journal of Research, 20*(1), 61–82.

Levine, M. D. (1987). *Developmental variation and learning disorders.* Cambridge, MA: Educators Publishing Service.

Losche, G. (1990). Sensorimotor and action development in autistic children from infancy to early childhood. *Journal of Child Psychology and Psychiatry and Allied Disciplines, 31*, 749–761.

Losse, A., Henderson, S. E., Elliman, D., Hall, D., Knight, E., & Jongmans, M. (1991). Clumsiness in children—Do they grow out of it? A 10-year follow-up study. *Developmental Medicine and Child Neurology, 33*, 55–68.

May-Benson, T. (1999). *Preliminary validity evidence on the Test of Ideational Praxis.* Unpublished interim paper. Boston University, Sargent College, Boston.

Miller, L. (1993). *First STEP: Screening Test for Evaluating Preschoolers.* San Antonio, TX: Psychological Corporation.

Missiuna, C., & Polatajko, H. (1995). Developmental dyspraxia by any other name: Are they all just clumsy children? *American Journal of Occupational Therapy, 49*(7), 619–627.

Morrison, C., Metzger, P., & Pratt, P. N. (1996). In J. Case-Smith, A. Allen, & P. N. Pratt (Eds.), *Occupational therapy for children* (p. 461–503). St. Louis: Mosby.

Moyers, P. (1999). The guide to occupational therapy practice. *American Journal of Occupational Therapy, 53*(3), 247–322.

O'Dwyer, S. (1987). Characteristics of highly and poorly co-ordinated children. *Irish Journal of Psychology, 8*(1), 1–8.

Oetter, P., Richter, E., & Frick, S. (1988). *M. O. R. E.: Integrating the mouth with sensory and postural functions.* Hugo, MN: PDP Press.

Orton, S. T. (1937). *Reading, writing and speech problems in children.* New York: Norton.

OTA-Watertown, P. C. (1998a). *Classroom accommodations.* Watertown, MA: Occupational Therapy Associates-Watertown, P. C.

OTA-Watertown, P. C. (1998b). *Home accommodations.* Watertown, MA: Occupational Therapy Associates-Watertown, P. C.

Paine, R. (1968). Minimal cerebral dysfunction. *Pediatric Clinics of North America, 15*(3), 611–616.

Parham, D. (1986). Assessment: The preschooler with suspected dyspraxia. *Sensory Integration Special Interest Newsletter, 9*(1), 1–3.

Piaget, J. (1963). *Play, dreams and imitation in childhood.* New York: W. W. Norton.

Piek, J., & Edwards, K. (1997). The identification of children with developmental coordination disorder by class and physical education teachers. *British Journal of Educational Psychology, 67,* 55–67.

Polatajko, H., Fox, M., & Missiuna, C. (1995). An international consensus on children with developmental coordination disorder. *Canadian Journal of Occupational Therapy, 62,* 3–6.

Puderbaugh, J., & Fisher, A. (1992). Assessment of motor and process skills in normal young children and children with dyspraxia. *Occupational Therapy Journal of Research, 12*(4), 195–215.

Reilly, M. (1974). *Play as exploratory learning.* Beverly Hills, CA: Sage Publications.

Reuben, R., & Bakwin, H. (1968). Developmental clumsiness. *Pediatric Clinics of North America, 15*(3), 601–610.

Schoemaker, M., & Kalverboer, A. (1994). Social and affective problems of children who are clumsy: How early do they begin? *Adapted Physical Activity Quarterly, 11,* 130–140.

Shepherd, J., Proctor, S., & Coley, I. (1996). Self-care and adaptations for independent living. In J. Case-Smith, A. Allen, & P. N. Pratt (Eds.), *Occupational therapy for children* (pp. 461–503). St. Louis: Mosby.

Taber, C. (1997). *Taber's cyclopedic medical dictionary* (18th ed.). Philadelphia: F. A. Davis.

Touwen, B. (1993). Longitudinal studies on motor development: Developmental neurological considerations. In A. F. Kalverboer, B. Hopkins, & R. Geuze (Eds.), *Motor development in early and later childhood: Longitudinal approaches.* Cambridge: Cambridge University Press.

Visser, J., Geuze, R., & Kalverboer, A. (1998). The relationship between physical growth, the level of activity and the development of motor skills in adolescence: Differences between children with DCD and controls. *Human Movement Science, 17,* 573–608.

Wall, A. E., McClements, J., Bouffard, M., Findlay, H., & Taylor, M. J. (1985). A knowledge-based approach to motor development: Implications for the physically awkward. *Adapted Physical Activity Quarterly, 2,* 21–42.

Wall, A., Reid, G., & Paton, J. (1990). The syndrome of physical awkwardness. In G. Reid (Ed.), *Problems in movement control* (pp. 283–316). New York: North-Holland.

Walton, J., Ellis, E., & Court, S. (1962). Clumsy children: Developmental apraxia and agnosia. *Brain, 85*, 603–612.

Wright, H., & Sugden, D. (1996). A two-step procedure for the identification of children with developmental co-ordination disorder in Singapore. *Developmental Medicine and Child Neurology, 38*, 1099–1105.

World Health Organization. (1997). *ICIDH-2: International classification of impairments, activities, and participation. A manual of dimensions of disablement and functioning. Beta-1 draft for field trials.* Geneva: World Health Organization.

Zero to Three. (1994). *Diagnostic classification: 0–3.* Arlington, VA: Zero to Three National Center for Clinical Infant Programs.

CHAPTER 10

Alston, J., & Taylor, J. (1987). *Handwriting: Theory, research and practice.* New York: Nichols.

Ayres, A. J. (1965). Patterns of perceptual-motor dysfunction in children: A factor analytic study. *Perceptual and Motor Skills, 20,* 335–368.

Ayres, A. J. (1972). *Southern California Test of Sensory Integration.* Los Angeles: Western Psychological Corporation.

Ayres, A. J. (1977). Cluster analysis of measures of sensory integration. *American Journal of Occupational Therapy, 31,* 362–366.

Ayres, A. J. (1989). *The Sensory Integration and Praxis Tests Manual.* Los Angeles, CA: Western Psychological Services.

Ayres, A. J., Mailloux, Z. K., & Wendler, C. L. W. (1987). Developmental dyspraxia: Is it a unitary function? *Occupational Therapy Journal of Research, 7,* 94–110.

Bairstow, P. J., & Laszlo, J. I. (1981). Kinaesthetic sensitivity to passive movements and its relationship to motor development and motor control. *Developmental Medicine and Child Neurology, 23,* 606–616.

Beery, K. (1989). *Developmental Test of Visual-Motor Integration (VMI).* Cleveland, OH: Modern Curriculum Press.

Benbow, M. (1995). Principles and practices of teaching handwriting. In A. Henderson & C. Pehoski (Eds.), *Hand function in the child: Foundations for remediation* (pp. 255–281). St. Louis, MO: Mosby.

Berninger, V., & Rutberg, J. (1992). Relationship of finger function to beginning writing: Application to diagnosis of writing disabilities. *Developmental Medicine and Child Neurology, 34,* 198–215.

Case-Smith, J. (1993). Comparison of in-hand manipulation skills in children with and without fine motor delays. *Occupational Therapy Journal of Research, 13,* 87–100.

Cermak, S. (1991). Somatodyspraxia. In A. G. Fisher, E. A. Murray, & A. C. Bundy (Eds.), *Sensory integration: Theory and practice* (pp. 137–165). Philadelphia: F. A. Davis.

Connolly, K., & Dalgleish, M. (1989). The emergence of a tool-using skill in infancy. *Developmental Psychology, 25,* 894–912.

Copley, J., & Ziviani, J. (1990). Kinesthetic sensitivity and handwriting ability in grade one children. *Australian Occupational Therapy Journal, 37*, 39–43.

Cornhill, H., & Case-Smith, J. (1996). Factors that relate to good and poor handwriting. *American Journal of Occupational Therapy, 50*, 732–739.

Cunningham Amundson, S. (1992). Handwriting: Evaluation and intervention in school settings. In J. Case-Smith & C. Pehoski (Eds.), *Development of hand skills in the child* (pp. 63–78). Rockville, MD: American Occupational Therapy Association.

Deuel, R. K. (1995). Developmental dysgraphia and motor skill disorders. *Journal of Child Neurology, 10*, 57–58.

Eliasson, A. C. (1995). Sensorimotor integration of normal and impaired development of precision movement of the hand. In A. Henderson & C. Pehoski (Eds.), *Hand function in the child: Foundations for remediation* (pp. 40–54). St. Louis, MO: Mosby.

Ellis, A. W. (1982). Spelling and writing (and reading and speaking). In A. W. Ellis (Ed.), *Normality and pathology in cognitive function* (pp. 113–146). London: Academic Press.

Ellis, A. W. (1988). Normal writing processes and peripheral acquired dysgraphias. *Language and Cognitive Processes, 3*, 99–127.

Exner, C. E. (1992). In hand manipulation skills. In J. Case-Smith & C. Pehoski (Eds.), *Development of hand skills in the child* (pp. 35–46). Rockville, MD: American Occupational Therapy Association.

Exner, C. E. (2000). Development of hand skills. In J. Case-Smith (Ed.), *Occupational therapy for children* (4th ed.) (pp. 289–328). St. Louis, MO: Mosby.

Folio, R., & Fewell, R. (2000). *Peabody Developmental Motor Scales* (2nd ed.). Austin, TX: Pro-Ed.

Gesell, A., Halverson, H. M., Thompson, H., Ilg, F. L., Castner, B. M., Ames, L. B., & Amatruda, C. S. (1940). *The first five years of life: A guide to the study of the preschool child*. New York: Harper & Brothers.

Goodgold-Edwards, S., & Cermak, S. (1990). Integrating motor control and motor learning concepts with neuropsychological perspectives on apraxia and developmental dyspraxia. *American Journal of Occupational Therapy, 44*, 431–439.

Haron, M., & Henderson, A. (1985). Active and passive touch in developmentally dyspraxic and normal boys. *Occupational Therapy Journal of Research, 5*, 101–112.

Henderson, S. E., & Sugden, D. A. (1992). *Movement Assessment Battery for Children*. London: Psychological Corporation.

Hill, E. L., & Wing, A. M. (1998). Developmental disorders and the use of grip force to compensate for inertial forces during voluntary movement. In K. J. Connolly (Ed.), *Psychobiology of the hand* (pp. 199–212). London: Mac Keith Press.

Hulme, C., Biggerstaff, A., Moran, G., & McKinley, I. (1982). Visual, kinaesthetic and cross-modal judgements of length by normal and clumsy children. *Developmental Medicine and Child Neurology, 24*, 461–471.

Hulme, C., Smart, A., Moran, G., & Raine, A. (1983). Visual, kinaesthetic and cross-modal development: Relationship to motor skill development. *Perception, 12*, 477–483.

Laszlo, J. I., & Bairstow, P. J. (1984). Handwriting: Difficulties and possible solutions. *School Psychology International, 5*, 207–213.

Laszlo J. I., & Bairstow, P. J. (1985a). *Perceptual motor behavior: Developmental assessment and therapy*. London: Holt, Rinehart & Winston.

Laszlo, J. I., & Bairstow, P. J. (1985b). *Test of kinesthetic sensitivity*. Eastbourne, England: Holt, Rinehart & Winston.

Laszlo, J. I., Bairstow, P. J., Bartrip, J., & Rolfe, U. T. (1989). Process oriented assessment and treatment of children with perceptuo-motor dysfunction. *British Journal of Developmental Psychology, 7*, 251–273.

Lederman, S. J., & Klatzky, R. L. (1998). The hand as a perceptual system. In K. J. Connolly, (Ed.), *The psychobiology of the hand* (pp. 16–35). London: Mac Keith Press.

Levine, J. (1987). *Developmental variation and learning disorders*. Toronto, Canada: Educators Publishing Service.

Levine, M. D., Oberklaid, F., & Meltzer, L. (1981). Developmental output failure: A study of low productivity in school aged children. *Pediatrics, 67*, 18–25.

Lord, R., & Hulme, C. (1982). Visual perception and drawing ability in clumsy and normal children. *British Journal of Developmental Psychology, 6*, 1–9.

Lord, R., & Hulme, C. (1987). Kinaesthetic sensitivity of normal and clumsy children. *Developmental Medicine and Child Neurology, 29*, 720–725.

Lundy-Ekman, L., Ivry, R., Keele, S., & Woollacott, M. (1991). Timing and force control deficits in clumsy children. *Journal of Cognitive Neuroscience, 3*, 367–376.

Mæland, A. F. (1992). Handwriting and perceptual-motor skills in clumsy, dysgraphic, and "normal" children. *Perceptual and Motor Skills, 75*, 1207–1217.

Margolin, D. I. (1984). The neuropsychology of writing and spelling: Semantic, phonological, motor, and perceptual processes. *Quarterly Journal of Experimental Psychology, 36*, 459–489.

Meulenbroek, R. G. J., & van Galen, G. P. (1988). The acquisition of skilled handwriting: Discontinuous trends in kinematic variables. In A. M. Colley & J. R. Beech (Eds.), *Cognition and action in skilled behavior* (pp. 273–281). Amsterdam: Elsevier Science.

Meulenbroek, R. G. J., & van Galen, G. P. (1990). Perceptual-motor complexity of printed and cursive letters. *Journal of Experimental Education, 58*, 95–110.

Mon-Williams, M. A., Wann, J. P., & Pascal, E. (1999). Visual-proprioceptive mapping in children with developmental coordination disorder. *Developmental Medicine and Child Neurology, 41*, 247–254.

Mulligan, S. (1998). Patterns of sensory integration dysfunction: A confirmatory factor analysis. *American Journal of Occupational Therapy, 54*, 819–828.

Pehoski, C. (1995). Object manipulation in infants and children. In A. Henderson & C. Pehoski (Eds.), *Hand function in the child: Foundations for remediation* (pp. 136–153). St. Louis, MO: Mosby.

Piek, J. P., & Coleman-Carman, R. (1995). Kinaesthetic sensitivity and motor performance of children with developmental coordination disorder. *Developmental Medicine and Child Neurology, 37*, 976–984.

Rogers, J. (1999). The relationships of handwriting and keyboarding to visual-motor integration, finger kinesthesia and fine motor speed and dexterity. Unpublished master's thesis, Ohio State University, Columbus, Ohio.

Rosblad, B., & von Hofsten, C. (1994). Repetitive goal-directed arm movements in children with developmental coordination disorders: Role of visual information. *Adapted Physical Activity Quarterly, 11*, 190–202.

Schneck, C. (1991). Comparison of pencil-grip patterns in first graders with good and poor writing skills. *American Journal of Occupational Therapy, 45*, 701–706.

Smyth, M. M., & Mason, U. C. (1997). Planning and execution of action in children with and without developmental coordination disorder. *Journal of Child Psychology and Psychiatry, 38*, 1023–1034.

Smyth, M. M., & Mason, U. C. (1998). Direction of response in aiming to visual and proprioceptive targets in children with and without developmental coordination disorder. *Human Movement Science, 17*, 515–539.

Smyth, T. R. (1991). Abnormal clumsiness in children: A defect of motor programming? *Child: Care, Health and Development, 17*, 283–294.

Smyth, T. R. (1994). Clumsiness in children: A defect of kinaesthetic perception. *Child: Care, Health and Development, 20*, 29–35.

Smyth, T. R., & Glencross, D. J. (1986). Information processing deficits in clumsy children. *Australian Journal of Psychology, 38*, 13–22.

Thomassen, A. J. W. M., & Teulings, H. L. H. M. (1983). The development of handwriting. In M. Martlew (Eds.), *The psychology of written language* (pp. 179–213). New York: John Wiley.

Tseng, M. H., & Cermak, S. A. (1993). The influence of ergonomic factors and perceptual-motor abilities in handwriting performance. *American Journal of Occupational Therapy, 47*, 919–926.

Tseng, M. H., & Murray, E. A. (1994). Differences in perceptual motor measures in children with good and poor handwriting. *Occupational Therapy Journal of Research, 14*, 19–36.

Van der Meulen, J. H. P., Denier van der Gon, J. J., Gielen, C. C. A. M., Gooskens, R. H. J. M., & Willemse, J. (1991). Visuomotor performance of normal and clumsy children. II: Arm-tracking with and without visual feedback. *Developmental Medicine and Child Neurology, 33*, 118–129.

Van Galen, G. P. (1991). Handwriting: Issues for a psychomotor theory. *Human Movement Science, 10*, 165–191.

Van Galen, G. P., Meulenbroek, R., & Hylkema, H. (1986). On the simultaneous processing of words, letters, and strokes in handwriting: Evidence for a mixed linear and parallel model. In H. Kao, G. P. van Galen, & R. Hoosain (Eds.), *Graphonomics: Contemporary research in handwriting* (pp. 199–211). Amsterdam: Elsevier Science.

Weil, M. J., & Cunningham Amundson, S. J. (1994). Relationship between visual motor and handwriting skills of children in kindergarten. *American Journal of Occupational Therapy, 48*, 982–988.

Weintraub, N., & Graham, S. (2000). The contribution of orthographic, fine-motor and visual-motor processes to the prediction of handwriting status. *Occupational Therapy Journal of Research, 20*, 121–140.

Wilson. P. H., & McKenzie, B. E. (1998). Information processing deficits associated with developmental coordination disorder: A meta-analysis of research findings. *Journal of Child Psychology and Psychiatry, 39*, 829–840.

Ziviani, J. (1995). The development of graphomotor skills. In A. Henderson & C. Pehoski (Eds.), *Hand function in the child* (pp. 184–195). St. Louis, MO: Mosby.

CHAPTER 11

ACHPER. (1996). *Australian Fitness Education Award*. Richmond, South Australia: Author.

Armstrong, N., & Simons-Morton, B. (1994). Physical activity and blood lipids in adolescents. *Pediatric Exercise Science, 6*, 381–405.

Bailey, D. A., & Martin, A. D. (1994). Physical activity and skeletal health in adolescents. *Pediatric Exercise Science, 6*, 330–347.

Bar-Or, O. (1983). *Pediatric sports medicine for the practitioner*. New York: Springer-Verlag.

Bar-Or, O. (1987). The Wingate Anaerobic Test: An update on methodology reliability and validity. *Sports Medicine, 4*, 381–394.

Bar-Or, O., Foreyt, J., Bouchard, C., Brownell, K. D., Deitz, W. H., Ravussin, E., Salbe, A. D., Schwenger, S., St. Jeor, S., & Torun, B. (1998). Physical activity, genetic, and nutritional considerations in childhood weight management. *Medicine and Science in Sport and Exercise, 30*(1), 2–10.

Beyer, R. (1993). *Motor proficiency of males with attention deficit hyperactive disorder and males with learning difficulties*. Ann Arbor, MI: UMI.

Bouffard, M., Watkinson, E. J., Thompson, L. P., Causgrove Dunn, J. L., & Romanow, S. K. E. (1996). A test of the activity deficit hypothesis with children with movement difficulties. *Adapted Physical Activity Quarterly, 13*, 61–73.

Bruininks, R. H. (1978). *Bruininks-Oseretsky Test of Motor Proficiency*. Circle Pines, MN: American Guidance Service.

Butcher, J. E., & Eaton, W. O. (1989). Gross and fine motor proficiency in preschoolers: Relationships with free play behavior and activity level. *Journal of Human Movement Studies, 16*, 27–36.

Calfas, K. J., & Taylor, W. C. (1994). Effects of physical activity on psychological variables in adolescents. *Pediatric Exercise Science, 6*, 406–412.

Casperson, C. J., Powell, K. E., & Christenson, G. M. (1985). Physical activity, exercise and physical fitness: Definitions and distinctions for health-related research. *Public Health Reports, 100*(2), 126–131.

Charney, E., Goodman, H. C., McBride, M., Lyon, B., & Pratt, R. (1976). Childhood antecedents of adult obesity: Do chubby infants become obese adults? *New England Journal of Medicine, 295*, 6–9.

Chianas, A. K., Reid, G., & Hoover, M. L. (1998). Exercise effects on health-related fitness of individuals with an intellectual disability: A meta-analysis. *Adapted Physical Activity Quarterly, 15*, 119–140.

Cureton, K. J., & Warren, B. L. (1990). Criterion-referenced standards for youth health-related fitness tests: A tutorial. *Research Quarterly for Exercise and Sport, 61*, 7–19.

Deschenes, A. (1994). *The physical fitness and gross motor performance of children with developmental coordination disorder*. Ann Arbor, MI: UMI.

Dwyer, T., & Gibbons, L. E. (1994). The Australian Schools Health and Fitness Survey: Physical fitness related to blood pressure but not lipoproteins. *Circulation*, *89*, 1539–1544.

Freedson, P. S. (1991). Electronic motion sensors and heart rate as measures of physical activity in children. *Journal of School Health*, *61*, 220–223.

Gutin, B., & Owens, S. (1999). Role of exercise intervention in improving body fat distribution and risk profile in children. *American Journal of Human Biology*, *11*, 237–247.

Hammond, J. (1995). *Investigation into the characteristics of children with motor difficulties: An holistic approach.* Unpublished doctoral disertation, University of New England, Armidale, NSW, Australia.

Harvey, W. J., & Reid, G. (1997). Motor performance of children with attention-deficit hyperactivity disorder: A preliminary investigation. *Adapted Physical Activity Quarterly*, *14*, 189–202.

Kuiper, D., Reynders, K., & Rispens, P. (1997, May). *Leisure time physical activity in children with movement difficulties: A pilot study.* Poster presented at the 11th International Symposium of Adapted Physical Activity ISAPA, Quebec, Canada.

Larkin, D., & Hoare, D. (1991). *Out of step: Coordinating kids' movement.* The University of Western Australia, Nedlands, West Australia: Active Life Foundation.

Larkin, D., Hoare, D., & Kerr, G. (1989, June). *Structure/function interactions: A concern in the movement impaired child.* Poster presented at the 7th ISAPA International Symposium, Berlin.

Li, X. J., & Dunham, P. (1993). Fitness load and exercise time in secondary physical education classes. *Journal of Teaching Physical Education*, *12*, 180–187.

Manitoba Department of Education. (1980). *Manitoba physical fitness performance test manual and fitness objectives.* Ottawa, Ontario: CAPHER.

Marshall, J. D., & Bouffard, M. (1997). The effects of quality daily physical education on movement competency in obese versus nonobese children. *Adapted Physical Activity Quarterly*, *14*, 222–237.

McKay, H. A., Petit, M. A., Schutz, R. W., Prior, J. C., Barr, S. I., & Khan, K. M. (2000). Augmented trochanteric bone mineral density after modified physical education classes: A randomized school-based exercise intervention study in prepubescent and early pubescent children. *Journal of Pediatrics*, *136*, 156–162.

Moore, L. L., Nguyen, U., Rothman, K. J., Cupples, L. A., & Ellison, R. C. (1995). Preschool physical activity level and changes in body fatness in young children. *American Journal of Epidemiology*, *142*, 982–988.

O'Beirne, C., Larkin, D., & Cable, T. (1994). Coordination problems and anaerobic performance in children. *Adapted Physical Activity Quarterly*, *11*, 141–149.

O'Beirne, C., & Larkin, D. (1991, August). *Fitness characteristics of clumsy children.* Poster presented at the 8th IFAPA International Symposium, Miami, Florida.

Orchard, T. J., Donahue, R. P., Kuller, L. H., Hodge, P. N., & Drash, A. L. (1983). Cholesterol screening in childhood: Does it predict adult hypercholesterolemia? The Beaver County experience. *Journal of Pediatrics*, *103*, 687–691.

Pate, R. R., Baranowski, T., Dowda, M., & Trost, S. G. (1996). Tracking of physical activity in young children. *Medicine and Science in Sports and Exercise*, *28*(1), 92–96.

Pate, R. R., Dowda, M., & Ross, J. G. (1990). Associations between physical activity and physical fitness in American children. *American Journal of Diseases in Children, 144,* 1123–1129.

Pyke, J. E. (1986). *Australian School Fitness Test for students aged 7–15.* Parkside, South Australia: ACHPER Publications.

Raitakari, O. T., Porkka, K. V., & Taimela, S. (1994). Effects of persistent physical activity and inactivity on coronary risk factors in children and young adults: The cardiovascular risk in young Finns study. *American Journal of Epidemiology, 140,* 195–205.

Rarick, G. L., & McKee, R. (1949). A study of twenty third-grade children exhibiting extreme levels of achievement on tests of motor proficiency. *Research Quarterly, 20,* 142–152.

Raudsepp, L., & Jurimae, T. (1998). Physical activity, aerobic fitness and fatness in preadolescent children. *Sports Medicine, Training and Rehabilitation, 8*(2), 123–131.

Raynor, A. J. (1989). *The running pattern of seven-year-old children—coordination and gender differences.* Unpublished honors thesis, The University of Western Australia, Nedlands, Australia.

Rintala, P., Lyytinen, H., & Dunn, J. M. (1990). Influence of a physical activity program on children with cerebral palsy: A single subject design. *Pediatric Exercise Science, 2,* 57–64.

Rowland, T. W. (1990). *Exercise and children's health.* Champaign, IL: Human Kinetics.

Safrit, M., & Wood, T. M. (1995). *Introduction to measurement in physical education and exercise science* (3rd ed.). St Louis, MO: Mosby.

Sallis, J. F., & McKenzie, T. L. (1991). Physical education's role in public health. *Research Quarterly for Exercise and Sport, 62,* 124–137.

Simons-Morton, B. G., O'Hara, N. M., Simons-Morton, D. G., & Parcel, G. S. (1987). Children and fitness: A public health perspective. *Research Quarterly for Exercise and Sport, 58,* 295–302.

Stratton, G., & Armstrong, N. (1991). The relationship between physical activity levels and motor ability during physical education lessons. *Journal of Sports Sciences, 9*(4), 432.

Thompson, L. P., Bouffard, M., Watkinson, E. J., & Causgrove Dunn, J. L. (1994). Teaching children with movement difficulties: Highlighting the need for individualized instruction in regular education. *Physical Education Review, 17*(2), 152–159.

Vaccaro, P., & Mahon, A. D. (1989). The effects of exercise on coronary heart disease risk factors in children. *Sports Medicine, 8,* 139–153.

Visser, J. (1998). *Clumsy adolescents: A longitudinal study on the relationship between physical growth and sensorimotor skills of boys with and without DCD.* Groningen: Author.

Visser, J., Geuze, R. H., & Kalverboer, A. F. (1998). The relationship between physical growth, the level of activity and the development of motor skills in adolescence: Differences between children with DCD and controls. *Human Movement Science, 17,* 573–608.

Ward, D. S. (1994). Exercise for children with special needs. In R. R. Pate & R. C. Hohn (Eds.), *Health and fitness through physical education* (pp. 99–111). Champaign, IL: Human Kinetics.

Wasmund-Bodenstedt, U. (1988). High and low achievers in primary school physical education. *International Journal of Physical Education, 15,* 13–19.

Williams, D. P., Going, S. G., Lohman, T. G., Harsha, D. W., Webber, L. S., & Bereson, G. S. (1992). Body fatness and the risk of elevated blood pressure, total cholesterol and serum lipoprotein ratios in children and youth. *American Journal of Public Health, 82,* 358–363.

Woynarowska, B., Mukherjee, D., Roche, A. F., & Siervogel, R. M. (1985). Blood pressure changes during adolescence and subsequent blood pressure level. *Hypertension, 7,* 695–701.

CHAPTER 12

American Psychiatric Association (1994). *Diagnostic and statistical manual of mental disorders* (4th ed.). Washington, DC: Author.

Ames, C. (1984). Competitive, cooperative, and individualistic goal structures: A motivational analysis. In R. E. Ames & C. Ames (Eds.), *Research on motivation in education. Vol 1: Student motivation* (pp. 177–207). New York: Academic Press.

Ames, C. (1992). Achievement goals, motivational climate, and motivational processes. In G. C. Roberts (Ed.), *Motivation in sport and exercise* (pp. 161–176). Champaign, IL: Human Kinetics.

Ames, C., & Ames, R. (1984a). Goal structures and motivation. *Elementary School Journal, 85,* 39–52.

Ames, C., & Ames, R. (1984b). Systems of student and teacher motivation: Toward a qualitative definition. *Journal of Educational Psychology, 76,* 535–556.

Ames, C., & Archer, J. (1988). Achievement goals in the classroom: Students' learning strategies and motivation processes. *Journal of Educational Psychology, 80,* 260–267.

Bouffard, M. (1993). The perils of averaging data in adapted physical activity research. *Adapted Physical Activity Quarterly, 10,* 371–391.

Bouffard, M., Watkinson, E. J., Thompson, L. P., Causgrove Dunn, J. L., & Romanow, S. K. E. (1996). A test of the activity deficit hypothesis with children with movement difficulties. *Adapted Physical Activity Quarterly, 13,* 61–73.

Butler, R. (1993). Effects of task- and ego-achievement goals on information seeking during task engagement. *Journal of Personality and Social Psychology, 65,* 18–31.

Cantell, M. H., Smyth, M. M., & Ahonen, T. P. (1994). Clumsiness in adolescence: Educational, motor, and social outcomes of motor delay detected at 5 years. *Adapted Physical Activity Quarterly, 13,* 115–129.

Causgrove Dunn, J. (1997). *Individual differences in personal and situational factors related to motivation and achievement behaviour in physically awkward children.* Unpublished doctoral dissertation, University of Alberta, Edmonton, Alberta, Canada.

Causgrove Dunn, J. (2000). Goal orientations, perceptions of the motivational climate, and perceived competence of children with movement difficulties. *Adapted Physical Activity Quarterly, 17,* 1–19.

Causgrove Dunn, J., & Watkinson, E. J. (1994). A study of the relationship between physical awkwardness and children's perceptions of physical competence. *Adapted Physical Activity Quarterly, 11,* 275–283.

Cavaliere, N. L. I. (1999). *Exploring the perceptions of goal structures and achievement motivation of children in badminton class*. Unpublished master's thesis, University of Alberta, Edmonton, Alberta, Canada.

Chase, M. A., & Dummer, G. M. (1992). The role of sports as a social status determinant for children. *Research Quarterly for Exercise and Sport, 63*, 418–424.

Clifford, L. D. (1985). *A profile of the leisure pursuits of seven physically awkward children*. Unpublished master's thesis, University of Alberta, Edmonton, Alberta, Canada.

Coopersmith, S. (1967). *The antecedents of self-esteem*. San Francisco: W. H. Freeman.

Cratty, B. J. (1979). *Perceptual and motor development in infants and children*. Englewood Cliffs, NJ: Prentice-Hall.

Cratty, B. J. (1994). *Clumsy child syndromes: Description, evaluation and remediation*. Langhorne, PA: Harwood.

Davis, W. E., & Burton, A. W. (1991). Ecological task analysis: Translating movement behavior theory into practice. *Adapted Physical Activity Quarterly, 8*, 154–177.

Davis, W. E., & van Emmerick, R. E. A. (1995a). An ecological task analysis approach for understanding motor development in mental retardation: Philosophical and theoretical underpinnings. In A. Vermeer & W. E. Davis (Eds.), *Physical and motor development in mental retardation* (pp. 1–32). Basel, Switzerland: Karger.

Davis, W. E., & van Emmerick, R. E. A. (1995b). An ecological task analysis approach for understanding motor development in mental retardation: Research questions and strategies. In A. Vermeer & W. E. Davis (Eds.), *Physical and motor development in mental retardation* (pp. 33–66). Basel, Switzerland: Karger.

Duda, J. L. (1987). Toward a developmental theory of children's motivation in sport. *Journal of Sport Psychology, 9*, 130–145.

Duda, J. L., & Hom, H. L. (1993). Interdependencies between the perceived and self-reported goal orientations of young athletes and their parents. *Pediatric Exercise Science, 5*, 234–241.

Duda, J. L., Olson, L. K., & Templin, T. J. (1991). The relationship of task and ego orientation to sportsmanship attitudes and the perceived legitimacy of injurious acts. *Research Quarterly for Exercise and Sport, 62*, 79–87.

Dunn, J. G. H., & Causgrove Dunn, J. (1999). Goal orientations, perceptions of aggression, and sportspersonship in elite male youth ice hockey players. *Sport Psychologist, 13*, 183–200.

Dweck, C. S. (1986). Motivational processes affecting learning. *American Psychologist, 41*, 1040–1048.

Dwyer, S. A. (1999). *Exploring children's goals for recess engagement*. Unpublished master's thesis, University of Alberta, Edmonton, Alberta, Canada.

Ebbeck, V., & Becker, S. L. (1994). Psychosocial predictors of goal orientations in youth soccer. *Research Quarterly for Exercise and Sport, 65*, 355–362.

Eccles, J. S., Adler, T. F., Futterman, R., Goff, S. B., Kaczala, C. M., Meece, J., & Midgley, C. (1983). Expectancies, values and academic behaviors. In J. T. Spence (Ed.), *Achievement and achievement motives* (pp. 75–146). San Francisco: W. H. Freeman.

Eccles, J. S., Barber, B., & Jozefowicz, D. (1999). Linking gender to educational, occupational, and recreational choices: Applying the Eccles et al. model of achievement-related choices. In W. B. Swann, J. H. Langlois, & L. A. Gilbert (Eds.), *Sexism and stereotypes in modern society: The gender science of Janet Taylor Spence* (pp. 153–192). Washington, DC: American Psychological Association.

Eccles, J. S., Wigfield, A., Harold, R. D., & Blumenfeld, P. (1993). Age and gender differences in children's self- and task perceptions during elementary school. *Child Development, 64*, 830–847.

Eccles, J., Wigfield, A., & Schiefele, U. (1998). Motivation to succeed. In W. Damon & N. Eisenberg (Eds.), *Handbook of child psychology* (5th ed., Vol. 3). New York: Wiley.

Evans, J., & Roberts, G. C. (1987). Physical competence and the development of children's peer relations. *Quest, 39*, 23–35.

Frey, K. S., & Ruble, D. N. (1990). Strategies for comparative evaluation: Maintaining a sense of competence across the life span. In R. J. Sternberg & J. Kolligian (Eds.), *Competence considered* (pp. 167–189). New Haven, CT: Yale University Press.

Gibson, J. J. (1979). *An ecological approach to visual perception.* Boston: Houghton-Mifflin.

Harter, S. (1978). Effectance motivation reconsidered: Toward a developmental model. *Human Development, 21*, 34–64.

Harter, S. (1981). The development of competence motivation in the mastery of cognitive and physical skills: Is there a place for joy? In G. C. Roberts & D. M. Landers (Eds.), *Psychology of Motor Behaviour and Sport*—1980 (pp. 3–29). Champaign, IL: Human Kinetics.

Harter, S. (1985). *Manual for the self-perception profile for children.* Denver, CO: University of Denver.

Hilton, S. (2000). *Children's perceived competence and participation in recess activities.* Unpublished master's thesis, University of Alberta, Edmonton, Alberta, Canada.

Hom, H. L., Duda, J. L., & Miller, A. (1993). Correlates of goal orientations among young athletes. *Pediatric Exercise Science, 5*, 168–176.

Horn, T. S., & Hasbrook, C. A. (1987). Psychological characteristics and the criteria children use for self-evaluation. *Journal of Sport & Exercise Psychology, 9*, 208–221.

Hulme, C., & Lord, R. (1986). Clumsy children—A review of recent research. *Child: Care, Health and Development, 12*, 257–269.

Johnson, D. W., & Johnson, R. T. (1985). Motivational processes in cooperative, competitive, and individualistic learning situations. In C. Ames & R. Ames (Eds.), *Research on motivation in education. Vol 2: The classroom milieu* (pp. 249–286). Orlando, FL: Academic Press.

Kalverboer, A. F., de Vries, H. J., & van Dellen, T. (1990). Social behaviour in clumsy children as rated by parents and teachers. In A. F. Kalverboer (Ed.), *Developmental biopsychology: Experimental and observational studies in children at risk* (pp. 257–269). Ann Arbor: University of Michigan Press.

Kavussanu, M., & Roberts, G. C. (1996). Motivation in physical activity contexts: The relationship of perceived motivational climate to intrinsic motivation and self-efficacy. *Journal of Sport & Exercise Psychology, 18*, 264–280.

Kirchner, G., & Fishburne, G. (1998). *Physical education for elementary school children*. Boston: McGraw-Hill.

Maehr, M. L., & Nicholls, J. G. (1980). Culture and achievement motivation: A second look. In N. Warren (Ed.), *Studies in cross-cultural psychology* (pp. 221–267). New York: Academic Press.

Markus, H., Cross, S., & Wurf, E. (1990). The role of the self-system in competence. In J. R. Sternberg & J. Kolligian (Eds.), *Competence considered* (pp. 205–225). New Haven, CT: Yale University Press.

Martinek, T., & Karper, W. (1984). The effects of noncompetitive and competitive instructional climates on teacher expectancy effects in elementary physical education classes. *Journal of Sport Psychology, 6*, 408–421.

Martinek, T., & Karper, W. (1986). Motor ability and instructional contexts: Effects on teacher expectation and dyadic interactions in elementary physical education classes. *Journal of Classroom Interaction, 21*, 16–25.

Newton, M., & Duda, J. L. (1993). Elite adolescent athletes' achievement goals and beliefs concerning success in tennis. *Journal of Sport & Exercise Psychology, 13*, 437–448.

Nicholls, J. G. (1978). The development of the concepts of effort and ability, perception of own attainment, and the understanding that difficult tasks require more ability. *Child Development, 49*, 800–814.

Nicholls, J. G. (1984). Conceptions of ability and achievement motivation. In R. E. Ames & C. Ames (Eds.), *Research on motivation in education. Vol. 1: Student motivation* (pp. 39–73). Orlando, FL: Academic Press.

Nicholls, J. G. (1989). *The competitive ethos and democratic education*. Cambridge, MA: Harvard University Press.

Nicholls, J. G. (1990). What is ability and why are we mindful of it? A developmental perspective. In R. Sternberg & J. Kolligian (Eds.), *Competence considered* (pp. 11–40). New Haven, CT: Yale University Press.

Nicholls, J. G. (1992). The general and the specific in the development and expression of achievement motivation. In G. C. Roberts (Ed.), *Motivation in sport and exercise* (pp. 31–56). Champaign, IL: Human Kinetics.

Nyisztor, D., & Rudicle, E. S. (1995). *Moving to learn: A guide to psychomotor development in early childhood*. Toronto, Canada: Harcourt Brace & Company.

O'Beirne, C., Larkin, D., & Cable, T. (1994). Coordination problems and anaerobic performance in children. *Adapted Physical Activity Quarterly, 11*, 141–149.

Papaioannou, A. (1995). Differential perceptual and motivational patterns when different goals are adopted. *Journal of Sport & Exercise Psychology, 17*, 18–34.

Papaioannou, A., & Macdonald, A. I. (1993). Goal perspectives and purposes of physical education as perceived by Greek adolescents. *Physical Education Review, 16*, 41–48.

Portman, P. A. (1995). Who is having fun in physical education classes? Experiences of sixth-grade students in elementary and middle schools. *Journal of Teaching in Physical Education, 14*, 445–453.

Roberts, G. C. (1992). Motivation in sport and exercise: Conceptual constraints and convergence. In G. C. Roberts (Ed.), *Motivation in sport and exercise* (pp. 3–29). Champaign, IL: Human Kinetics.

Roberts, G. C., Kleiber, A. D., & Duda, J. L. (1981). An analysis of motivation in children's sport: The role of perceived competence in participation. *Journal of Sport Psychology, 3*, 206–216.

Roberts, G. C., & Treasure, D. C. (1992). Children in sport. *Sport Science Review, 1*, 46–64.

Roberts, G. C., Treasure, D. C., & Hall, H. K. (1994). Parental goal orientation and beliefs about the competitive-sport experience of their child. *Journal of Applied Social Psychology, 24*, 631–645.

Roberts, G. C., Treasure, D. C., & Kavussanu, M. (1996). Orthogonality of achievement goals and its relationship to beliefs about success and satisfaction in sport. *Sport Psychologist, 10*, 398–408.

Rose, B., Larkin, D., & Berger, B. G. (1997). Coordination and gender influences on the perceived competence of children. *Adapted Physical Activity Quarterly, 14*, 130–140.

Schoemaker, M., & Kalverboer, A. (1994). Social and affective problems of children who are clumsy: How early do they begin? *Adapted Physical Activity Quarterly, 11*, 130–140.

Seifriz, J. J., Duda, J. L., & Chi, L. (1992). The relationship of perceived motivational climate to intrinsic motivation and beliefs about success in basketball. *Journal of Sport & Exercise Psychology, 14*, 375–391.

Sherrill, C. (1993). *Adapted physical activity, recreation and sport: Crossdisciplinary and lifespan* (4th ed.). Dubuque, IA: Brown & Benchmark.

Smyth, T. R. (1992). Impaired motor skill (clumsiness) in otherwise normal children: A review. *Child: Care, Health and Development, 18*, 283–300.

Stanne, M. B., Johnson, D. W., & Johnson, R. T. (1999). Does competition enhance or inhibit motor performance: A meta-analysis. *Psychological Bulletin, 125*, 133–154.

Thompson, L. P., Bouffard, M., Watkinson, E. J., & Causgrove Dunn, J. (1994). Teaching children with movement difficulties: Highlighting the need for individualised instruction in regular physical education. *Physical Education Review, 17*, 152–159.

Treasure, D. C., & Roberts, G. C. (1994). Cognitive and affective concomitants of task and ego goal orientations during the middle school years. *Journal of Sport & Exercise Psychology, 16*, 15–28.

Treasure, D. C., & Roberts, G. C. (1995). Applications of achievement goal theory to physical education: Implications for enhancing motivation. *Quest, 47*, 475–489.

Ulrich, B. (1987). Perception of physical competence, motor competence, and participation in organized sport: Their relationships in young children. *Research Quarterly for Exercise and Sport, 58*, 57–67.

van Rossum, J. H. A., & Vermeer, A. (1990). Perceived competence: A validation study in the field of motoric teaching. *International Journal of Disability Development and Education, 37*, 71–81.

Wall, A. E. (1982). Physically awkward children: A motor development perspective. In J. P. Das, R. F. Mulcahy, & A. E. Wall (Eds.), *Theory and research in learning disabilities* (pp. 253–268). New York: Plenum Press.

Wall, A., Reid, G., & Paton, J. (1990). The syndrome of physical awkwardness. In G. Reid (Ed.), *Problems in movement control* (pp. 283–315). New York: Elsevier.

Walling, M. D., & Duda, J. L. (1995). Goals and their associations with beliefs about success in and perceptions of the purposes of physical education. *Journal of Teaching in Physical Education, 14,* 140–156.

Watkinson, E. J., & Causgrove Dunn, J. (2000). [Children's perceptions of task difficulty of selected playground activities]. Unpublished raw data.

Watkinson, E. J., Causgrove Dunn, J., Calzonetti, K., Cavaliere, N., Wilhelm, L., Dwyer, S., & Covey, J. (2001). Engagement in playground activities as a criterion for diagnosing Developmental Coordination Disorder. *Adapted Physical Activity Quarterly, 18,* 18–34.

Watkinson, E. J., Causgrove Dunn, J., Calzonetti, K., Spencer, N., Wilhelm, L., Dwyer, S., & Covey, J. (1997, October). *What's being done at recess, and why isn't everyone doing it?* Symposium conducted at the North American Federation of Adapted Physical Activity 1998 Symposium, Minneapolis, MN.

Watkinson, E. J., Causgrove Dunn, J., & Cavaliere, N. (2000). *The role of perceptions of competence and activity value in children's choices to take part in playground activities?* Manuscript in preparation.

Watkinson, E. J., Dwyer, S., & Nielsen, A. B. (2000). *Children theorizing about recess: Testing Eccles' expectancy-value theory.* Manuscript submitted for publication.

Weiss, M., & Duncan, S. (1992). The relationship between physical competence and peer acceptance in the context of children's sport participation. *Journal of Sport & Exercise Psychology, 14,* 177–191.

Weiss, M. R., Ebbeck, V., & Horn, T. S. (1997). Children's self-perceptions and sources of physical competence information: A cluster analysis. *Journal of Sport & Exercise Psychology, 19,* 52–70.

White, S. A., & Zellner, S. R. (1996). The relationship between goal orientation, beliefs about the causes of sport success, and trait anxiety among high school, intercollegiate, and recreational sport participants. *The Sport Psychologist, 10,* 58–72.

Wigfield, A. (1994). Expectancy-value theory of achievement motivation: A developmental perspective. *Educational Psychology Review, 6,* 49–78.

Wigfield, A., & Eccles, J. S. (1992). The development of achievement task values: A theoretical analysis. *Developmental Review, 12,* 265–310.

Wright, J. C., Giammarino, M., & Parad, H. W. (1986). Social status in small groups: Individual-group similarity and the social "misfit. " *Journal of Personality & Social Psychology, 50,* 523–536.

Yun, J., & Ulrich, D. A. (1997). Perceived and actual physical competence in children with mild mental retardation. *Adapted Physical Activity Quarterly, 14,* 314–326.

CHAPTER 13

Abbie, M. H., Douglas, H. M., & Ross, K. E. (1978). The clumsy child: Observations in cases referred to the gymnasium of the Adelaide children's hospital over a three-year period. *The Medical Journal of Australia, 1,* 65–69.

Ahern, K. (1995). *Family systems factors and the diagnostic process of movement difficulties in children.* Unpublished doctoral dissertation, Department of Human Movement and Exercise Science, The University of Western Australia, Nedlands, Australia.

Anderssen, N., & Wold, B. (1992). Parental and peer influences on leisure-time physical activity in young adolescents. *Research Quarterly of Exercise and Sport, 63*, 341–348.

Brown, W., & Barrera, I. (1999). Enduring problems in assessment: The persistent challenges of cultural dynamics and family issues. *Infants and Young Children, 12*(1), 34–42.

Brustad, R. J. (1993). Who will go out and play? Parental and psychological influences on children's attraction to activity. *Pediatric Exercise Science, 5*, 210–223.

Cantell, M., Larkin, D., & Hands, B. (1999, October). *Unigym: A case study of an intervention programme for children with DCD*. Poster presentation at DCD-IV Developmental Coordination Disorder: From Research to Practice, 4th Biennial Workshop, Groningen, Holland.

Chesson, R., McKay, C., & Stephenson, E. (1990). Motor/learning difficulties and the family. *Child: Care, Health and Development, 16*, 123–138.

Chia, S. H. (1997). The child, his family, and dyspraxia. *Professional Care of Mother & Child, 7*(4), 105–107.

Cintas, H. L. (1995). Cross-cultural similarities and differences in developmental and the impact of parental expectations on motor behavior. *Pediatric Physical Therapy, 7*, 103–111.

Cohn, E. S. (2001). Parent perspectives of occupational therapy using a sensory integration approach. *American Journal of Occupational Therapy, 55*(3), 285–294.

Cohn, E. S., & Cermak, S. A. (1998). Including the family perspective in sensory integration research. *American Journal of Occupational Therapy, 52*, 540–546.

Cohn, E. S., Miller, L. J., & Tickle-Degnen, L. (2000). Parental hopes for therapy outcomes: Children with sensory modulation disorders. *American Journal of Occupational Therapy, 54*, 36–43.

Dyspraxia Foundation. (1998). Member's questionnaire—June 1997 awareness and diagnosis. (http://www. emmbrook. demon. co. uk/dysprax/report. html)

Fox, A. M., & Lent, B. (1996). Clumsy children: A primer on developmental coordination disorder. *Canadian Family Physician, 42*, 1965–1971.

Gibson, R. C. (1996). The effects of dyspraxia on family relationships. *British Journal of Therapy and Rehabilitation, 3*, 101–105.

Gubbay, S. S. (1975). *The clumsy child: A study in developmental apraxic and agnosic ataxia*. London: W. B. Saunders.

Henderson, A. (1995). Self-care and hand skill. In A. Henderson & C. Pehoski (Eds.), *Hand function in the child* (pp. 164–183). St. Louis, MO: Mosby.

Hoare, D. (1991). *Classification of movement dysfunctions in children: Descriptive and statistical approaches*. Unpublished doctoral dissertation, University of Western Australia, Nedlands, Western Australia, Australia.

Hopkins, B., & Westra, T. (1989). Maternal expectations of their infants' development: Some cultural differences. *Developmental Medicine and Child Neurology, 31*, 384–390.

Humphry, R., & Case-Smith, J. (2000). Working with families. In J. Case-Smith (Ed.), *Occupational therapy for children* (4th ed., pp. 95–135). St. Louis, MO: Mosby.

Larkin, D., & Parker, H. E. (1996). [Parent reports and questionnaires about physical activity]. Unpublished raw data.

Larkin, D., & Parker, H. E. (1999). Physical activity profiles of adolescents who experienced motor learning difficulties. In D. Drouin, C. Lepine, & C. Simard (Eds.), *Proceedings of the 11th International Symposium for Adapted Physical Activity* (pp. 175–181). Quebec City, Canada: International Federation of Adapted Physical Activity (IFAPA).

Lawlor, M. C., & Mattingly, C. F. (1998). The complexities embedded in family-centered care. *American Journal of Occupational Therapy, 52,* 259–267.

Levine, M. D., Brooks, R., & Shonkoff, J. P. (1980). *A pediatric approach to learning disorders.* New York: John Wiley.

Miller, L. J., & Hanft, B. E. (1998). Building positive alliances: Partnerships with families as the cornerstone of developmental assessment. *Infants and Young Children, 11*(1), 49–60.

Rarick, G. L., & McKee, R. (1949). A study of twenty third-grade children exhibiting extreme levels of achievement on tests of motor proficiency. *Research Quarterly, 20,* 142–152.

Reuben, R. N., & Bakwin, H. (1968). Developmental clumsiness. *Pediatric Clinics of North America, 15*(3), 601–610.

Revie, G., & Larkin, D. (1993). Looking at movement: Problems with teacher identification of poorly coordinated children. *ACHPER National Journal, 40,* 4–9.

Schoemaker, M., & Kalverboer, A. F. (1994). Social and affective problems of children who are clumsy: How early do they begin? *Adapted Physical Activity Quarterly, 11,* 130–140.

Seligman, M., & Darling, R. B. (1997). *Ordinary families, special children: A systems approach to childhood disability* (2nd ed.). New York: Guilford Press.

Short, H., & Crawford, J. (1984). Last to be chosen: The awkward child. *Pivot, 2,* 32–36.

Sprinkle, J., & Hammond, J. (1997). Family, health, and developmental background of children with developmental coordination disorder. *Australian Educational and Developmental Psychologist, 14*(1), 55–62.

Stephenson, E., & McKay, C. (1989). A support group for parents of children with motor-learning difficulties. *British Journal of Occupational Therapy, 52*(5), 181–183.

Stephenson, E., McKay, C., & Chesson, R. (1990). An investigative study of early developmental factors in children with motor/learning difficulties. *British Journal of Occupational Therapy, 53*(1), 4–6.

Stephenson, E., McKay, C., & Chesson, R. (1991). The identification and treatment of motor/learning difficulties: Parent's perceptions and the role of the therapist. *Child: Care, Health and Development, 17,* 91–113.

Taylor, M. J. (1990). Marker variables for early identification of physically awkward children. In G. Doll-Tepper, C. Dahms, B. Doll, & H. von Selzam (Eds.), *Adapted physical activity* (pp. 379–386). Berlin: Springer-Verlag.

Thursfield, D. (1980). Psychiatry. In N. Gordon & I. McKinlay (Eds.), *Helping clumsy children* (pp. 154–164). Edinburgh: Churchill Livingstone.

CHAPTER 14

Arendt, R. E., MacLean, W. E., & Baumeister, A. A. (1988). Critique of sensory integration therapy and its application in mental retardation. *American Journal on Mental Retardation, 92,* 401–411.

Ayres, A. J. (1965). Patterns of perceptual-motor dysfunction in children: A factor analytic study. *Perceptual and Motor Skills, 20,* 335–368.

Ayres, A. J. (1966a). Interrelations among perceptual-motor abilities in a group of normal children. *American Journal of Occupational Therapy, 20,* 288–292.

Ayres, A. J. (1966b). Interrelations among perceptual-motor abilities in children. *American Journal of Occupational Therapy, 20,* 68–71.

Ayres, A. J. (1969). Deficits in sensory integration in educationally handicapped children. *Journal of Learning Disabilities, 2*(3), 160–168.

Ayres, A. J. (1972a). *Sensory integration and learning disorders.* Los Angeles: Western Psychological Services.

Ayres, A. J. (1972b). *Southern California Sensory Integration Tests Manual.* Los Angeles: Western Psychological Services.

Ayres, A. J. (1972c). Improving academic scores through sensory integration. *Journal of Learning Disabilities, 5,* 338–343.

Ayres, A. J. (1977). Cluster analyses of measures of sensory integration. *American Journal of Occupational Therapy, 31,* 362–366.

Ayres, A. J. (1978). Learning disabilities and the vestibular system. *Journal of Learning Disabilities, 11*(1), 30–41.

Ayres, A. J. (1979). *Sensory integration and the child.* Los Angeles: Western Psychological Services.

Ayres, A. J. (1985). *Developmental dyspraxia and adult-onset apraxia.* Torrance, CA: Sensory Integration International.

Ayres, A. J. (1989). *Sensory Integration and Praxis Tests.* Los Angeles: Western Psychological Services.

Burke, J. P. (1998). Play: The life role of the infant and young child. In J. Case-Smith (Ed.), *Pediatric occupational therapy and early intervention* (2nd ed., pp. 189–206). Boston: Butterworth-Heinemann.

Cermak, S. (in press). Developmental dyspraxia and clumsiness in children. In D. Tupper (Ed.), *Developmental neuropsychology and soft neurological signs: An update. Special issue of Developmental Neuropsychology.*

Cermak, S. A. (1991). Somatodyspraxia. In A. Fisher, E. Murray, & A. Bundy (Eds.), *Sensory integration: Theory and practice* (pp. 137–165). Philadelphia: F. A. Davis.

Cermak, S. A., & Henderson, A. (1989). The efficacy of sensory integration procedures. Part I. *Sensory Integration Quarterly, 17*(1), 1–5.

Clark, F. A., Mailloux, Z., & Parham, D. (1989). Sensory integration and children with learning disabilities. In P. N. Pratt & A. S. Allen (Eds.), *Occupational therapy for children* (2nd ed.), (pp. 457–507). St. Louis, MO: C. V. Mosby.

Dunbar, W. B. (1999). A child's occupational performance: Considerations of sensory processing and family context. *American Journal of Occupational Therapy, 53,* 231–235.

Dunn, W. (1999). *The Sensory Profile examiner's manual.* San Antonio, TX: Psychological Corporation.

Fisher, A. G., & Murray, E. A. (1991). Introduction to Sensory Integration Theory. In A. G. Fisher, E. A. Murray, & A. C. Bundy (Eds.), *Sensory integration theory and practice* (pp. 3–26). Philadelphia: F. A. Davis.

Fisher, A. G., Murray, E. A., & Bundy, A. C. (1991). *Sensory integration theory and practice*. Philadelphia: F. A. Davis.

Hoehn, T. P., & Baumeister, A. A. (1994). A critique of the application of sensory integration therapy to children with learning disabilities. *Journal of Learning Disabilities, 27*, 338–350.

Kimball, J. G. (1988). The emphasis is on integration, not sensory. *American Journal on Mental Retardation, 92*(5), 423–424.

Kimball, J. G. (1993). Sensory integrative frame of reference. In P. Kramer & J. Hinojosa (Eds.), *Frames of reference for pediatric occupational therapy* (pp. 87–169). Baltimore: Williams & Wilkins.

Kimball, J. G. (1999). Sensory integrative frame of reference. In P. Kramer & J. Hinojosa (Eds.), *Frames of reference in pediatric occupational therapy* (pp. 87–176). Baltimore: Williams & Wilkins.

Kimball, J. G. (2000). When individuals with high IQ experience sensory integration of sensory systems modulation problems. In K. Kay (Ed.), *Uniquely gifted: Identifying and meeting the needs of the twice exceptional student*. Gilsum, NH: Avocus Publishing.

McIntosh, D. N., Miller, L. J., Shyu, V., & Dunn, W. (1999). Overview of the Short Sensory Profile. In W. Dunn (Ed.), *The Sensory Profile Examiner's Manual* (pp. 59–73). San Antonio, TX: Psychological Corporation.

McIntosh, D. N., Miller, L. J., Shyu, F., & Hagerman, R. J. (1999). Sensory modulation disruption, electrodermal responses, and functional behaviors. *Developmental Medicine and Child Neurology, 41*, 608–615.

Miller, L. J. (1988). *Miller Assessment for Preschoolers Manual—1988 revision*. San Antonio, TX: Psychological Corporation.

Miller, L. J., & Kinnealey, M. (1993). Researching the effectiveness of sensory integration. *Sensory Integration Quarterly, 21*(2), 1–7.

Miller, L. J., McIntosh, D. N., McGrath, J., Shyu, V., Lampe, M., Taylor, A. K., Tassone, F., Neitzel, K., Stackhouse, T., & Hagerman, R. (1999). Electrodermal responses to sensory stimuli in individuals with Fragile X syndrome: A preliminary report. *American Journal of Medical Genetics, 83*(4), 268–279.

Missiuna, C., & Polatajko, H. (1995). Developmental dyspraxia by any other name: Are they still just clumsy children? *American Journal of Occupational Therapy, 49*(7), 57–71.

Ottenbacher, K. (1982). Sensory integration: Affect or effect. *American Journal of Occupational Therapy, 36*, 573–578.

Ottenbacher, K. (1991). Research in sensory integration: Empirical perceptions and progress. In A. G. Fisher, E. A. Murray, & A. C. Bundy (Eds.), *Sensory integration: Theory and practice* (pp. 387–399). Philadelphia: F. A. Davis.

Parham, D. (1987). Evaluation of praxis in preschoolers. In Z. Mailloux (Ed.), *Sensory integration approaches to occupational therapy* (pp. 23–26). New York: Haworth Press.

Parham, L. D., & Mailloux, Z. (1996). Sensory integration. In J. Case-Smith, A. Allen, & P. N. Pratt (Eds.), *Occupational therapy for children* (2nd ed.). St. Louis, MO: Mosby.

Parham, L. D., & Mailloux, Z. (2001). Sensory integration. In J. Case-Smith (Ed.), *Occupational therapy for children* (3rd ed., pp. 329–381) St Louis, MO: Mosby.

Polatajko, H. J., Kaplan, B. J., & Wilson, B. N. (1992). Sensory integration for children with learning disabilities: Its status 20 years later. *Occupational Therapy Journal of Research, 12,* 323–341.

Schaeffer, R. (1984). Sensory integration therapy with learning disabled children: A critical review. *Canadian Journal of Occupational Therapy, 51,* 73–77.

Spitzer, S., Roley, S., Clark, F., & Parham, D. (1996). Sensory integration: Current trends in the United States. *Scandinavian Journal of Occupational Therapy, 3,* 123–138.

Stallings-Sahler, S. (1998). Sensory integration: Assessment and intervention with infants and young children. In J. Case-Smith (Ed.), *Pediatric occupational therapy and early intervention* (2nd ed., pp. 223–254). Boston: Butterworth-Heinemann.

Vargas, S., & Camilli, G. (1999). A meta-analysis of research on sensory integration treatment. *American Journal of Occupational Therapy, 53,* 189–198.

Wilbarger, P., & Wilbarger, J. (1991). *Sensory defensiveness in children 2–12.* Santa Barbara, CA: Avanti Education Programs.

CHAPTER 15

Adams, J. A. (1971). A closed-loop theory of motor learning. *Journal of Motor Behavior, 3,* 111–150.

Adams, J. A. (1987). Historical review and appraisal of research on the learning, retention and transfer of human motor skills. *Psychological Bulletin, 101,* 41–74.

Ayres, A. J. (1985). *Developmental dyspraxia and adult-onset dyspraxia.* Torrance, CA: Sensory Integration International.

Bernstein, N. (1967). *The coordination and regulation of movements.* London: Pergamon Press.

Blanche, E. I. (1998). Intervention for motor control and movement organization disorders. In J. Case-Smith (Ed.), *Pediatric occupational therapy and early intervention* (2nd ed., pp. 255–276). Boston: Butterworth-Heinemann.

Bouffard, M., Watkinson, E. J., Thompson, L. P., Causgrove Dunn, J. L., & Romanow, S. K. E. (1996). A test of the activity deficit hypothesis with children with movement difficulties. *Adapted Physical Activity Quarterly, 13,* 61–73.

Burton, A. W., & Davis, W. E. (1996). Ecological task analysis: Utilizing intrinsic measures in research and practice. *Human Movement Science, 15,* 285–314.

Burton, A. W., & Miller, D. E. (1998). *Movement skill assessment.* Champaign, IL: Human Kinetics.

Colley, A. M. (1989). Learning motor skills: Integrating cognition and action. In A. M. Colley & J. R. Beech (Eds.), *Acquisition and performance of cognitive skills* (pp. 167–186). New York: John Wiley and Sons.

Colley, A. M., & Beech, J. R. (1989). *Acquisition and performance of cognitive skills.* New York: John Wiley and Sons.

Davis, W. E., & Burton, A. W. (1991). Ecological task analysis: Translating movement behavior theory into practice. *Adapted Physical Activity Quarterly, 8,* 154–177.

Denckla, M. (1984). Developmental dyspraxia: The clumsy child. In M. D. Levine & P. Satz (Eds.), *Middle childhood: Development and dysfunction* (pp. 245–260). Baltimore, MD: University Park Press.

Eliasmith, C. (1998). The third contender: A critical examination of the dynamicist theory of cognition. In P. Thagard (Ed.), *Mind readings: Introductory selections on cognitive science* (pp. 303–333). Cambridge, MA: MIT Press.

Fitts, P. M. (1964). Perceptual motor skill learning. In A. W. Melton (Ed.), *Categories of human learning* (pp. 243–285). New York: Academic Press.

Fitts, P. M., & Posner, M. I. (1967). *Human performance*. Belmont, CA: Brooks/Cole Publishing.

Gentile, A. M. (1998). Implicit and explicit processes during acquisition of functional skills. *Scandinavian Journal of Occupational Therapy, 5*, 7–16.

Goodgold-Edwards, S. A., & Cermak, S. A. (1990). Integrating motor control and motor learning concepts with neuropsychological perspectives on apraxia and developmental dyspraxia. *American Journal of Occupational Therapy, 44*, 431–439.

Henderson, S., & Sugden, D. (1992). *Movement Assessment Battery for Children*. London: Psychological Corporation.

Kamm, K., Thelen, E., & Jensen, J. L. (1990). A dynamical systems approach to motor development. *Physical Therapy, 70*, 763–775.

Larin, H. (1998). Motor learning: A practical framework for paediatric physiotherapy. *Physiotherapy Theory and Practice, 14*, 33–47.

Lee, T. D., Swanson, L. R., & Hall, A. L. (1991). What is repeated in a repetition? Effects of practice conditions on motor skill acquisition. *Physical Therapy, 71*, 150–156.

Lee, T. D., Swinnen, S. P., & Serrien, D. J. (1994). Cognitive effort and motor learning. *Quest, 46*, 328–344.

Lefebvre, C., & Reid, G. (1998). Prediction in ball catching by children with and without a developmental coordination disorder. *Adapted Physical Activity Quarterly, 15*, 299–315.

Luria, A. (1961). *The role of speech in the regulation of normal and abnormal behaviour*. New York: Pergamon Press.

Ma, H., Trombly, C. A., & Robinson-Podolski, C. (1999). The effect of context on skill acquisition and transfer. *American Journal of Occupational Therapy, 53*, 138–144.

Magill, R. A. (1998). *Motor learning: Concepts and applications* (5th ed.). Boston: McGraw-Hill.

Mandich, A. (1997). *Cognitive strategies and motor performance*. Unpublished master's thesis, University of Western Ontario, London, Ontario, Canada.

Mandich, A., Polatajko, H., Missiuna, C., & Miller, L. (2001). Cognitive strategies and motor performance in children with developmental coordination disorder. *Physical and Occupational Therapy in Pediatrics, 20*(2/3), 125–143.

Marteniuk, R. G. (1986). Information processes in movement learning: Capacity and structural interference effects. *Journal of Motor Behavior, 18*, 55–75.

Meichenbaum, D. (1977). *Cognitive-behavior modification: An integrative approach*. New York: Plenum Press.

Miles Breslin, D. M. (1996). Motor learning theory and the neurodevelopmental treatment approach: A comparative analysis. *Occupational Therapy in Health Care, 10*, 25–40.

Miller, L., Polatajko, H., Missiuna, C., Malloy-Miller, T., & Mandich, A. (1999). *Cognitive intervention for children with DCD: Final report*. Toronto: Hospital for Sick Children Foundation.

Missiuna, C., Malloy-Miller, T., & Mandich, A. (1998). Mediational techniques: Origins and application to occupational therapy in pediatrics. *Canadian Journal of Occupational Therapy, 65,* 202–209.

Missiuna, C., Mandich, A., Polatajko, H., & Malloy-Miller, T. (2001). Cognitive orientation to daily occupational performance (CO-OP). Part I: Theoretical foundations. *Physical and Occupational Therapy in Pediatrics, 20*(2/3), 69–81.

Nicholson, D. E. (1996). Motor learning. In C. M. Fredericks & L. K. Saladin (Eds.), *Pathophysiology of the motor systems: Principles and clinical presentations* (pp. 238–254). Philadelphia: F. A. Davis Company.

O'Beirne, C., Larkin, D., & Cable, T. (1994). Coordination problems and anaerobic performance in children. *Adapted Physical Activity Quarterly, 11,* 141–149.

Polatajko, H. J., Mandich, A. D., Miller, L. T., & Macnab, J. J. (2001). Cognitive orientation to daily occupational occupational performance (CO-OP). Part II: The evidence. *Physical and Occupational Therapy in Pediatrics, 20*(2/3), 83–106.

Poole, J. L. (1991). Application of motor learning principles in occupational therapy. *American Journal of Occupational Therapy, 45,* 531–537.

Rose, B., Larkin, D., & Berger, B. G. (1998). The importance of motor coordination for children's motivational orientations in sport. *Adapted Physical Activity Quarterly, 15,* 316–327.

Schmidt, R. A. (1975). A schema theory of discrete motor skill learning. *Psychological Review, 82,* 225–260.

Schmidt, R. A. (1988). *Motor control and learning: A behavioral emphasis*. Champaign, IL: Human Kinetics.

Schmidt, R. A. (1991). *Motor learning and performance*. Champaign, IL: Human Kinetics.

Schoemaker, M. M., Hijlkema, M. G. J., & Kalverboer, A. F. (1994). Physiotherapy for clumsy children: An evaluation study. *Developmental Medicine and Child Neurology, 36,* 143–155.

Shumway-Cook, A., & Woollacott, M. H. (1995). *Motor control: Theory and practical applications*. Baltimore, MD: Williams & Wilkins.

Sigmundsson, H., Pedersen, A. V., Whiting, H. T. A., & Ingvaldsen, R. P. (1998). We can cure your child's clumsiness: A review of intervention methods. *Scandinavian Journal of Rehabilitative Medicine, 30,* 101–106.

Singer, R. N. (1988). Strategies and metastrategies in learning and performing self-paced athletic skills. *Sport Psychologist, 2,* 49–68.

Singer, R. N., & Caraugh, J. H. (1984). Generalization of psychomotor learning strategies to related psychomotor tasks. *Human Learning, 3,* 215–225.

Sugden, D. A., & Sugden, L. (1990). *The assessment and management of movement skill problems*. Leeds, England: School of Education.

Thelen, E. (1995). Motor development: A new synthesis. *American Psychologist, 50,* 79–95.

Thelen, E., Kelso, J. A., & Fogel, A. (1987). Self-organizing systems and infant motor development. *Developmental Review, 7,* 39–65.

Toglia, J. P. (1991). Generalization of treatment: A multicontext approach to cognitive perceptual impairments in adults with brain injury. *American Journal of Occupational Therapy*, *45*, 505–516.

Ulrich, B. D. (1997). Dynamic systems theory and skill development in infants and children. In K. J. Connolly & H. Forssberg (Eds.), *Neurophysiology and neuropsychology of motor development* (pp. 319–345). Cambridge: Mac Keith.

Van Wieringen, P. C. W. (1988). Discussion: Self organisation or representation? Let's have both! In A. M. Colley & J. R. Beech (Eds.), *Cognition and action in skilled behaviour* (pp. 247–253). Amsterdam: North-Holland.

Wall, A. E., Reid, G., & Paton, J. (1990). The syndrome of physical awkwardness. In G. Reid (Ed.), *Problems in movement control* (pp. 283–315). Amsterdam: Elsevier Science.

Yang, J. J., & Porretta, D. L. (1999). Sport/leisure skill learning by adolescents with mild mental retardation: A four-step strategy. *Adapted Physical Activity Quarterly*, *16*, 300–315.

CHAPTER 16

Arend, S., & Higgins, J. R. (1976). A strategy for the classification, subjective analysis, and observation of human movement. *Journal of Human Movement Studies*, *2*, 36–52.

Bernstein, N. (1967). *The co-ordination and regulation of movement*. Oxford: Pergamon Press.

Bertalanffy, L. von. (1968). *General system theory*. New York: George Braziller.

Broer, M. (1955). Evaluation of a basic skills curriculum for women students of low motor ability at the University of Washington. *Research Quarterly*, *26*, 15–27.

Clark, J. E. (1995). On becoming skillful: Patterns and constraints. *Research Quarterly for Exercise and Sport*, *66*, 173–183.

Collier, D., & Reid, G. (1987). A comparison of two models designed to teach autistic children a motor task. *Adapted Physical Activity Quarterly*, *4*, 226–236.

Davis, W. E., & Burton, A. W. (1991). Ecological task analysis: Translating movement behavior theory into practice. *Adapted Physical Activity Quarterly*, *8*, 154–177.

Ellfeldt, L., & Methany, E. (1959). Comment—Movement and meaning: Development of a general theory. *Research Quarterly*, *30*(2), 244.

Gentile, A. M. (1972). A working model of skill acquisition with application to teaching. *Quest Monograph 17*, 3–23.

Gentile, A. M. (1987). Skill acquisition: Action, movement, and the neuromotor processes. In J. H. Carr, R. B. Shepherd, J. Gordon, A. M. Gentile, and J. M. Held (Eds.), *Movement science: Foundations for physical therapy in rehabilitation* (pp. 93–154). Rockville, MD: Aspen.

Gibson, J. J. (1966). *The senses considered as perceptual systems*. Boston: Houghton Mifflin.

Henderson, S. E., & Sugden, D. A. (1992). *Movement Assessment Battery for Children Manual*. Sidcup, Kent: The Psychological Corporation.

Higgins, J. (1977). *Human movement: An integrated approach*. St. Louis, MO: Mosby.

Hoare, D. (1994). Subtypes of developmental coordination disorder. *Adapted Physical Activity Quarterly, 11,* 158–169.

Kelly, L. E. (1989, August). Instructional time the overlooked factor in PE curriculum development. *Journal of Physical Education, Recreation and Dance, 60,* 29–32.

Lafuze, M. (1951). A study of the learning of fundamental skills by college freshman women of low motor ability. *Research Quarterly, 22,* 149–157.

Larkin, D., & Parker, H. E. (1998a). Teaching landing to children with and without developmental coordination disorder. *Pediatric Exercise Science, 10,* 123–136.

Larkin, D., & Parker, H. E. (1998b). Teaching children to land softly: Individual differences in learning outcomes. *ACHPER Healthy Lifestyles Journal, 45*(2), 19–24.

Leonard, C. T. (1998). *The neuroscience of human movement.* St. Louis, MO: Mosby.

Lippitt, L. C. (1926). *A manual of corrective gymnastics.* New York: Macmillan.

Magill, R. (1998). Knowledge is more than we can talk about: Implicit learning in motor skill acquisition. *Research Quarterly for Exercise and Sport, 69,* 104–110.

Marchiori, G. E., Wall, A. E., & Bedingfield, E. W. (1987). Kinematic analysis of skill acquisition in physically awkward boys. *Adapted Physical Activity Quarterly, 4,* 305–315.

Miyahara, M. (1996). A meta-analysis of intervention studies on children with developmental coordination disorder. *Corpus Psyche et Societas, 3,* 11–18.

Newell, K. M. (1986). Constraints on the development of coordination. In M. G. Wade & H. T. A. Whiting (Eds.), *Motor development in children: Aspects of coordination and control* (pp. 341–360). The Hague, The Netherlands: Nijhoff.

O'Beirne, C., Larkin, D., & Cable, T. (1994). Coordination problems and anaerobic performance in children. *Adapted Physical Activity Quarterly, 11,* 141–149.

Oslin, J. L., Stroop, S., & Siedentop, D. (1997). Use of component-specific instruction to promote development of the overarm throw. *Journal of Teaching Physical Education, 16,* 340–356.

Parker, H. (1992). Children's motor rhythm and timing: A dynamical approach. In J. J. Summers (Ed.), *Approaches to the study of motor control and learning* (pp. 163–194). Amsterdam: Elsevier Science.

Parker, H. E., & Blanksby, B. A. (1997). Starting age and aquatic skill learning in young children: Mastery of prerequisite water confidence and basic aquatic locomotion skills. *Australian Journal of Science and Medicine in Sport, 29*(3), 83–87.

Revie, G., & Larkin, D. (1993). Task specific intervention with children reduces movement problems. *Adapted Physical Activity Quarterly, 10,* 29–41.

Rose, B., Larkin, D., & Berger, B. (1994). Perceptions of social support in children of low, moderate and high levels of coordination. *ACHPER Healthy Lifestyles Journal, 41*(4), 18–21.

Rose, B., Larkin, D., & Berger, B. (1999). Athletic anxiety in boys and girls with low and high levels of coordination. *ACHPER Healthy Lifestyles Journal, 46*(2/3), 10–13.

Scholz, J. P. (1990). Dynamic pattern theory—some implications for therapeutics. *Physical Therapy, 70,* 827–843.

Shepherd, R., & Carr, J. (1991). An emergent or dynamical systems view of movement dysfunction. *Australian Journal of Physiotherapy, 37*(1), 5–6, 17.

Sigmundsson, H., Pedersen, A. V., Whiting, H. T. A., & Ingvaldsen, R. P. (1998). We can cure your child's clumsiness! A review of intervention methods. *Scandinavian Journal of Rehabilitation Medicine, 30,* 101–106.

Sporns, O., & Edelman, G. M. (1993). Solving Bernstein's problem: A proposal for the development of coordinated movement by selection. *Child Development, 64,* 960–981.

Sveistrup, H., Burtner, P. A., & Woollacott, M. H. (1992). Two motor control approaches that may help to identify and teach children with motor impairments. *Pediatric Exercise Science, 4,* 249–269.

Thelen, E., & Ulrich, B. D. (1991). *Hidden skills. Monographs of the Society for Research in Child Development, vol. 56, no. 1.* Chicago: University of Chicago Press.

Touwen, B. C. L. (1998). The brain and development of function. *Developmental Review, 18,* 504–526.

Wall, A. E., McClements, J., Bouffard, M., Findlay, H., & Taylor, M. J. (1985). A knowledge-based approach to motor development: Implications for the physically awkward. *Adapted Physical Activity Quarterly, 2,* 21–42.

Werner, P., & Rink, J. (1989). Case studies in teacher effectiveness in second grade physical education. *Journal of Teaching in Physical Education, 8,* 280–297.

Wright, H. C., & Sugden, D. A. (1996). The nature of developmental coordination disorder: Inter- and intragroup differences. *Adapted Physical Activity Quarterly, 13,* 357–371.

CHAPTER 17

Alston, J., & Taylor, J. (1987). *Handwriting: Theory, research and practice.* London: Croom Helm.

American Psychiatric Association. (1994). *Diagnostic and statistical manual of mental disorders* (4th ed.). Washington, DC: Author.

Beery, K. E. (1997). *Developmental Test of Visual-Motor Integration, VMI-4.* Los Angeles: Psychological Corporation.

Benbow, M. (1987). *Sensory and motor measurements of dynamic tripod skill.* Unpublished master's thesis, Boston University, Boston.

Benbow, M. (1990). *Loops and other groups. A kinesthetic writing system.* Tucson, AZ: Therapy Skill Builders.

Benbow, M. (1995). Principles and practices of teaching handwriting. In A. Henderson & C. Pehoski (Eds.), *Hand function in the child: Foundation for remediation* (pp. 255–281) St. Louis: Mosby.

Benbow, M. (1999). *Fine motor development. Activities to develop hand skills in young children.* Columbus, OH: Zaner-Bloser.

Benbow, M., Hanft, B., & Marsh, D. (1992). *Handwriting in the classroom: Improving written communication.* AOTA Self Study Series. Rockville, MD: AOTA Press.

Bushnell, S. (1970). *Surgery of the hand* (5th ed.). Philadelphia: J. B. Lippincott.

Capener, N. (1956). The hand in surgery. *Journal of Bone and Joint Surgery [Br], 38B*(1), 128–140.

Clough, C. (1999). Teaching cursive writing. *OT Practice, 4*(8), 41–42.

Connolly, K. J. (1973). *Factors influencing the learning of manual skills in children.* London: Academic Press.

Exner, C. (1997). Clinical interpretation of "In-hand manipulation in young children: Translation movements. " *American Journal of Occupational Therapy, 51,* 729–732.

Fitts, P. M., & Posner, M. I. (1967). *Human performance.* Belmont, CA: Brooks/Cole.

Getman, G. N. (1992). *Smart in everything . . . Except school.* Santa Ana, CA: Vision Extension.

Guiard, Y. (1987). Asymmetric division of labor in human skilled bimanual action: The kinematic chain as model. *Journal of Motor Behavior, 19,* 486–517.

Johansson, R. S., & Westling, G. (1987). Signals in tactile afferents from the fingers eliciting adaptive motor responses during precision grip. *Experimental Brain Research, 66,* 141–154.

Kapandji, I. A. (1982). *The physiology of the joints: Vol. 1. Upper limb* (5th ed.). Edinburgh: Churchill Livingstone.

Lamme, L. L. (1979). Handwriting in an early education curriculum. *Young Children, 35,* 20–27.

Levine, M. (1987). *Developmental variations and learning disorders.* Cambridge, MA: Educators Publishing Service.

Long, C., Conrad, M. S., Hall, E. A., & Furler, M. S. (1970). Intrinsic-extrinsic muscle control of the hand in power and precision handling. *Journal of Bone and Joint Surgery [Am], 52A,* 853–867.

McHale, K., & Cermak, S. (1992). Fine motor activities in elementary school: Preliminary findings and provisional implications for children with fine motor problems. *American Journal of Occupational Therapy, 46,* 898–903.

Moberg, E. (1958). Objective methods of determining the functional value of sensibility of the hand. *Journal of Bone and Joint Surgery, 40B,* 454–476.

Moberg, E. (1983). The role of cutaneous afferents in position sense, kinesthesia and motor function of the hand. *Hand, 106,* 1–19.

Rosenbloom, L., & Horton, M. E. (1971). The maturation of fine prehension in young children. *Developmental Medicine and Child Neurology, 13,* 3–8.

Schneck, C. (1991). Comparison of pencil-grip patterns in first graders with good and poor writing skill. *American Journal of Occupational Therapy, 45,* 701–706.

Tubiana, R. (1981). *The hand* (Vol. 1). Philadelphia: W. B. Saunders.

Weil, M., & Amundson, S. (1994). Relationship between visual motor and handwriting skills of children in kindergarten. *American Journal of Occupational Therapy, 48,* 982–988.

Wright, J., & Allen, E. (1975). Ready to write! *Elementary School Journal, 75,* 430–435.

Ziviani, J. (1987). Pencil grasp and manipulation. In J. Alston & J. Taylor (Eds.), *Handwriting: Theory, research and practice.* New York: Nichols Publishing.

Index

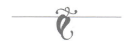